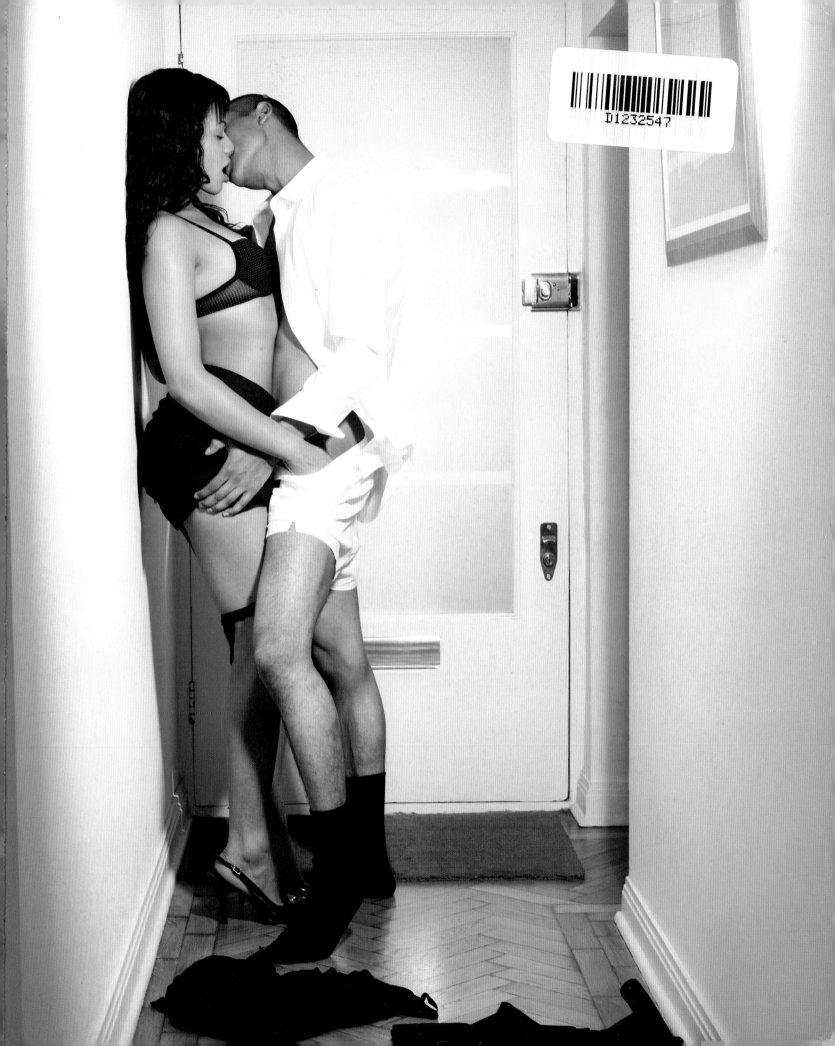

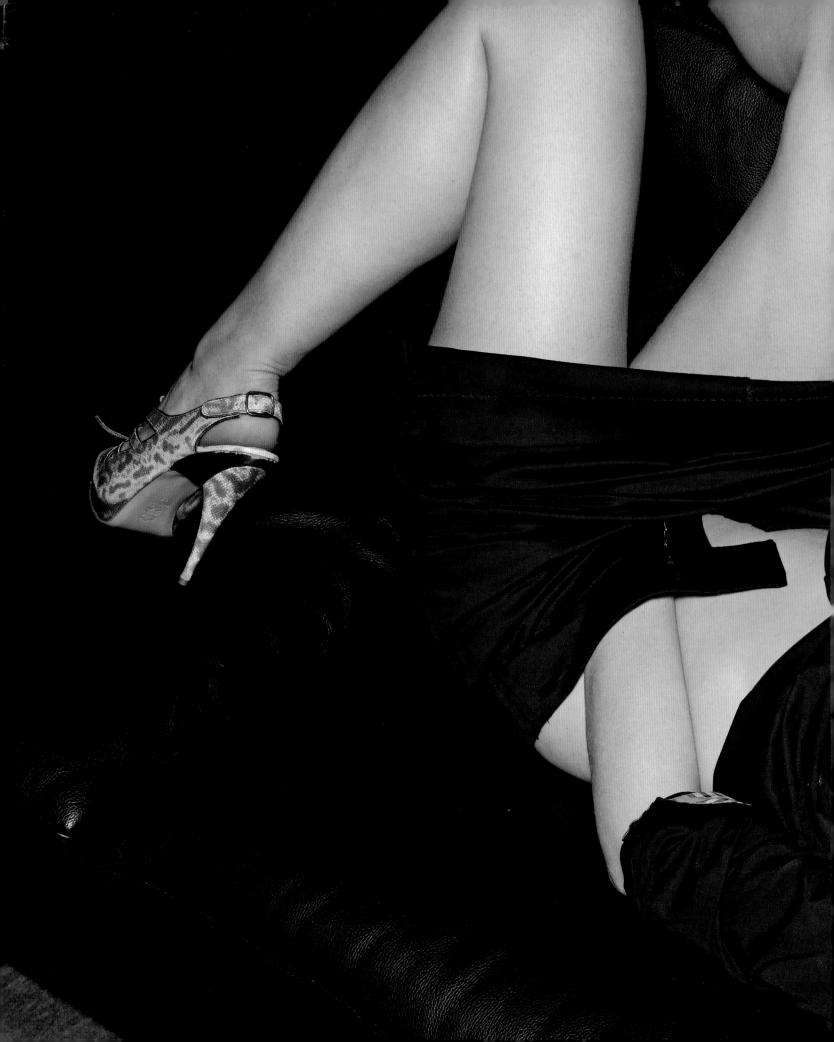

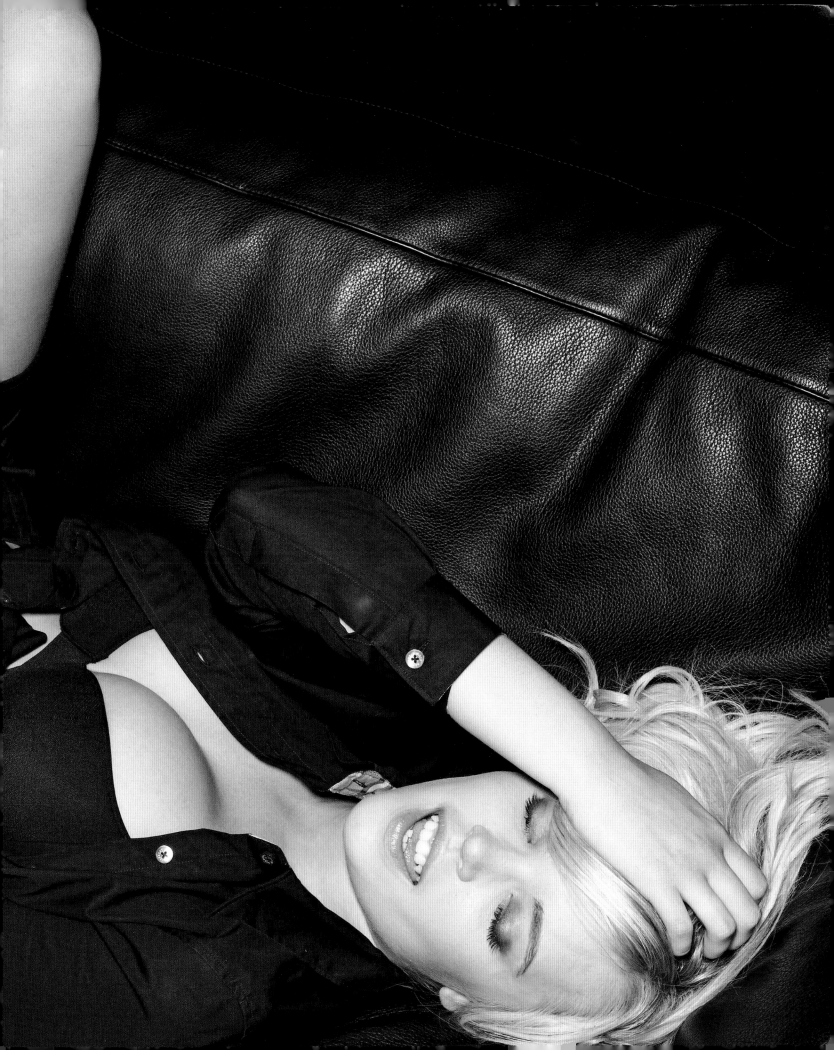

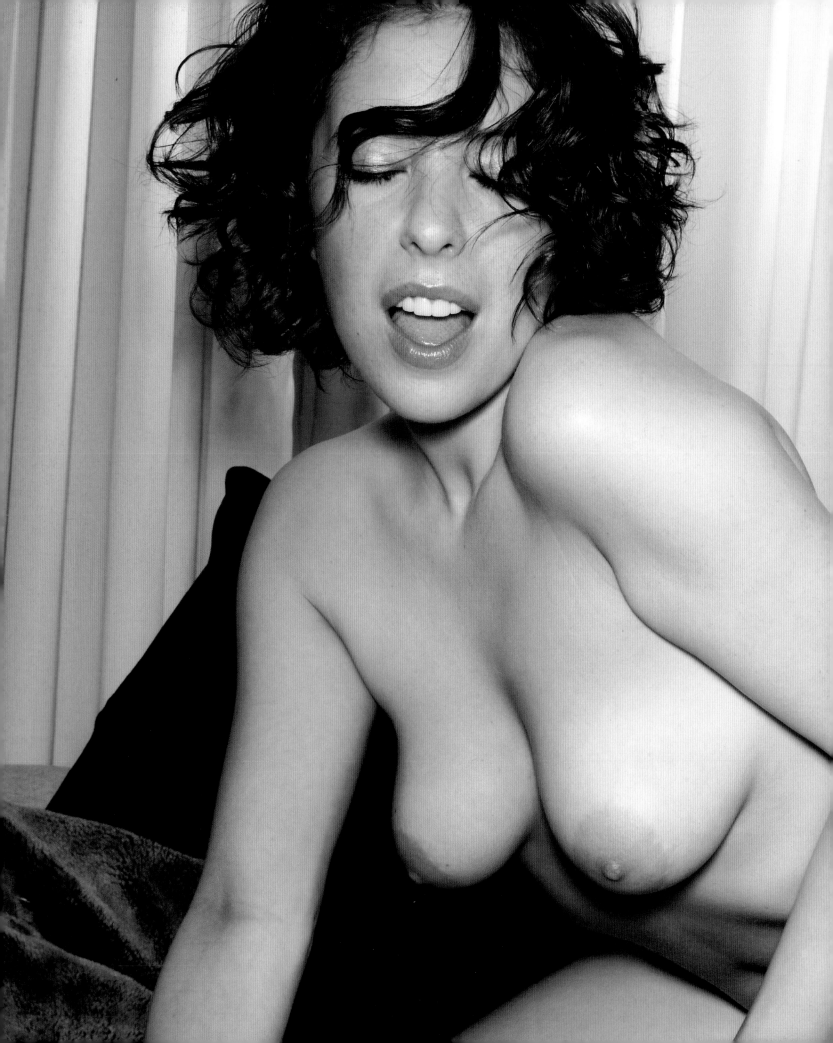

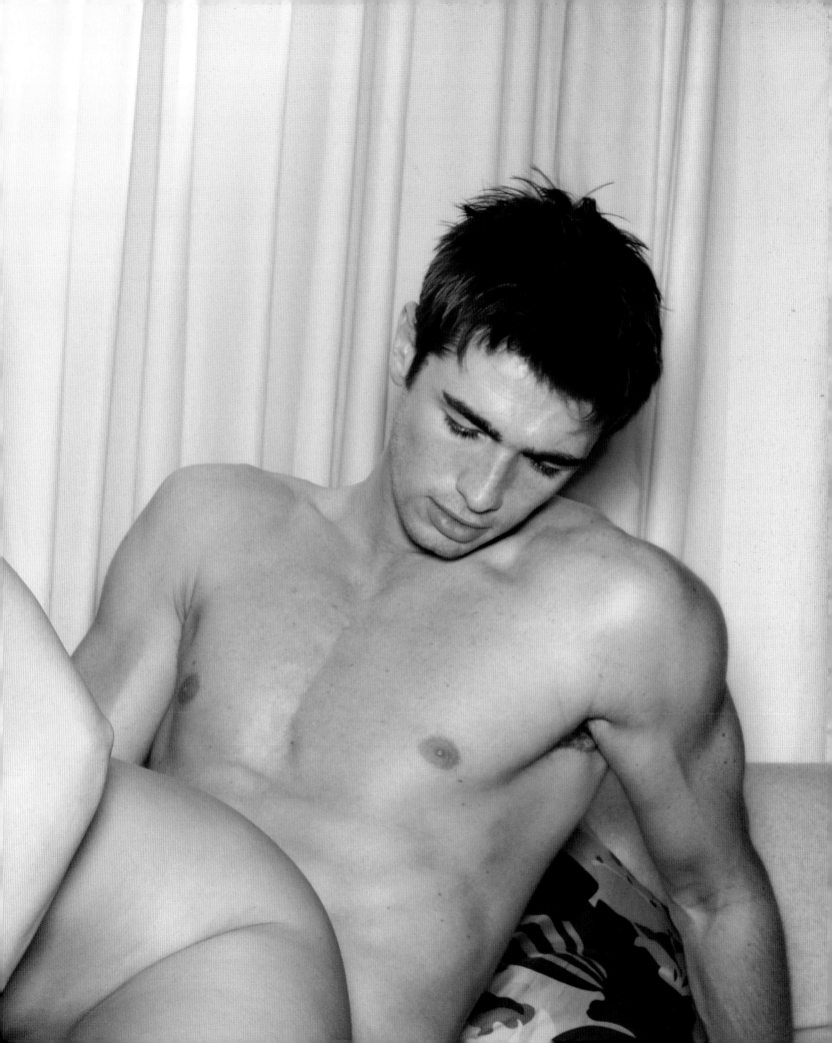

Sex—
how to do everything

Em & Lo

Contents—

Lawyers get hit up for free legal advice. Doctors are privy to their friends' aches and pains ("Does this look infected...?"). And if you're a sex columnist? Everyone asks for the key to better sex. Actually, first they ask what's the craziest agony aunt letter we've ever received and we tell them the one about the necrophiliac who worked in the morgue (another story for another book). And then they ask us how to improve their sex life.

But there's no one-size-fits-all answer. Over the years we've learned that orgasms and sexual preferences come in as many flavors as ice cream and jelly beans. As a sexual being, your sexual response is as unique as your orgasm face—what's sheer ecstasy to you may feel downright annoying to your best friend. If you're the glass-half-empty type, you could view this as being "high maintenance." If you're the glass-half-full type, you could see it as a sexy challenge.

Or you could just read this book. The next 182 pages won't tell you what sex is *supposed* to look, feel, or sound like for heterosexual couples—that's what the unrealistic expectations created by Hollywood sex scenes and porn flicks are for (the main difference between the two being good lighting). Rather, we want to arm you with the right combination of knowledge and naughty ideas so you can go exploring on your own.

A common misconception of sex manuals is that they take all the mystery out of sex. And that's true if you consider it "mysterious" not to know exactly how deep the clitoris runs or what particular kind of lube works best for a little backdoor loving.

If it ruins sex for you to be told which sex toys might move the earth for you and which will just irritate your sensitive bits, then go ahead and leave this book on the shelf. We're sure there's something interesting in the gardening aisle for you. But as for the

Introduction

for the real mystery of sex—how an orgasm can make you forget your own name, how the best sex can feel like two souls merging, how sex with a complete stranger can sometimes free you to be yourself, how bumping uglies can feel like anything but—well, we promise this book won't spoil any of that. Because, honestly, we don't fully understand that aspect of sex ourselves. And we kind of like it that way. Though we wouldn't mind if someone out there could enlighten us as to what, exactly, is the appeal of teabagging (Google it!).

Think of this book as your road atlas to the human body, full of short cuts, scenic routes, and landmarks of note. But don't wait until you're lost to crack it open. Because the most important thing to know about sex is that there's more than one way to be sexy, and there's usually more than one road to your happy place. There's a lot of pressure out there to fuck or look a certain way—but all that really matters is what makes you and your partner feel good. If you could use a bit of help figuring that out, then read on. Or if you'd like to know what else might make you and your partner feel really good, then read on. We can't guarantee you multiple orgasms on demand—that's just not in the cards for everyone (they're overrated anyway). What we *can* guarantee is more sexual pleasure and satisfaction—whether you just lost your virginity or have been married for 20 years.

Lastly, we'd like to think that this book is a hell of a lot sexier than a road atlas (or anything you might find in the gardening aisle, for that matter). So read it together. Read it in bed. Read it over a bottle of wine. It's not homework, it's foreplay. And if you never make it to the end of the book because you keep tearing each other's clothes off, we promise not to be offended. In fact, we'd be delighted.

—Em & Lo

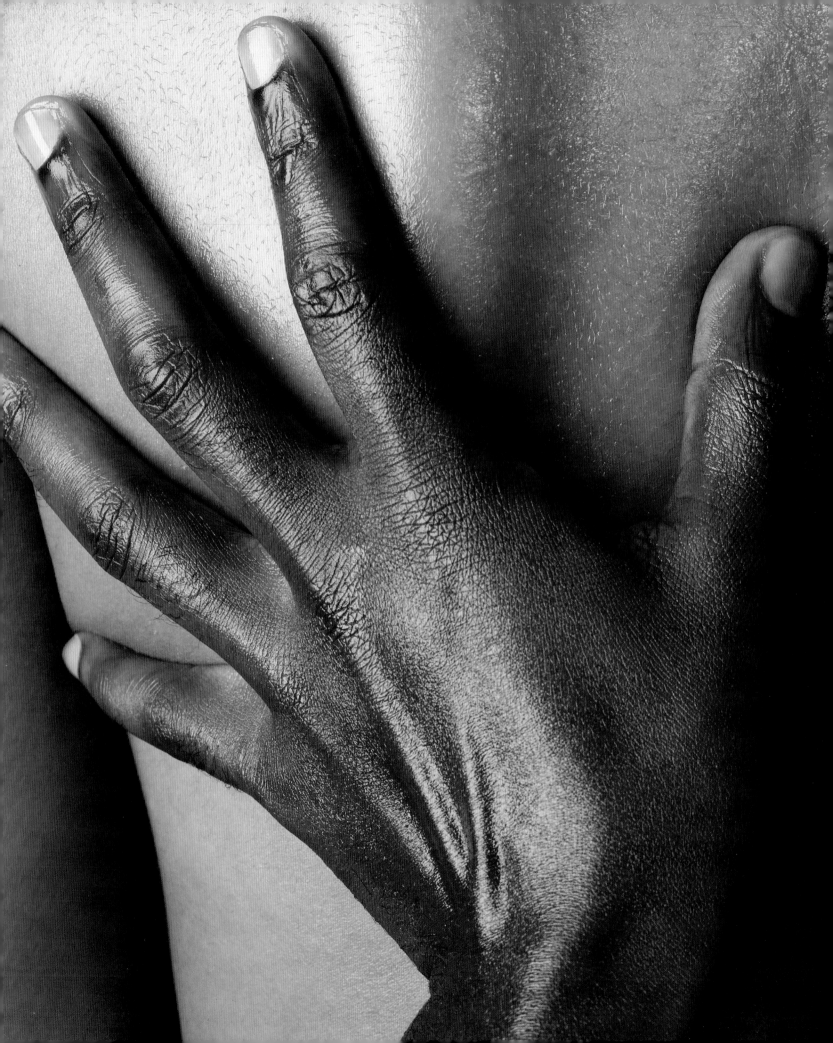

⁰¹ Seduction

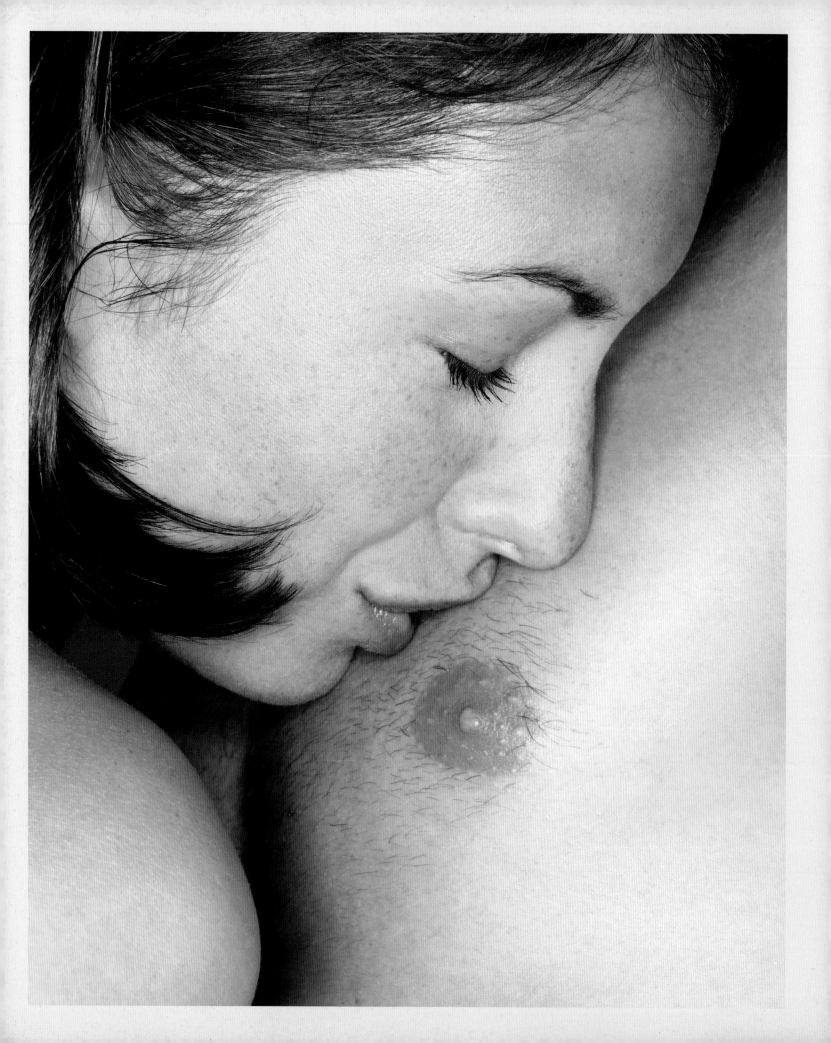

Redefining Foreplay

Foreplay is not an obligatory two minutes of making out, it's not purely physical, it's not a routine that automatically earns you intercourse, it's not just for women, and it doesn't always have to be candle-lit (though fluorescent overhead lights are *never* seductive). Sometimes it's about slowing down time, cultivating the senses, and setting a sex-conducive scene—think music, wine, a bubble bath, full-body massage, Chinese take-out on the best china, hours of kissing, teasing, and fondling on the couch, and, yes, candles. Other times it's about sharing a kinky secret over dinner ("Did I ever tell you how much it turns me on when…") or giving a gift that makes you both blush (pp.124–139 for shopping suggestions). Maybe it's sending a text message at noon with explicit (in both senses of the word) instructions for that evening: "be home @ 7, showered & naked on bed & I will… [*insert your own dirty promise*]". Or perhaps it's just forgoing the after-work small-talk and pulling your partner directly into the bedroom, rather than waiting until lights-out when they're expecting it. Foreplay can last all day, if not *days*—or it can just take a look. When you actively embrace the arts of seduction, relaxation, and even interior decorating, you can transform any night into an homage to love… or at least lust.

Seduction is unfairly reputed to be an art of trickery or deceit—convincing someone they want something that is wrong, or bad for them. (That'd be "*foreploy*, noun: Any misrepresentation about yourself for the purpose of getting laid.") No, true seduction is a mutual pursuit, an agreement between two consenting adults that paying attention to the details, and delaying gratification will heighten the pleasure ahead—whether that's making out for hours or just dropping a hint about what's to come hours before you see each other. It's an intermingling of words, touch, sound, sight, scent, and taste. It can be love (or lust) letters, elbows brushing, suggestive whispering over dessert, the outline of a shoulder beneath draped fabric, breathing in each other's skin, tracing the outline of each other's bodies with kisses, or even laughing together at a truly terrible joke.

All these delights have long been assigned to the beginning of a relationship, when you're driven by longing for what you haven't yet had. You draw each other in and then pull apart, torn between wanting this pining to last forever, and convinced that you simply can't bear another minute of it. Dinners last for hours, kissing for hours more, and every new sensual act is an act of unveiling. Or at least that's how it should be in a new relationship. If not, then you're doing it wrong: you're rushing, you're a cynic, or you just don't care. Slow down and *invest* in the lovin'.

And if you're in a not-so-new relationship? Ask yourself why you left all that good stuff behind. Do you really have to sacrifice that yearning simply because the one you yearn for wakes up next to you each morning? In a word, no.

Whether you're with a new lover or a familiar one, making and keeping sex special is not unthinkable or impossible as long as you make time for seduction, and accept that it won't always come naturally. Just because something takes a bit of effort, doesn't mean it's out of place in the bedroom. At the start of a relationship, you seduce in order to entice someone into your bed—you need to woo them away from all others, into your arms and your arms alone. Later, you seduce your lover to remind them why they are there, why they once longed to be there. Instead of wooing them away from others your job is to entice them away from everyday distractions, wandering thoughts, lingering to-do lists, and rote bonking. You'd be a fool to take someone's presence in your bed for granted at *any* time—seduce deliberately and with good intentions and you'll show them that you don't.

It's a rare treat when your sex life exceeds your own expectations, and thus the art of seduction—setting a scene and getting in the mood—lies in avoiding routine so your expectations are not so limited. The following pages will give you plenty of ideas on how exactly to expand your sensual—and ultimately your sexual—horizons.

Getting in the Mood

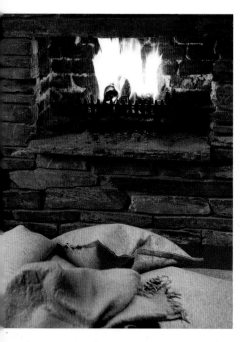
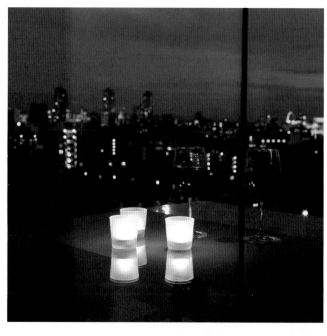
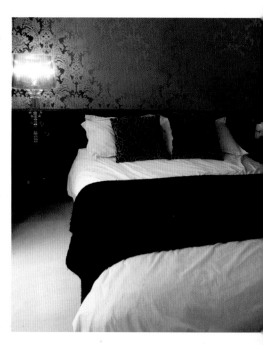

Decor

Sometimes sex is no more than a mood you create. The space you find yourself in, the air you breathe, the lights you dim, the furniture you lounge upon, the music you choose to play (no Barry White or his ilk, please)—all these things can serve to ignite your passion… or snuff it out.

First, learn to revere and respect sex—if not nightly, then at least often enough that you remember how. Just as you would decorate and straighten up before having platonic company over for dinner, so should you decorate and straighten up for more intimate guests. Pull the drapes across the windows as if to say, "this evening is for our eyes only." Or if you're feeling saucy, leave the drapes open just a sliver so that your misbehaving shadows catch the eyes of passersby. Extinguish harsh overhead lights in favor of dim, flattering lighting (installing dimmer switches is a great trick; so is floorlamp lighting tucked in corners and behind furniture). When you switch to candlelight, it's clear that no more bills will be paid, no more dishes will be scrubbed, no more magazines will be skimmed, and no more phones will be answered. (But if you light enough candles to be a fire hazard, you've overdone it.) Instead, you'll be poring over each other's bodies, admiring how light falls on skin, and how the flickering flames dramatize your partner's curves or sinews. Aw yeah.

Remember, it's not just the bedroom that can sustain a sensual mood. A sexy night can begin the moment you or your partner walks in the door, and every room you move through can play a part. So remove the day's mail from the coffee table and replace it with an orchid plant or a blush-worthy gift (see Sweet Somethings, p.20). Ignore any furniture that isn't built for two, so that even if you're just dozing in front of a movie, you're doing so with your legs intertwined. Or sprawl on a *faux*-fur rug, surrounded by copious cushions, so that even if you're doing the crossword, you're in each other's arms—sometimes a few hours of this "might-not-go-anywhere" body contact is all the seduction you need. If you're lucky enough to have a fireplace, then light a damn fire every now and then. If the fire grows dim (or you don't have a fireplace to begin with), snuggle up under a blanket.

Ultimately, you'll be drawn to the bedroom. Kiss as you go. Open the window to let the long curtains waft in the breeze (or to give the nosy neighbors something to listen to). The lights should be, yes, dimmed. There should be no clutter, no mess, no unsexy piles of work, laundry, or bills (if this means shoving all your crap under the bed with the dust bunnies, so be it). Slide your limbs between satin sheets (or at least sheets with a decent thread count). Consider moving the standing mirror closer to the bed for later kinky use.

And if the satin sheets are in the wash? Sometimes, changing your usual sex venue is all you need to reinvigorate the usual sex ritual. There's no rule book that says good lovin' must take place in the bedroom each and every time (see Marking Your Territory on p.110 for inspiration). A new five-star hotel in town is an excuse to dress up for a night, indulge in oysters at the bar, and later press each other against the thick glass door of the shower in your well-appointed room. A sleazy budget motel rented for a lunch-hour might bring out the taboo in you. A lavish soirée may give you the opportunity to part, flirt with others until you "accidentally" bump into each other, introduce yourselves as if you've never met before, and eventually abscond to a nearby stairwell to lock lips (see the Fantasy chapter on page 140 for more ideas like this). Or a romantic picnic in a remote corner of the park might inspire you to commune on the long grass.

You certainly don't need a lot of money to set a sexy mood, only a willingness to invest a little time, effort, and imagination. In the end, if you can both keep your eyes open and still get and stay in the right head space for fantastic sex, you've succeeded. We'd give you a medal, but in this case the fantastic sex is its own reward. Plus, we're all out of medals.

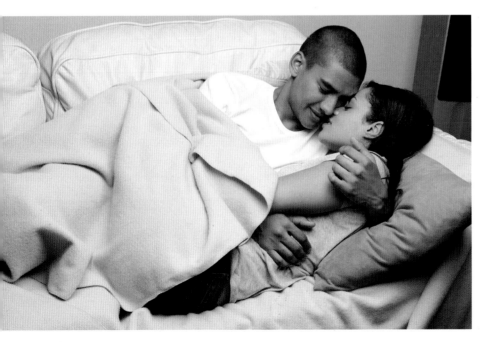

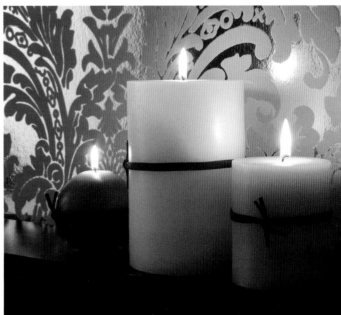

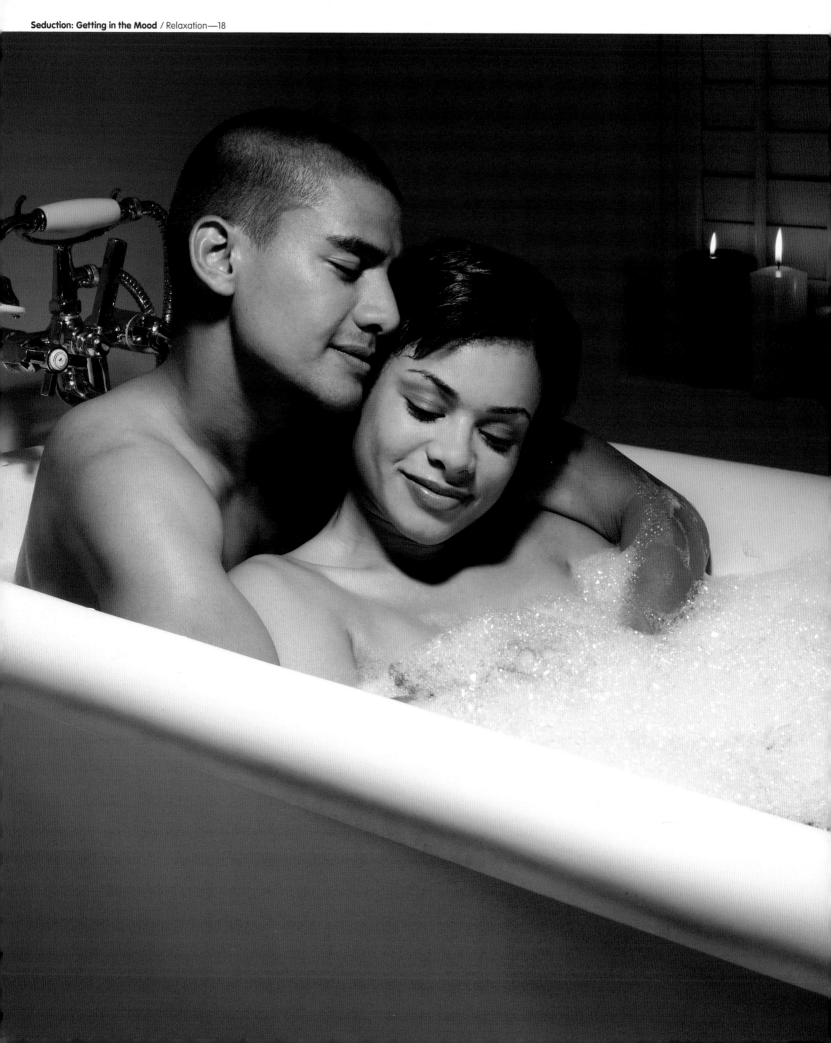

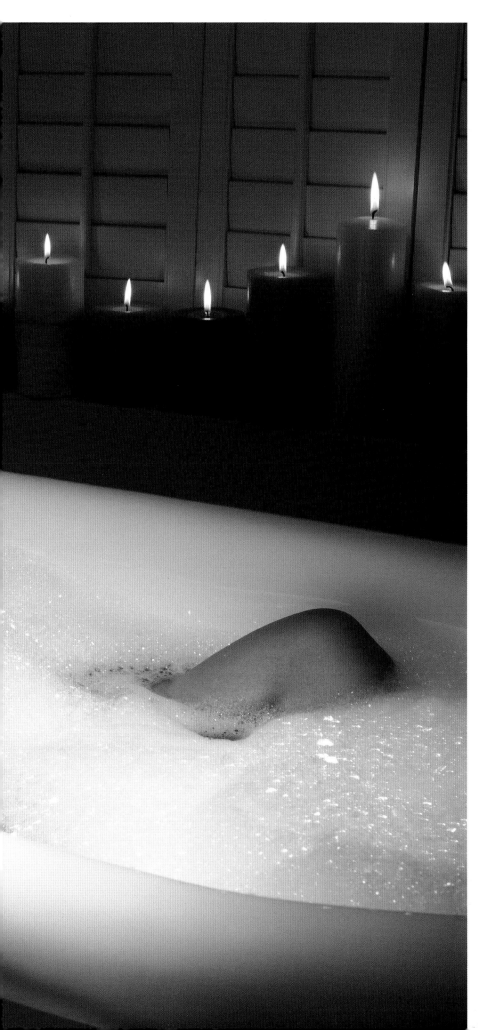

Relaxation

Good sex is no endeavor for the weary—and this is especially true, it must be said, for women. Alas, the world—a frenetic, kinetic, frantic, and frenzied place— often makes you so. Your senses are bombarded daily by unpleasantries (think rush-hour commute), so you've got to take care to heal them with beautiful sights, soothing sounds, aromatic scents, delectable tastes, and rejuvenating touch. Not only do you deserve regular respite, you *require* it. After all, it's only when you care for yourself that you're truly able to care for your loved ones.

First, give yourself the time and space to relax. If you can steal an hour or two for yourself (or an entire day if you're lucky), embrace the opportunity without guilt. No time spent caring for your body and soul is wasted. Scout out or create a reliable sanctuary that you can retreat to whenever you need it: a meditation space, a chaise longue by a window with a view, a spacious bathtub, a neighborhood spa, a gym sauna, a favorite country inn amenable to last-minute reservations… hell, even a quiet broom closet where you can chill out will do.

Wherever you are, learn how to shut out sounds that threaten to drag you back into the stresses of the day: turn down your phone, turn off the news, and drown out the outside world with music that clears your mind of to-do lists (death metal is probably not ideal for sensual relaxation rituals).

Then light a votive lavender or jasmine candle and breathe deeply like you do in yoga class. If that's too precious for you, pick up some freshly cut gardenias from the florist on the corner, put them in water, and let their subtle scent fill the room (guys, your girlfriends will love that you're secure enough in your masculinity to appreciate fresh flowers). Even something as simple as freshly baked rosemary bread from the corner bakery slowly warming in the oven can fill your space with the scent of comfort and well-being. Put on a pot of handcrafted blended tea, break open a pomegranate, or indulge in a few French chocolate ganaches. Soon your senses will remember their primary purpose: to be indulged.

If you can, seek out the healing touch of a professional— massage therapy can do wonders for your stress levels. (A very *un*professsional erotic massage—we mean one from your partner—is an even better form of pre-sex relaxation.) Or simply soothe your muscles with a ritualistic hot bath, filled with rich bubbles or soothing scented oils, or a pulsating shower that has no time limit (until the hot water runs out or your inner Al Gore starts berating you for waste). Not only will a warm washing ease tension, it'll make you feel more confident to eventually have all your nooks and crannies intimately explored (hey, the less you have to worry about, the better the sex). Afterward, when you're calmed yet invigorated, moisturize all over, lightly perfume or apply a nice deodorant, mist or dust yourself with the balm of your choice—basically, anoint your body as an act of self-love.

If you're not convinced you need to retreat to any kind of "special place" to get in the mood for sex, don't be so sure about your other half—maybe the art of seduction in this case is creating that place for your partner (hello, spa day) and joining them a few hours later. And, of course, any or all of the above can be done *with* a partner for simultaneous relaxation and foreplay. It's killing two birds with one pumice stone!

Connecting

How well you connect and communicate outside the bedroom will affect how well you connect and communicate inside the bedroom. Sure, people who hate each other can sometimes have intensely amazing, clothes-ripping, hair-pulling sex. But generally speaking, you've got to establish a solid foundation of mutual respect and interest that you can screw on—a foundation that can withstand all your tossing and turning and rocking and knocking in the throes of passion. Especially if you'd like the sexual relationship to last longer than one drunken evening.

Body Language—Whether you're wooing a stranger across the bar or a long-term partner whose body you've already charted, inch by inch, it all starts by catching their eye. Put down your drink or your book and look up; with your eyes, trace the face that you've known for a moment or for months. Make direct eye contact. The longer you've known the person, the longer you can hold their gaze; obviously, staring contests with complete strangers may have the opposite effect you're going for, so use discretion.

Once in conversation, on a date, or at home together, turn your body toward the object of your affection, maintain eye contact (no looking over their shoulder or around the room), lean in, touch their arm casually in agreement. Pay attention with your body without invading their personal space (i.e. going straight for the boobs).

The Art of Conversation—You've heard it before, we'll say it again: the best way to convey romantic interest (and fuel sexual interest) is to ask questions of your partner. *And actually pay attention to the answers.* In fact, the most important aspect of the art of conversation is simply listening. This does not mean you should not talk about yourself, discuss politics, goof around, or tell jokes—your partner should want to know you better, hear your thoughts, and be entertained by you, too. Smart talk and a sense of humor can be just as sexy as a cute bum. It's all about creating conversational balance. Simply put: be present.

Putting Pen to Paper—Write letters to each other, not just on your anniversary or special occasions, but on, say, Wednesday. The only reason you need to write is to express your affection—and thus pave the way for better sex (hey, affection, sex… it's all interconnected). Such letters don't always have to be sweeping declarations of love—sometimes one or two lines about what you thought as you watched them sleep that morning can say more than a book's worth of poetry. Perhaps it's a recollection of an early date, an invitation to a meaningful restaurant, an instruction to wear a favorite item of clothing this evening, or a dirty thought you had about them while at work. Of course, stealing from the pro's is entirely acceptable, too (just be sure to give e.e. cummings credit when it's due). Balance the romantic with the salacious. And while the handwritten note (whether on scented paper or a post-it) left somewhere for your partner to secretly discover cannot be beat for its old-fashioned novelty, the sweet email or naughty text should be employed whenever the spirit moves you. Better yet, they should be employed whenever you think it would move your partner. (For the record, gals, one dirty text that you actually follow up on is probably better than three hours of candlelit foreplay for most guys.)

Sweet Somethings—When words feel clumsy or inadequate, a gift can do the talking for you. Seducers are famously distracted by the object of their affection, and sensual gifts are a reminder that, early on or years later, the object of your affection is or remains a formidable distraction. The gifts say, I spent my time away from you planning how to please you. But choose wisely: gifts don't have to be expensive, they don't have to be traditional, but they should suit the recipient and complement their wants and desires. A 12-inch strap-on may not be at the top of your beloved's Christmas list. (Then again…) If you're going for a sex-related present, opt for the upscale if possible. As with food, when it comes to sex toys, it's all about the presentation: a black box with a satin ribbon will probably set the mood for seriously good sex way better than a cheap plastic box decorated with cheesy porn stars. (See pp.124–139 for inspiration.) And though we're sure we don't have to say it: never give a gift with the expectation that you'll automatically receive some oral attention in return.

Dirty Talk—You can also use your voice as a tool of seduction and variety. The same lustful command triumphantly exclaimed while standing in four-inch, Swarovski-encrusted heels or a three-piece suit will sound like another language when whispered pleadingly in your partner's ear as you lie alongside them, stripped bare. You can read aloud to each other from the ancient sex poetry of Ovid or Sappho for kicks (and ideas). Talk about what you're currently doing to your partner, what you plan to do next, and what you would really like to do. If the two of you employ refined language in your daily life, then inside the bedroom embrace words that make you blush. Quietly whisper something completely inappropriate when out in public together. In the heat of the moment, don't be afraid to admit what works for you: just be sure to speak in positive suggestions rather than criticisms. And sometimes, of course, say nothing at all—the longing conveyed in one heartfelt sigh can speak volumes. (For more on talking dirty and sharing fantasies, see pp.144–145.)

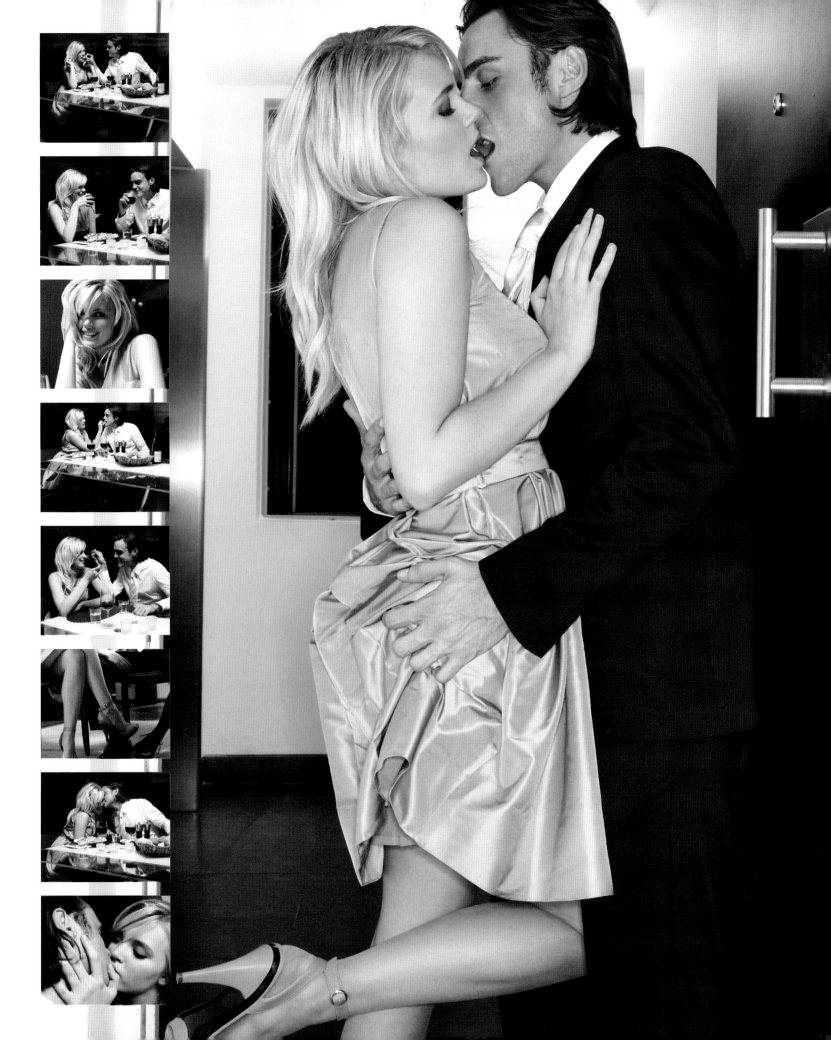

Saving something for later isn't just for prudes anymore. In fact, delayed gratification is one of the best forms of foreplay around. Love and sex are always more satisfying when there are obstacles to achieving them—you feel like you've really earned them. That's why taking your time, prolonging the inevitable, and touching everything but can be great for couples who know they're a sure thing for each other: it creates the *illusion* of adversity and challenge. Plus, it makes the eventual orgasm that much more satisfying.

Start with a hot and heavy make-out session before leaving the house for dinner and save the sex for your return (you might want to skip the dessert). Wear something sexy your partner will want to rip off you… but can't until much later. Let your hands wander during the opening credits next time you're at the movies (though please consider your fellow theater-goers' delicate sensibilities). When you get home, pretend you're 16 again and your parents might walk in at any second. Make undressing a deliberate, suspenseful act. Give each other a full-body massage. Kiss—just kiss—for at least an hour (okay, at least 15 minutes). The possibilities are only limited by your imagination… and your self control.

Teasing & Tantalizing

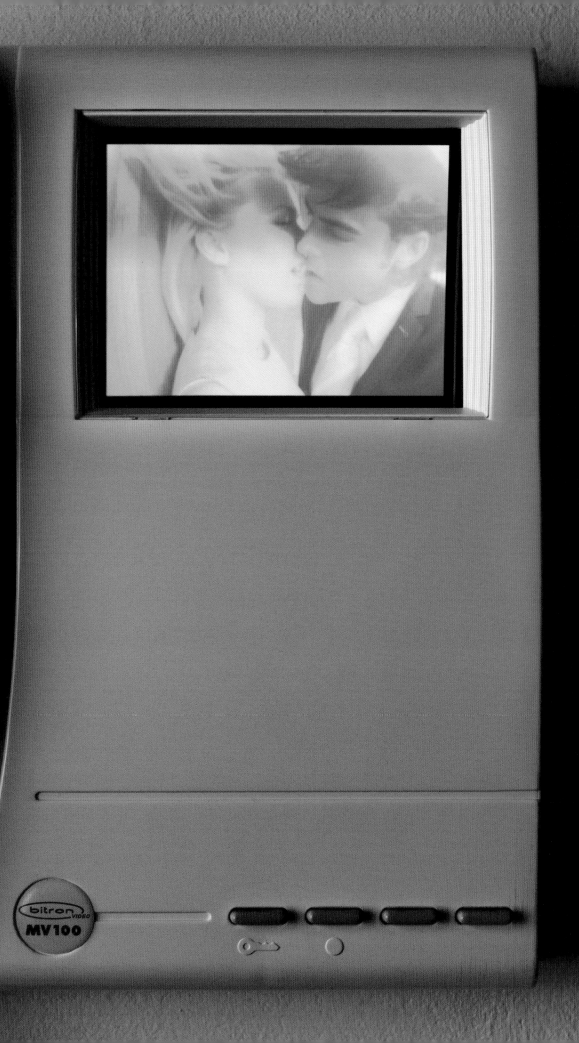

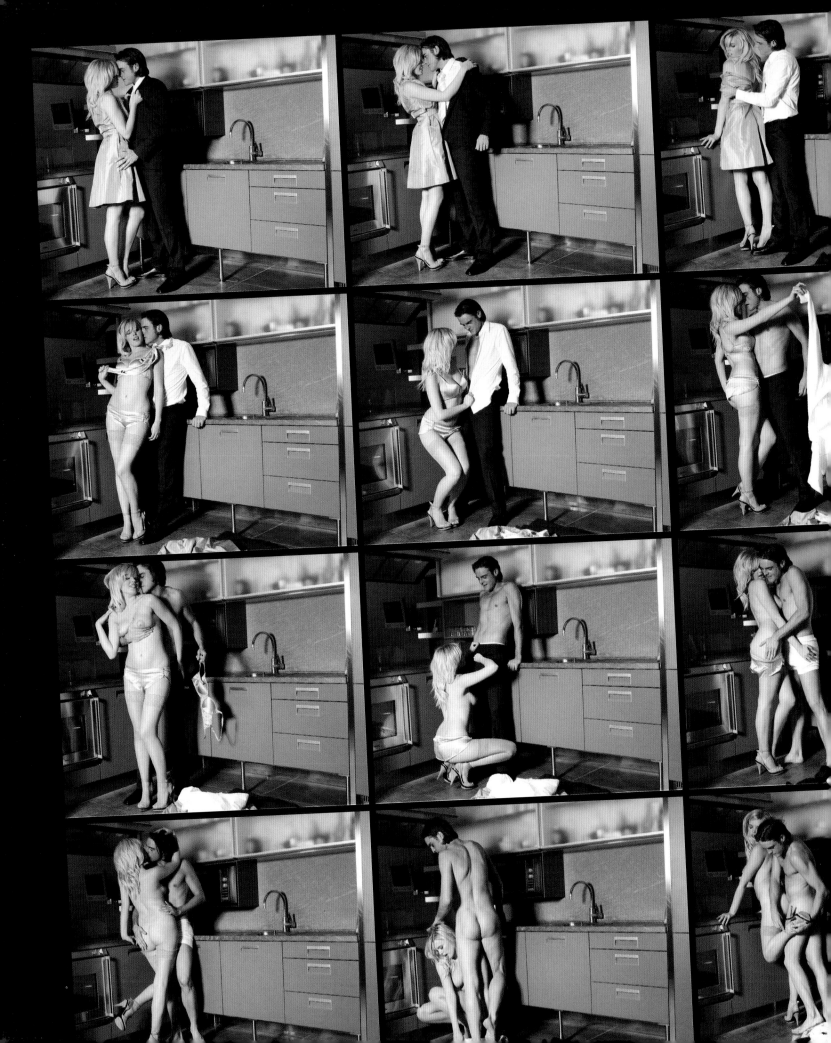

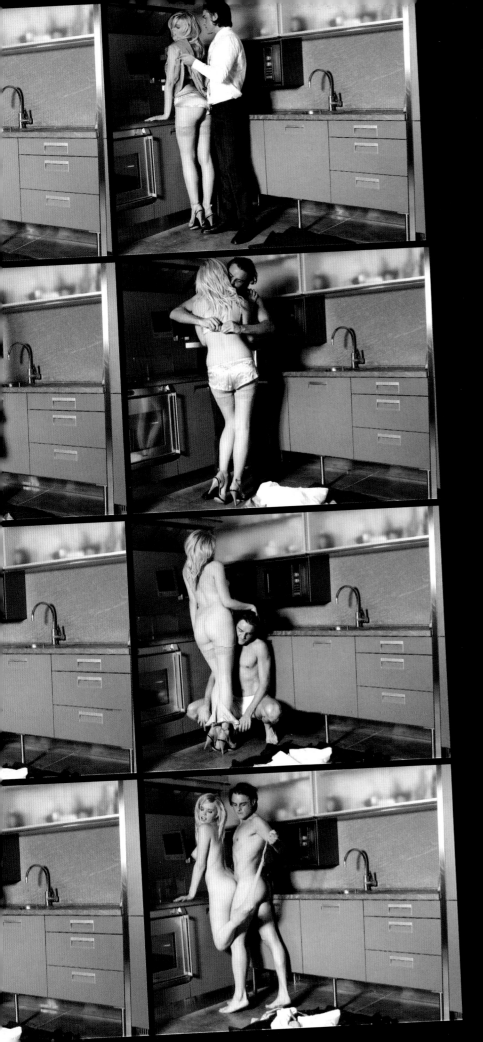

Adornment

What you put on and how you take it off can mean the difference between sex that's just a habit and sex that's an *event*.

Dressing for Sex—If you think you only get *un*dressed for sex, then you're missing out on half the fun. And we're not talking about cheap polyester lingerie or any other ensemble that makes you feel awkward, embarrassed, or itchy. Getting dolled up and dressed for sex is supposed to turn you *both* on—meaning that it should feel as good as it looks. The right outfit—whatever that is for you—should empower as it flatters.

You've probably worn such an outfit early on in a relationship, when you were hoping for sex with a new partner. But why primp and prep only for near strangers? Commitment is not a free pass to slovenliness. You should consider your appearance a part of extended foreplay in any relationship —not every hour of every day, but enough to show you care about looking good to and for your partner and yourself, at least occasionally. (Men, this applies to you too.)

Prefacing sex with a nice night out on the town should inspire you to get decked out. But even if you're spending a quiet evening at home together, think twice before stripping off your suit and grabbing that stained sweatshirt. Why not shower first, like you would for a second date? And then put on something that's comfortable *and* alluring: cleavage you'd never dare reveal in public, a soft fitted tee that hugs your biceps just so, a dress that's indecently sheer, a silk robe with a sash that will handily double as a blindfold later, soft fabrics that beg to be touched, a dab of your partner's favorite scent. Or, comfort be damned: wear the tight jeans or racy corset you've always been too shy to leave the house in and reinvent yourself for the night. You've got an audience of one, so play to it!

Undressing Each Other—Everyone loves a good tear-off-the-clothes quickie, but what makes a quickie hot is how feverish and urgent it feels. If you *always* tear off your clothes (your partner's or your own), then a quickie will become the norm— and there's nothing feverish or urgent about the norm. So the next time you undress, slow things way down for a change. Take it in turns, piece by piece: she takes off his jacket, he unzips her dress, she unbuttons his shirt, he pushes her bra straps off her shoulders and kisses her clavicle, she traces his lips with her fingertips while unzipping his fly… Appreciate the effect of each item's removal. And here's a hint: start with the shoes. Because nothing spoils an intimate undressing more than getting your trousers stuck around your ankles, causing you to fall to the floor with the grace of an overweight amateur ice skater.

Undressing Yourself—If you *really* want to control the pace of the unveiling, you'll have to take matters into your own hands—literally. Undress your partner completely without letting them near so much as a button of your own, and then undress in front of them like you've got all day—lean in to tease, but never let them get close enough to touch. They may cry "torture," but they're loving it really. Or undress yourself completely and *then* start on them, but insist they keep their hands to themselves until the last layer is off. It's like a striptease but without all that "Do I look ridiculous?" anxiety. (If you think you can overcome those fears, turn to pp.150–151 to learn how the pros do it.)

Kissing

Hollywood movies don't get a lot right when it comes to sex—in fact, we hold them responsible for 54 percent of the orgasm-faking in this world, thanks to the unrealistic expectations they create—but we'll give them this: they know kissing. On the big screen, the right kiss can make the characters swoon—and that's not unbelievable cinematic hyperbole, people, that's just good kissing. Hell, even just watching those smooches can induce a swoon.

It's time to learn a thing or two from the matinee idols. You might think you don't need a refresher course, but we heard otherwise. Because, while everyone thinks they're a good kisser, everyone can't be right (think about it: how many bad kissers have *you* known? See? Everyone can't be right). The pure excitement of first pecks can sometimes offset any egregious osculation errors, but still, the kiss can make or break successful seduction. And while it's one thing to kiss someone for the first time, it's quite another to make someone weak at the knees a thousand kisses later.

So next time you kiss your partner hello or goodbye, kiss as if this were all there was in the world, as if this were more than you had ever hoped for, as if you might win an Oscar for it. Stop to kiss outside the front door before letting yourselves inside, kiss before opening the mail, kiss before asking, "How was your day, dear?" Hold each other's faces, run your hands through each other's hair. Let your lips brush ears, cheeks, shoulder blades, the soft inside of the wrists. And, for Cupid's sake, *swoon*.

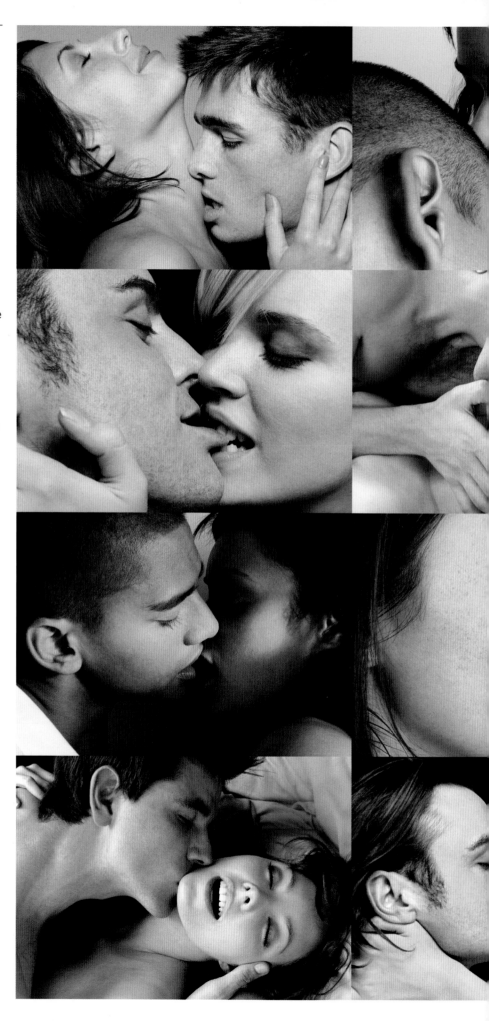

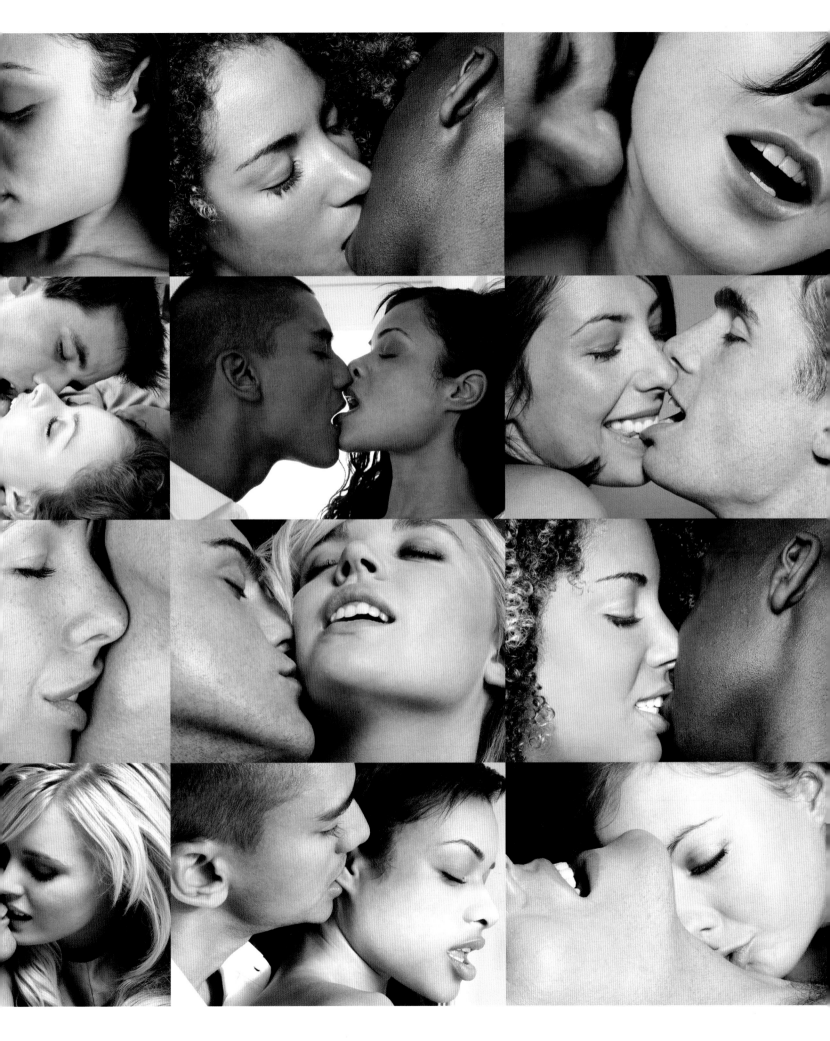

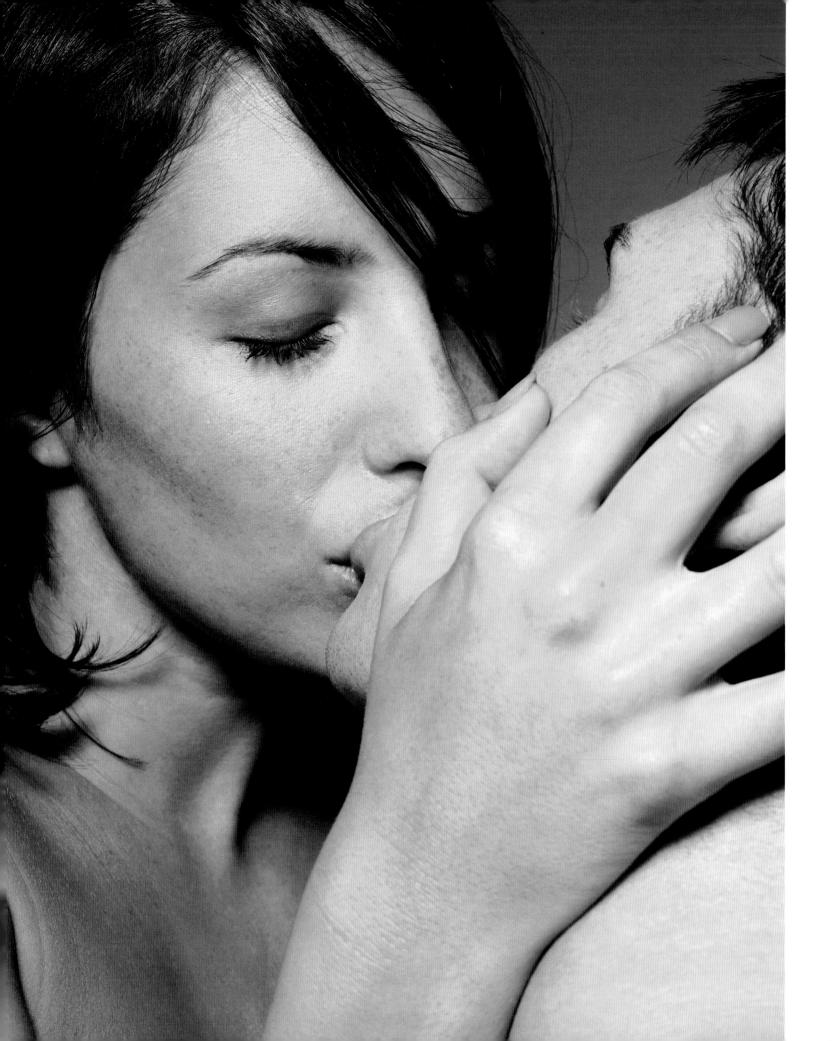

23 Calls to Lip Action

01 Brush your tongue as well as your teeth, floss regularly (no whining), and keep mints handy for emergency touch-ups, because bad breath makes every other tip on this list moot.

02 Moisturize—chapped lips are a bummer.

03 But don't lick your lips when going in for a kiss, lest you look like the Big Bad Wolf sizing up his next meal.

04 Go easy on the gloss, because three coats of red lipstick or thick sticky goo make you about as kissable as a bulldog with gum disease.

05 Use restraint when it comes to tongue (i.e. don't ever think of kissing as "tonsil hockey").

06 Create a crescendo by starting with no tongue at all, progressing to one tongue, and advancing to two—but only if you can follow rule 5.

07 Keep your tongue soft and flat, not pointy like an eel.

08 Cradle your partner's face, neck, or head in your hands.

09 Entwine your fingers in their hair.

10 Pull gently on that hair if things get really heated.

11 Kiss everywhere above the shoulders: the side of their neck, their forehead, their closed eyes, the front of their neck at the base where the collarbones meet, behind the ears, the earlobes (but never the canal).

12 Push aside their collar to kiss a bare shoulder and then cover it up again.

13 Barely brush their lips as you kiss with yours slightly parted.

14 Gently suck or even nibble their lower lip or the fleshy part of an earlobe, but only for a few seconds.

15 Do not run your tongue along their upper and lower gums as if trying to dislodge dentures.

16 If you'd like them to kiss you a bit more aggressively, tease them with your tongue and keep pulling back.

17 Suck on their tongue—gently, and with prudence: not everyone's a fan.

18 Keep your salivation in check—sloppiness does not equate to passion.

19 Make out on the couch during commercial breaks.

20 Push your partner against a wall and kiss them (unless they're on their way to the loo).

21 Whisper sweet (or dirty) nothings into their mouth instead of their ear, so your lips brush theirs as you speak.

22 Tell them you can't wait to go down on them, but then make them wait for it longingly while you kiss for a bit longer, as a sort of preview of things to come.

23 Remember that while kissing goes well with everything else, everything else doesn't necessarily go with kissing: savor the smooching and save the boob groping and crotch grabbing for a little later.

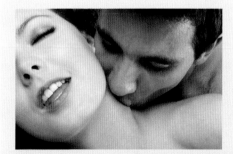

The Lovebite

When you're freshly post-pubescent, the lips are the gateways to all pleasure. Just touching two sets together releases the floodgates below. And once the mouth begins exploring other areas, no publicly exposed skin is safe—along the clavicle, behind the knees, in the armpits, even. Unsure of how far you can go, but hungry for more and more, you end up snogging like a Dyson. That's why lovebites are so popular with the kids—they're a way to be bad and bold without taking off so much as a watch. Then you grow up and start having adult sex. But dismissing the lovebite rules out a whole slew of sexual play even grown-ups can enjoy. For a start, it takes you back to simpler times, when you were young with bad skin and worse haircuts, when sex was new and, most importantly, fun. At any age, giving or receiving a lovebite taps into your animal instincts— that toothy grip of the lion on the back of his mate's neck, that lingering vampire fantasy. (However, for safety's sake, never break the skin!) And if you're on the receiving end of someone's suction cup, the hickey serves as a dirty little reminder of what you've been up to. You wake up the next day, the previous evening's romp a happy blur, and look in the mirror to see an imprint the size of Belgium on your neck.

Sure, on the one hand it gets you some ribbing at the office—which reminds us: never administer a visible lovebite until you know the recipient is up for it—but on the other it's proof that, even though you're no longer 18, you're still getting some.

Massage

There's no better foreplay. It creates a moat between the day's stresses and the evening's hanky-panky, forces you to slow down, gives your partner the perfect excuse to start moaning, and awakens nerve endings they forgot they had (don't laugh or we'll talk about your chakras).

Get Ready—You need massage oil (body lotion gets absorbed too quickly) or, at the very least, soft hands; a warm room with low lighting; peace and quiet or mellow-but-sexy music (not "world music"); a soft but firm surface. If yours is a water bed, try a well-padded floor with nice carpeting or blankets (and consider upgrading to a bed from *this* decade). If you opt for the oil, lay down a soft towel to absorb any excess.

Get Set—Remember, your goal is to seduce, not work out knots. No professional distance necessary! That said, don't forget about symmetry: you could be giving the most erotic massage of your life, but if you ignore your partner's left side after working on their right, it'll spoil the whole damn thing. And be prepared to coach your partner into rag-doll relaxation—they should not be lifting their own body parts to help you out.

Get Naked—*Both* of you. Consider a relaxing candle-lit bubble bath first—you'll be glad you did when you get to the toes. If your partner lies perpendicular to the edge of the bed, you'll have better access and the option of sitting on the bed *or* standing beside it for some of the moves. Finally, before you begin, warm the oil between your hands; to be *really* nice, run the bottle under warm water or keep it within arm's reach in a bowl of hot water.

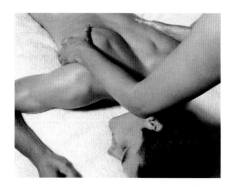

Sexy Back—Your partner lies face down. From over their head, lean in and glide your palms down their back; as you reach the haunches, spread your hands in opposite directions like the breast stroke and pull back toward you, cupping each side of their body. Repeat, using long, slow, smooth strokes—your hands should barely leave your partner's body (unless it's to reapply oil). Trace the same path with light fingertips or fingernails and then palms again, alternating between a strong rub and a gentle caress. Then, straddle your partner's legs and use two strong then feathery fingertips to trace a line up either side of the spine (never directly on the spine), from tailbone to neck.

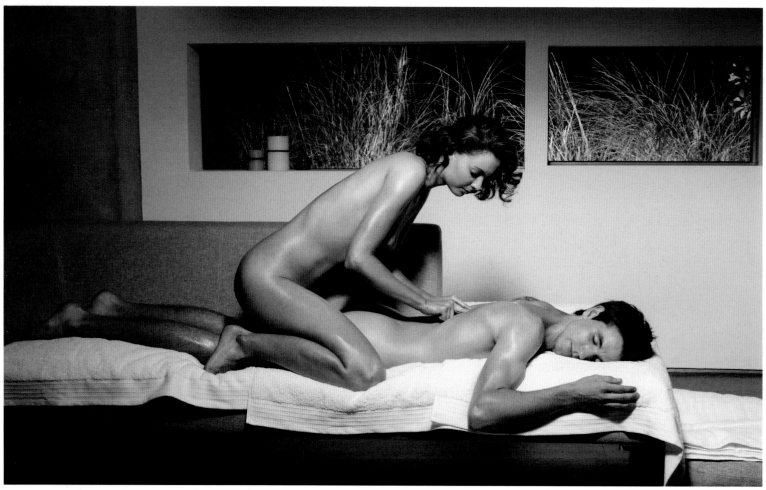

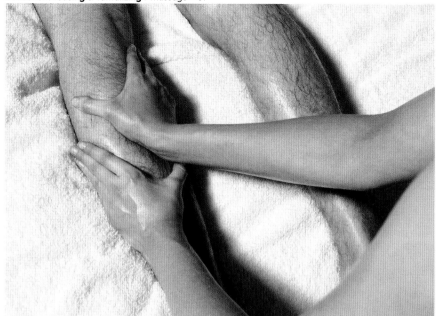

Legs that Go All the Way Up—Place both hands at the back of an ankle so that each forms a V between thumb and index finger, then glide your hands forward as far as you dare. Then play footsie—turn your partner over, perhaps placing a rolled towel or pillow under their knees, calves, and/or ankles like the pros (it's more comfortable on their back). Roll your knuckles or press your thumbs into the soles of their feet, then focus on the pads and heels. Squeeze the tip of each toe between your fingertips. For a truly naughty sensation, slide your fingers back and forth between their toes!

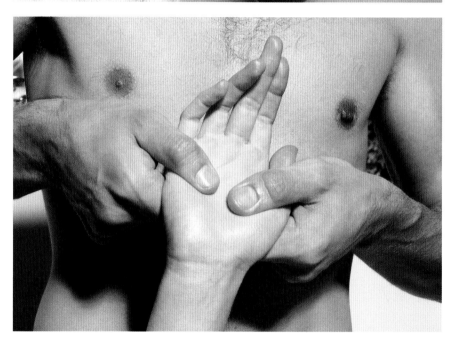

Give Me A Hand—Stand or kneel beside your partner and hold one of their arms up and out from their body at just under a 45-degree angle, using one of your hands for support under their upper arm, the other near their wrist. Now pull your hands, one after the other, toward your own body along the length of your partner's arm, like pulling a length of rope, except very, very gently—dislocated shoulders are not sexy. Next: support your partner's arm against your body (relish the skin contact) and massage their palm with both your hands, especially your thumbs. Try those moves above we suggested for the feet.

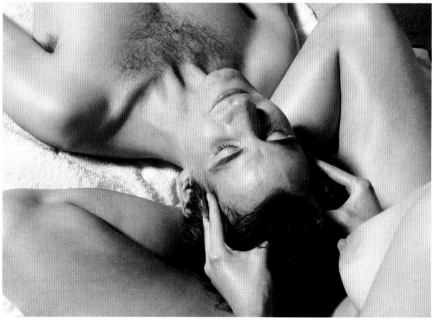

Head Rush—Cradle your partner's head on your thighs or lap and rub a few drops of tingly peppermint oil into the scalp with your fingertips (no nails). For the face, switch to a light lotion and gently smooth your fingers from the center out toward their ears, focusing on their forehead, eyelids, cheeks, and chin. Rub—but don't tug on—their earlobes. Definitely *don't* "steal their nose." Steal a kiss instead.

A Note on Touching Tatas—Erotic massage is a great time to discover how your partner likes to have their chest, breasts, and nipples touched. Remember that most boobs welcome focused touch only once their owner is aroused. Assuming your partner likes to have them touched in *some* way, try mixing things up: soft stroking, squeezing (but not like a teenager), licking, sucking (but not like an infant), and the occasional hard nipple tweak. Don't always go straight for the nips. In fact, the side-boob is a highly underrated, under-touched area full of nerve-endings. And try to avoid anything that resembles a breast exam.

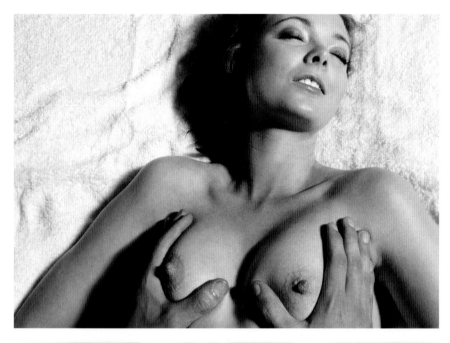

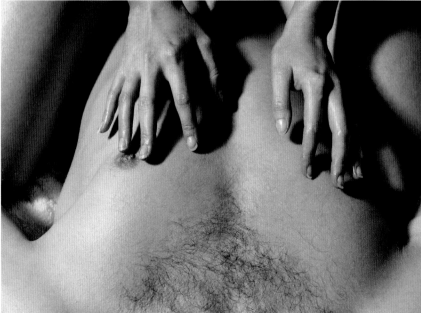

Her Breasts—Ready for the grown-up portion of your massage? Start by massaging up between her breasts, then around the outsides, cupping them gently before moving back down to her stomach so that each hand makes an oval, avoiding the nipples for now. Next, place a palm, fingers splayed, on the underside of each breast; massage upwards, gently closing in on each nipple between your index fingers and thumbs. Then either continue your upward motion, passing over her nipples toward her chest, or gently squeeze up and away from her body at her nipples (no vise clamps please). Or cup each breast and slowly pull your fingers toward the nipple, tweaking *gently* as you draw your fingers into a point (don't attempt to tune in Tokyo).

His Chest—A male friend once told us, "My breasts are like flowers. Women never send me flowers. They should. Women never suck and touch my chest and nipples. They should." If your fellow is a fan (not all of them are), then straddle him and gently tickle and stroke his entire front torso with feathery fingertips, making little tapping motions. Move into the nipple zone: again, some men love the outlying-area attention but will flinch if you hit an actual nip nerve (bless their delicate sensibilities). Assuming your partner is like our friend, have him close his eyes, then lean in and circle each nipple with your tongue—you're the inappropriate masseuse, remember!

Happy Endings—An erotic massage isn't meant to lure the recipient into sex (unlike all those backrubs you gave in college). It's something you do when sex is already a given. Nevertheless, you've got to commit to the massage and agree to *at least* 20 minutes of sensual stroking before you hump on your makeshift massage table. Oils are not latex-safe, so if you've been using oil on or near the genitals, use a polyurethane condom or just rub 'n' tug your way to a happy ending. Also, to be safe, please don't ever push down hard on any vital organs! And bear in mind that after receiving an hour of blissful massage culminating in a massive, quivering O, the last thing your partner will be in the mood for is doling out a return massage—if they have to reciprocate immediately, it'll be half-hearted at best. Decide in advance that reciprocation will take place on another day. Because, while it may not be karmically kosher to admit it, nothing spoils the joy of giving a good erotic massage like getting shortchanged on the return.

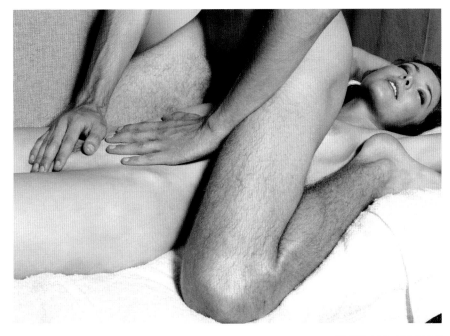

The Goods (Hers)—Where does erotic massage end and manual sex begin? It's all about context— and lube. Oil is not meant for internal massage: it can irritate sensitive vaginas or even lead to an infection, so stay out on the front porch for now (if you really want to go inside, switch to a *water-based* lube and turn to p.59). Cup the mons with your fingers pointing down and pull up from the perineum in long strokes. Draw things out by moving from the center of her universe down to her toes and across to her fingertips, or up between her breasts and back again, repeatedly.

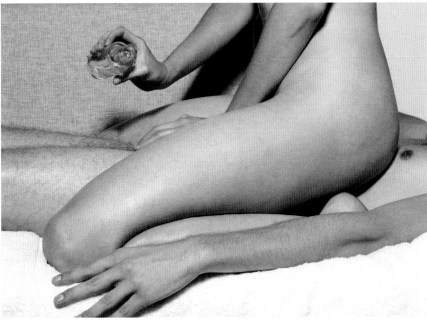

The Goods (His)—This is your basic handjob (p.62), but without the acceleration. His parts are hardier, so oil away—just don't forget that oils can break latex condoms and may irritate your own gal parts, if intercourse is on the menu. Rest your hand on his package and pour *warm* oil through your fingers. Cup his balls, slide up and down his shaft, and massage his perineum. Keep your strokes long and steady, and if it all gets too hot too soon, massage his legs, arms, or chest to cool him down. If he's a backdoor friend, you can throw in a little "prostate massage" (p.119). But if he's new to the male G-spot thing, do this *only* by prior arrangement. Otherwise, the muscles you just relaxed might tense up like rigor mortis.

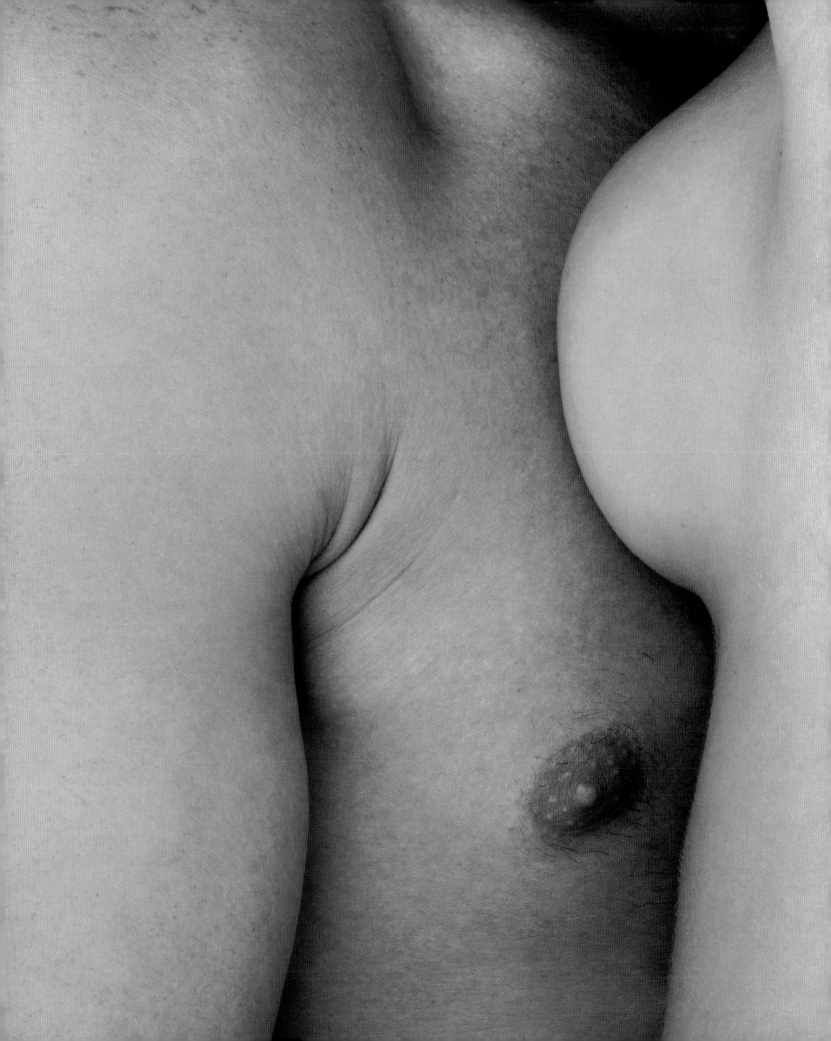

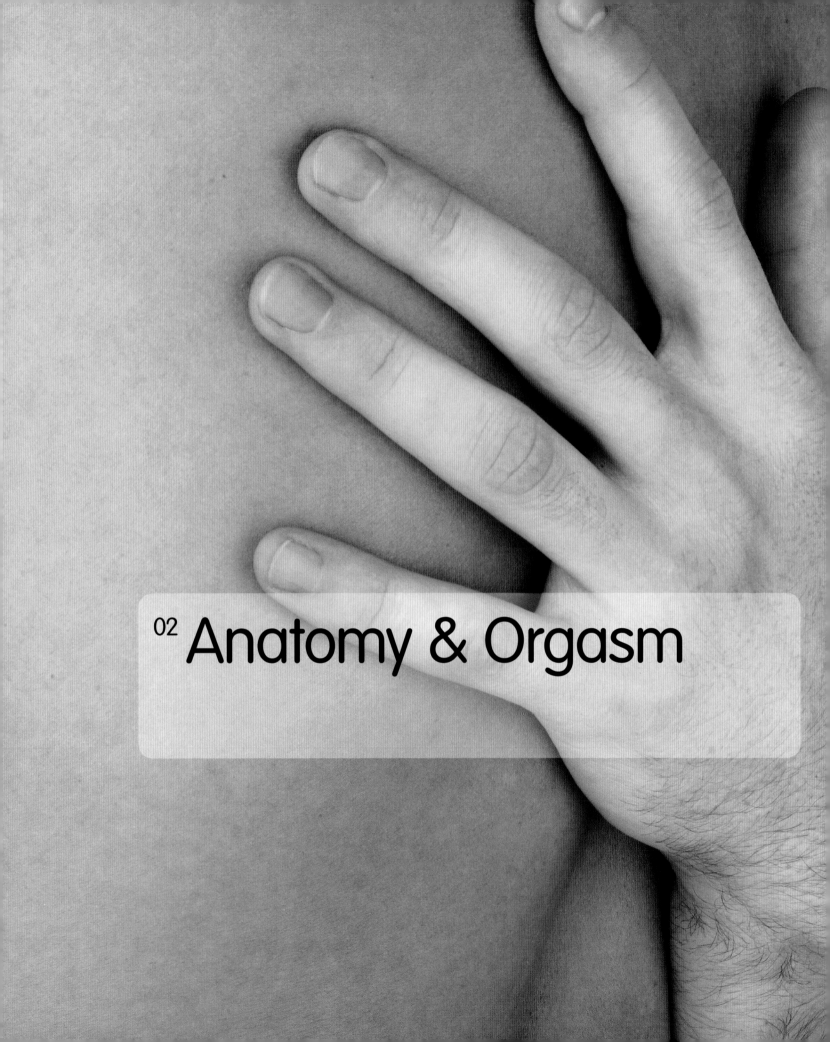

02 Anatomy & Orgasm

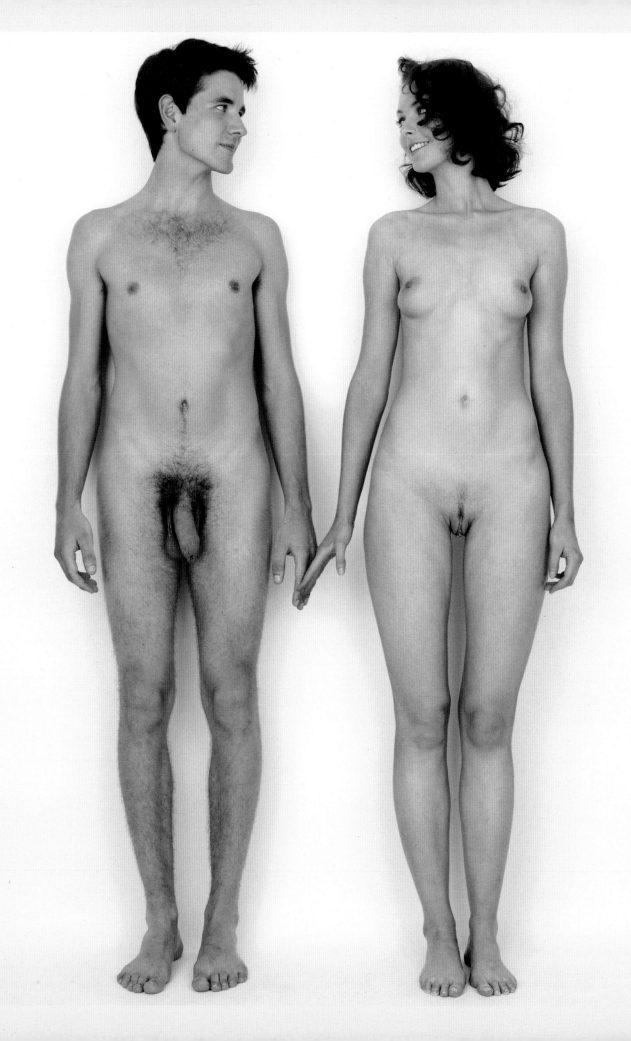

Getting To Know You

Before you can create a masterpiece, you have to understand your medium. Knowledge is power, *especially* when it comes to sex. When you know the anatomy of women and men (as well as the variations among us), when you can name and pinpoint parts, then everything becomes much less mysterious and intimidating; you realize men and women aren't that different after all, which puts you and your partner on an equal playing field; and you can better manipulate your bodies at will to get the pleasurable responses you desire.

There's much more to your genitals than what you learned back in middle school sex-ed. And info on the Internet is often either too clinical, too out-dated, or too just plain wrong. So familiarize yourself with the new-and-improved biology lesson on the following pages. But don't stop there: take time to know thyself—thy physical self. Explore your genitals with your eyes and hands before, during, and after arousal. Get an up close and personal view of your parts. Use a hand-mirror. Use your fingers to feel what you can't see. Notice how arousal affects their shape and color. (Men definitely have a head-start here, as more of his parts are external, but guys can still benefit from a more deliberate assessment of cause and effect.) Once you've familiarized yourself with your own anatomy, do the exact same thing with your partner—make it a kinky doctor's exam, if you like.

Self-exploration may sound hippy-dippy, but people used to say that about yoga, too. We encourage you to get off your asses, stop relying on instinct alone, and take an active interest in your machinery and how it works. Not only will it get you orgasms, it will get you *improved* orgasms. The better you know your body, the better you know your partner's, the more you like and accept yourself, the more you believe you're entitled to sexual pleasure, the more confident you are in bed, the better shot you have at a screaming good time. So be patient. Masturbate on a regular basis. Show and tell your partner what you like. Vow never to fake again. Don't chase your or your partner's orgasm with a blind vengeance. But don't give up on it either.

There's a lot more than meets the eye when it comes to her sexual anatomy: the waters of her pleasure system run way deep. (And we're not just talking about the vaginal canal here.) Her parts are not inferior, miniature versions of his, but rather equitable, albeit more internal, sexual structures that enjoy stimulation just as much as his. They just need the right kind of stimulation. Understanding those structures—and understanding how each part compares to his bits and pieces—is the first step in learning how to provide this stimulation.

Mons Pubis—The mons or mons pubis is the area less formally known as your bikini triangle: it's the padded tissue that protects your pubic bone and would be covered in pubic hair if we weren't all such manic groomers. Some women enjoy having this area stimulated, especially if they actually have hair here that you can run your fingers through.

Vulva—The external, visible parts of the female genitalia. When people say vagina, they often actually mean vulva, as the latter term includes not just the vaginal opening but also the inner and outer lips, the clitoral head, the urinary opening, and the mons.

Clitoris, a.k.a. the Female Penis—Contrary to popular belief, the clitoris is more than just that little nubbin you see or feel protruding near the top of the labia—that's just the tip of the iceberg. No, the clitoris is actually a complex organ of nerve-rich erectile tissue (just like the penis) extending throughout the genital area. We're talking four inches long (one inch shy of the average penis, but proportional to her body size) in the shape of a wishbone. During arousal, this tissue becomes engorged and erect, just like the penis—it's just more difficult to notice in women because most of the erection occurs internally. Another difference in erections: a woman's has a better chance of lasting long after orgasm, hence her ability to have subsequent orgasms more easily than a man. And here's a bit of trivia for your next cocktail party: the clitoris is the only organ in the human body—in either men or women—that exists solely for sexual pleasure.

Clitoral Head, Tip, or Glans—The little "handle" of the wishbone that protrudes externally at the junction where the top of the labia connect—what most people usually think of when they think "clitoris." Some clitoral heads extend out like an erect nipple, while shyer ones hide under the hood. (The more aroused she becomes, the more retracted the clitoral head may become as the ligament supporting it tightens with sexual tension.) One of the best ways to arouse the entire clitoris is to provide stimulation to this head/tip, not only because it's external, but because it contains more nerve endings than any other part of the body, male or female. (See clittage, p.58.)

Clitoral Hood—The female equivalent of foreskin: the clitoral shaft runs under it and the clitoral head sticks out of it. The hood is created by the junction of the outer edges of the inner lips meeting above the clitoral head.

Clitoral Shaft—You can often feel the short (i.e., less than an inch long) shaft of the clitoris underneath the hood as it burrows into the genitalia, first in the direction of the pubic mound, before it turns sharply back downward and splits into two long wishbone legs.

Female Anatomy

Clitoral Legs—The two slim prongs of the clitoral wishbone that run underneath the labia and flank either side of the urethra, the urethral sponge, and the vagina (p.41). Like the clitoral head and shaft, the legs are made of erectile tissue that stiffens during arousal.

Clitoral Bulbs—As well as the wishbone, there are two eggplant-shaped bulbs that run along the inside of the clitoral legs, beneath the inner labia and around the sides of the urethra, the urethral sponge, and the vagina (p.41). This erectile tissue also becomes engorged during arousal, puffing up even more than the legs, and making the inner labia balloon.

Outer Labia or Lips, a.k.a. the Female Scrotum—Developed from the same embryonic tissue that becomes the scrotal sack in men, the outer labia are the two hairy pads of fatty tissue that pocket the inner labia, clitoral head, and the urethral and vaginal openings. While sensitive to touch, the outer labia—unlike the clitoris and the inner labia—don't have a very rich concentration of nerves, nor do they change in shape or color much during arousal. The outer lips, which are usually covered in pubic hair, are sometimes referred to as the *labia majora*, though we tend to avoid this term as it implies that the outer lips always protrude further, which is not necessarily the case.

Inner Labia or Lips—The two, moist, hairless, inner folds of tissue that connect at the top around the clitoral head (forming the clitoral hood and the frenulum), run along either side of the urethral and vaginal openings, and connect at the bottom just under the vagina (forming the fork). Despite what porn and labiaplasty docs might have you believe, there is great—not to mention totally normal—variation in their appearance from woman to woman: light or dark, trim or long, smooth or wrinkled, turned inward or flared outward, one side larger than the other… And during arousal, a woman's lips will often change in appearance, swelling and darkening from increased blood flow to the area. Due to their sensitivity and role in arousal, the inner labia are often considered an extension of the external part of the clitoris. The inner lips are sometimes referred to as the *labia minora*, though again we prefer not to use this term, as it's quite common for a woman's inner lips to protrude further than the outer lips. And given the number of nerve endings in the inner lips compared to the outer, this can actually be quite a good thing, so don't let anyone tell you otherwise.

Frenulum, a.k.a. Bridle—The junction of the inner edges of the two inner lips, usually just below the clitoral head, which, like a man's frenulum, is sensitive to stimulation. It may also be considered a part of the external clitoris.

Urethra—The short thin tube running from the bladder to the small opening between the clitoral head and the vaginal opening through which urine and, in some women, female ejaculate is eliminated.

Urethral Sponge, a.k.a. the Female Prostate—The spongy erectile tissue surrounding the length of the urethra that consists of glands, known as paraurethral glands, which produce an alkaline fluid similar to that produced by the male prostate (i.e., it's not urine). This fluid may be expelled into and then out of the urethra and out of the paraurethral ducts in a process known as female ejaculation; this may occur in spurts, in a rush of fluid, or in such insignificant amounts as to be undetectable. The embryonic tissue that develops into the prostate gland in male fetuses is the same tissue that develops into the urethral sponge in female fetuses.

U-spot—The external area surrounding the urethral opening. Like the area right around the penis's urethral opening, this nerve-rich spot is sensitive to touch and may be an undiscovered erogenous zone for her, because you are indirectly stimulating one end of the urethral sponge (similarly, with G-spot probing, you are stimulating one side of the

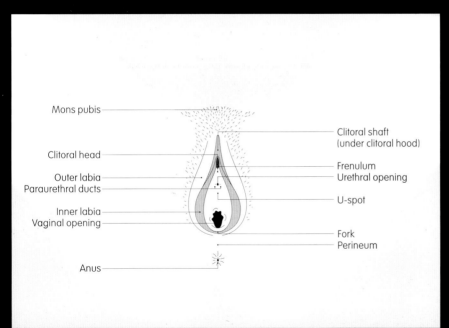

Mons pubis

Clitoral head

Outer labia
Paraurethral ducts

Inner labia
Vaginal opening

Anus

Clitoral shaft
(under clitoral hood)

Frenulum
Urethral opening

U-spot

Fork
Perineum

External Female Anatomy

urethral sponge). Stimulation of the U-spot is often a happy accident of nearby clitoral head and vaginal orifice stimulation. Upon arousal, it may protrude a bit and take on the appearance of an acorn top (like the external tip of a penis).

G-spot—The area of the urethral sponge (or female prostate) that can be felt and stimulated through the top wall of the vagina by inserting a finger, fingers, penis, or sex toy a few inches inside and pressing up toward the navel or the back of the pubic bone (p.59). The texture of this area is often rougher and more ridged than the other, smoother vaginal walls. Some women find this stimulation incredibly pleasurable, some find it necessary for orgasm, some find it enables female ejaculation, and some find it uncomfortable, a sort of painful pressure reminiscent of a urinary tract infection.

Paraurethral Glands & Ducts—Prostatic-fluid-producing glands (usually about 30) embedded in the urethral sponge. Upon arousal, they fill with this fluid, which may, during G- or U-spot stimulation or orgasm, drain (i.e., gush, spurt, or dribble) out into and then from the urethra as well as out of the two external openings embedded in the U-spot known as the paraurethral ducts (they're almost impossible to detect). This process is known as female ejaculation; depending on the size and number of glands you've got (every woman is different), and whether you enjoy G- and U-spot stimulation, you may spurt across the room, or not even notice any extra fluid emanating from this area (p.59).

Vagina, a.k.a. Vaginal Canal or Birth Canal—The canal that runs from the cervix (the door of the uterus or womb) to the orifice between the urethra and the anus. Penises, fingers, and sex toys can go in here; it's also where menstrual blood and perhaps babies come out. The clitoral legs, clitoral bulbs, the urethral sponge, the perineal sponge, and the pelvic floor muscles all surround the lower half of the vagina—during arousal, they become engorged and erect,

and then (and only then) can they be stimulated by vaginal penetration. The resulting tightening of the outer third of the vagina causes it to become sensitive to friction and pressure. (It could be argued that these other structures are what are really being stimulated during penetration, not the vagina). This is why girth and shallow penetration is often more effective for her pleasure than length and deep pelvic thrusting, and why penetration feels best once a woman is fully aroused or perhaps even has just had an orgasm.

While the vagina is self-lubricating (the pressure of increased blood to the genitals during arousal expresses a clear fluid that's filtered from the blood through the mucous-membrane walls of the vagina), don't rely on lubrication as her quintessential sign of arousal, as many factors can inhibit the natural flow of this wetness, even when she's turned on.

The vagina's fornices (fornix = singular) are the deepest recesses of the vagina created by the extension of the cervix into the vaginal canal. The A-spot (the anterior fornix) and the cul-de-sac (the posterior fornix), two other "vaginal hot spots," may be easier to reach and stimulate once she is fully aroused, as the uterus lifts and the back of the vagina balloons out. There's also the PS-spot directly opposite the G-spot (see "perineum" below). However, keep in mind that other as-of-yet unnamed hot spots may exist for her anywhere within the vaginal canal (for example, the sides of the canal), and it's a matter of exploring and experimenting with what feels right and nice. The vagina is often misconceptualized as the equivalent of the penis, and while there certainly is an undeniable ying-yang factor necessary for reproductive purposes, as far as sexuality and pleasure goes, the female equivalent of the penis is the clitoris.

A-spot, a.k.a. A-zone, Anterior Fornix, AFE Zone (Anterior Fornix Erotic or Erogenous Zone), or T-zone (for Trigone of the Urinary Bladder)—There are way too many names and way too many erroneous write-ups on the web about this particular vaginal zone. Put simply, it's the nerve-rich area deep inside the front (i.e., anterior or belly-side) wall of the vagina, next to the cervix (i.e., *past* the G-spot, beside, or even beyond the tip of the cervix). Think of it as stimulating one side of the bladder via the front wall of the vagina (just as you stimulate the urethral sponge via the front wall of the vagina when G-spotting). It's not always easy to stimulate the A-spot with typical intercourse and it's hard to reach with your own fingers, so squatting or pulling your knees up while having a partner reach for it with their finger(s) or using a G-spotter (a vibrator or dildo with a curved tip) with a long shaft may be better at determining your sensitivity there. Some people, like the Malaysian doc who "discovered" this zone in the early '90s, report that stimulating this area, especially with repetitive stroking that eventually incorporates the G-spot too, can help increase vaginal lubrication and orgasmic potential (p.44).

Cul-de-sac, a.k.a. Posterior Fornix—The nerve-rich area deep on the back (i.e., posterior or bum-side) wall of the vagina, beside and just past the cervix (named by Dr. Barbara Keesling in *Super Sexual Orgasm*). It may be difficult to reach, not only because of its depth, but because the cervix may block access to it, especially if the woman is not sufficiently aroused. During arousal, the uterus tends to lift up and the back of the vagina tents out, opening this area up for stimulation (pressure is often preferable to thrusting; p.59). However, if she's not fully aroused or she has a low-riding uterus, the thrusts of intercourse may just result in a less-than-pleasant cervix pounding, never reaching the cul-de-sac.

Fork, a.k.a. Fourchette—The junction where the bottoms of the two inner labia meet, just beneath the vaginal opening.

Perineum & the Perineal Sponge (a.k.a. PS-spot)—The perineum is the short bridge of tissue between the vaginal opening and the anus (p.39). Just beneath it is a tightly packed tangle of blood vessels alternately known as the perineal sponge, perineal body, or PS-spot. Like other erectile tissue, this mass fills with blood upon arousal and can be sensitive to massage and pressure via the perineum, the lower back wall of the vagina (opposite the G-spot), or the anus (see below).

Anus & Rectum—The rectum is the S-shaped tube that serves as the passage way for poo between the intestine and the final exit, the anus. This nerve-rich orifice—which consists of two, fairly snug, ring-like sphincter muscles—is surrounded on all sides by one layer of the pelvic floor muscles, which also surround the vagina and urethra. Nearby is the sensitive perineal sponge, as well. Thus, it makes sense that the anal area would respond to stimulation and can be an integral part of her genital pleasure and even orgasm. (For more important info on proper stimulation and penetration, see pp.114–123.)

Pelvic Floor Muscles—A series of muscles stretching from the pubic bone to the tailbone and running between, around, and beneath the various sexual structures which, if strong and healthy, provide a) support to these structures and other internal organs, b) urinary and fecal continence, and c) sexual pleasure: they contract in response to sexual stimulation, causing sexual tension, which may eventually get released during the involuntary contractions of orgasm. (To ensure yours are strong and healthy, see p.175 for important info on Kegel exercises.)

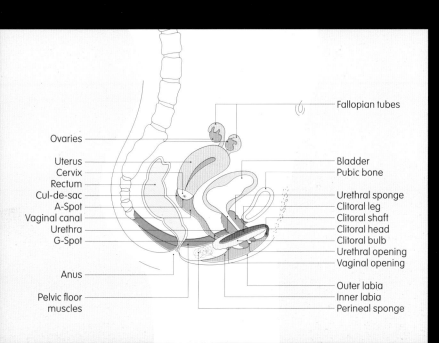

Ovaries
Uterus
Cervix
Rectum
Cul-de-sac
A-Spot
Vaginal canal
Urethra
G-Spot
Anus
Pelvic floor muscles

Fallopian tubes
Bladder
Pubic bone
Urethral sponge
Clitoral leg
Clitoral shaft
Clitoral head
Clitoral bulb
Urethral opening
Vaginal opening
Outer labia
Inner labia
Perineal sponge

Internal Female Anatomy (Cross Section)

Just because his sexual structures are a bit more, shall we say, obvious, does not mean you can forgo the anatomy lesson. There are important parallels between his and her sexual machinery that will help you both understand how to best to use what you've got on your own and with your partner. For instance, did you know he has a clitoris too?!

Penis, a.k.a. the male clitoris—The most valuable player of male sexual function. This very visible shaft is often considered the corresponding puzzle piece to the vagina. Understandable, but that often leads both men and women to discount the importance of her clitoris (especially when it doesn't seem to actively provide stimulation to his member). It's useful to know that the penis actually incorporates many of the same or similar sexual components that are key to female sexual functioning, including the clitoris. In his case, those components may be a little more efficiently organized and consolidated, at least when when you consider penetration: during intercourse, all the parts of his penis/clitoris are stimulated simultaneously, which is one reason why penetration tends to be a sure-fire method of orgasm for him; however, traditional intercourse stimulates only the sides of only some of her clitoral structures, making orgasm through mere penetration tricky (or even impossible) for many women.

Shaft—The long external neck of the penis that extends from the man's body to the penile glans.

Corpus Cavernosum—Within the penis runs this narrow wishbone-shaped erectile tissue much like the woman's clitoral wishbone, except in men the "handle" end is long, about four inches (running the length of the shaft, parallel to the urethra), and the two clitoral "Y" legs are short (splitting at the base near the pubic bone). Upon arousal, it fills with blood and becomes bigger, straighter, and more sensitive, i.e., erect, just like her clitoris.

Urethra—The tube that runs from the bladder, through the prostate gland and along the shaft (where it's surrounded by spongy erectile tissue), to the urethral opening at the penile tip, through which urine and ejaculate are expelled.

Urethral Sponge, a.k.a. Corpus Spongiosum—Like the female urethral sponge, this erectile tissue surrounds his urethra, responds to stimulation, and fills with blood upon arousal (though it remains much more pliable than the corpus cavernosum so the urethra doesn't get pinched closed, which would cut off ejaculation). Some consider this the single equivalent of the two clitoral bulbs in women, as it ends in one bulbous structure within his body just past the base (the "root" of the penis). At the other, outermost end, the corpus spongiosum forms the acorn-shaped head or glans, molded over the exterior end of the corpus cavernosum.

Penile Tip, a.k.a. U-spot—The sensitive, innervated skin around the urethral opening.

Penile Head or Glans—At the outermost end of the penile shaft, the corpus spongiosum forms the acorn-shaped head or glans which is molded over the rounded, exterior end of the corpus cavernosum. Many consider this the equivalent of the female clitoral glans (both the female and male hoods or foreskins protect these two "heads"). But by stimulating his glans, you're also stimulating the exterior end of the corpus cavernosum, which can also be considered an equivalent to her clitoral head, though in his case it's not external.

Foreskin—The retractable sheath of skin attached to the shaft of the penis via the frenulum that serves as a sort of

Male Anatomy

oversized turtleneck: it's pulled over most if not all of the penile glans when not erect (protecting the naturally moist mucous membrane of the glans), and pulled back during arousal (aiding in both his and her pleasure during penetration). It's the equivalent of the clitoral hood in women. If the foreskin is removed via circumcision, the membrane of the glans will become tougher and permanently dry, and he'll probably benefit from the addition of lube during manual sex, since his foreskin can't act as a natural moveable stimulation sheath.

Frenulum—A highly sensitive band of tissue on the underside of the penis, just under the glans, that keeps the foreskin in place. Whether the frenulum is left intact, partially removed, or fully removed during circumcision, the area tends to remain a particular pleasure point (albeit to varying degrees).

Prostate gland—The smooth, walnut-sized organ located behind his pubic bone, below the bladder, and above the perineum, through which the urethra runs. The prostate produces an alkaline fluid that constitutes up to a third of the contents of ejaculate which helps transport and protect sperm during and after ejaculation. The muscles of the prostate also help expel the ejaculate from the body. When you gently stimulate it via the front wall of the rectum, you'll feel it get bigger and firmer the closer he gets to climaxing (see p.119 for more info). Butt plugs, like the Aneros, are designed specifically for the pleasure and health of the prostate (p.136).

P-spot (for Prostate), a.k.a. the Male G-spot—The area of the prostate gland that can be felt and stimulated through the top, belly-side wall of the rectum by inserting a finger, fingers, dildo, or anal sex toy a few inches inside and pressing toward the navel or the back of the pubic bone. (To stimulate the gland indirectly, press up on the perineum.) Some men find this stimulation incredibly pleasurable, some find that it intensifies orgasm, and some find it downright uncomfortable. However, we suspect some of this discomfort is psychological

in nature, as many hetero men (mistakenly) feel that penetration is either too girly, too gay, or too unhygienic. Or else they're just not doing it right—to do it right, turn to p.118.

Testicles & Scrotum (a.k.a. the male labia)—Analogous to the egg- and estrogen-producing ovaries in women, the testicles are two reproductive organs which produce sperm and male hormones (like testosterone). The "balls" are inside the scrotum or scrotal sack, the equivalent of a woman's outer labia (both develop from the same embryonic tissue), which hang outside the body (behind the flaccid penis) and may similarly enjoy gentle stroking. Gently pulling the testicles during arousal may help delay ejaculation.

Perineum—The short bridge of tissue between the back of the testicles and the anus. Also known universally, but mostly for men, as the "taint" (it ain't the balls and it ain't the asshole). Perineal massage indirectly stimulates his prostate.

Anus & Rectum—The rectum is the S-shaped tube that serves as the passage way for poop between the intestine and the exit, the anus. This nerve-rich orifice—which consists of two, fairly snug, ring-like sphincter muscles—is surrounded on all sides by one layer of the pelvic floor muscles, which also surround his other sexual structures. And his prostate gland can be stimulated a few inches inside the anus via the front rectal wall. Thus, it makes sense that the anal area can be an integral part of his genital pleasure and even orgasm. (For important info on stimulation and penetration, see pp.114–123)

Pelvic Floor Muscles—A series of muscles stretching from the pubic bone to the tailbone and running between, around, and beneath the various sexual structures which, if strong and healthy, provide a) support to these structures and other internal organs, b) urinary and fecal continence, and c) sexual pleasure: they contract in response to stimulation, causing sexual tension, which may eventually get released during the involuntary contractions of orgasm. (To ensure yours are

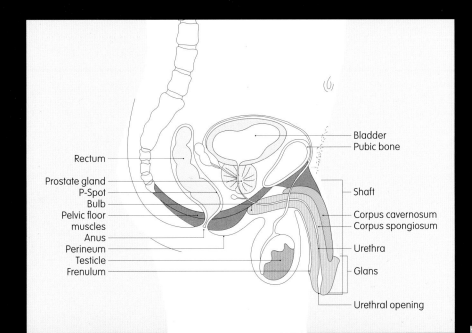

Rectum
Prostate gland
P-Spot
Bulb
Pelvic floor muscles
Anus
Perineum
Testicle
Frenulum

Bladder
Pubic bone
Shaft
Corpus cavernosum
Corpus spongiosum
Urethra
Glans
Urethral opening

His Internal Anatomy (Cross Section)

Some people wake the neighbors when they climax while others hold their breath, as if time itself were standing still. Some people say your name, others call out to God, and still others may yell things in a language unrecognizable as human. In other words, no two orgasms sound alike. That said, anatomically, all orgasms come from the same place, and understanding that can help us get there more often. So, let's find out: what are orgasms made of?

Sexual Response

The traditional (and male-centric) model of sexual response is linear: desire > sexual arousal > sexual excitement > climax > resolution. But recent studies suggest that some response cycles, especially women's, seem to be more complex and circuitous than originally thought. Rather than *sexual* desire, the cycle may start with an emotional desire (to be loved, found attractive, etc). Distracting thoughts can inhibit arousal and climax. Traditional physical indicators of arousal may not be reliable: you can be sexually aroused without your parts working in ways they're expected to, and you can be physically aroused without actually being mentally aroused. Climax of course is not guaranteed. And physical arousal can occur (from a physical or subliminal stimulus) before cognitive desire: i.e. you're turned on before you even know it.

So rather than just telling yourself to "get in the mood", it might be better to focus on the physical cues or activities that kickstart your sexual arousal. It should go without saying that

you should never do anything you don't want to. But most of the time it's not that we don't want to, it's just that we're too tired, too stressed, or too annoyed—so just doing it can get you over that hump, as it were. (It's like working out—the hardest part is just getting yourself to the gym. But once you're there, you're almost always glad you went.) Plus, the more sex you engage in, the more you want it, because sex increases your testosterone level, which actually increases your desire.

Other recent studies have also highlighted differences in male and female heterosexual desire: women's sexual tastes vary more, they're more likely to find homosexual content arousing (men are more black and white when it comes to preferences), men have a higher sex drive across the board while women span the full range (some have low libidos, others have skyscraper-high ones), and men may be more perpetually primed for sex while women are more cyclical in their desires.

But before we go segregating the sexes into Martians and Venusians, we should remember that age, experience, culture, context, and personality can affect sex in ways that make it unpredictable, no matter what your gender. We all have different sex drives, and different reasons for and expectations of sex. And there are plenty of grey areas and overlap. So acknowledge and respect your differences, but not at the expense of finding common ground to fuck on.

What Happens During Orgasm—In both women and men, the brain sends out sexual hormones and chemicals into the bloodstream. Heart rate and blood pressure increase. Pupils dilate. Blood rushes to the genitals and fills the erectile tissue, and hey, guess what? Erection occurs: his penis becomes stiffer, straighter, bigger, and longer; so does her entire clitoris (as a result, her labia balloon and the vaginal canal becomes constricted). Nerve cells in the area are awakened, and skin (particularly erogenous zones) becomes more sensitive. Lubrication may occur (pre-ejaculate in him; vaginal fluid in her). Pelvic muscles and ligaments tighten up, causing sexual

Orgasms!

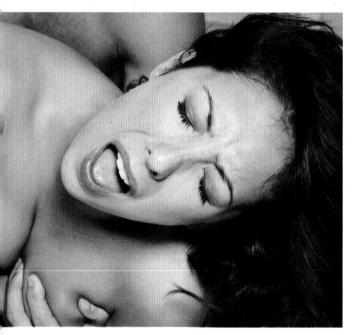
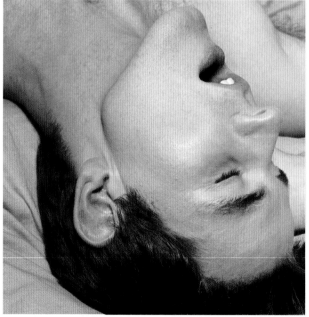
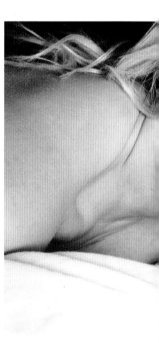

tension. His and her erectile tissue continue to become hypersensitive due to increased blood flow. Assuming the right kind of rhythmic stimulation is provided (whatever "right" means for the individual), and no distractions (mental or otherwise) get in the way, all these sensations ideally reach a crescendo and the sexual tension is released in a series of regular, involuntary contractions (from a few to 15) as blood leaves the area (more so in men) and more feel-good chemicals (like oxytocin) flood the body. For him, ejaculation (the mix of sperm from the testicles and prostatic fluid from the prostate) is usually released during orgasm. However, men can learn, through a series of techniques grounded in Eastern philosophy, to separate their orgasm from their ejaculation in order to retain energy and attain multiple orgasms themselves (see Resources on p.188 for information on how). For her, orgasm *may* result in prostatic fluid from the urethral sponge being expelled via the urethra and paraurethral ducts (though this is much less common—or at least less noticeable—than his ejaculation). Feelings of well-being and relaxation wash over both men and women, but while the former are more prone to a sleepy recovery phase of sexual disinterest, the latter are more likely to continue feeling sexual, energized, and ready for more— a great reason to adopt the "ladies first" rule in bed.

The Elusive Female O

Let's be honest here: women drew the short straw when it comes to achieving orgasm. Men's orgasms practically grow on trees—can you imagine a bunch of blokes sitting around the pub complaining about how hard it is to climax? (Sure, they've got other problems, like climaxing too soon—for that, turn to p.177.) The female struggle to O is a two-pronged problem. First, her orgasm, unlike his, is not necessary for reproduction, so there's no evolutionary pressure for women to climax. Exhibit A: her genitals are not as efficiently designed for penetration pleasure as his are—he could poke away all

day long, but if she's not appropriately aroused or they're not in exactly the right position, intercourse is not going to give her the kind of clitoral stimulation she probably needs to come. Secondly, and more importantly, our culture still perpetuates myths that keep women's orgasms from being a priority, such as: intercourse is the highest form of sex two people can engage in; women take forever to climax; men are naturally sexual takers while women are givers; quantity is better than quality; blah blah blah. Add to that the dearth of good information on female anatomy and decent research on female sexual function, and it's a wonder women climax at all.

The first key to unlocking the female orgasm is technical. You've got to get a grasp, as it were, on her anatomy (turn back a few pages). Once you understand the parts, you can better manipulate them via masturbation and manual sex, whether alone or in addition to intercourse, oral sex, or anal sex. Remember, it's not just a matter of supplying hours of stimulation, but rather supplying the right kind of stimulation. This usually means engaging some if not all of her clitoral network, perhaps in conjunction with a "hot-spot", via manual sex, and avoiding penetration until she's fully aroused. See Handwork on Her on pp.56–59 for specific techniques.

The second key is more mental. While anyone can be affected by cognitive inhibitors (and men can certainly benefit from the following advice, too), generally speaking, women tend to be more easily distracted from the sexual response process. Stress about a work deadline, annoyance over a partner failing to do the laundry, feelings of unattractiveness, sexual guilt from a religious upbringing, etc—all can work to sabotage enjoyment and ultimately orgasm. This may be why countless women's magazines talk about the importance of foreplay—not necessarily extended stimulation (since many women, once aroused, can bring themselves to orgasm within minutes), but rather a deliberate warming up to the idea and getting in the right headspace (since sex for women tends to be a full-body experience, which includes the mind).

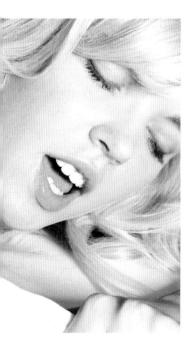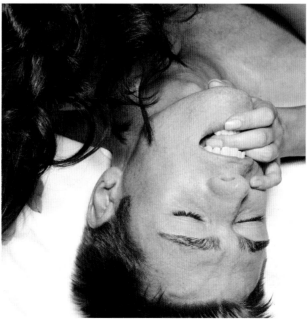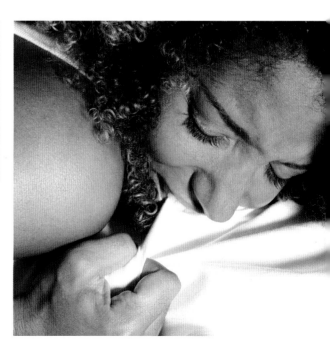

Gals are generally a lot more amenable to some hanky panky after 20 minutes of hair-stroking or back-rubbing in front of the TV, followed by sex that makes their pleasure a priority. Things like a sexy soundtrack, good lighting, and clean sheets can also help them stay focused on the road to their happy place (see Getting in the Mood in the previous chapter).

Of course, the music could be seductive, the lighting dim, the position comfortable, and the man gorgeous, but if her mind isn't present in the moment—for example, she starts stressing about why her office-mate didn't invite her to a cocktail party or, worse, she begins worrying why she hasn't climaxed yet—she won't get no satisfaction. So ladies, first, tell yourself, "I'm allowed to do anything except have an orgasm" in order to take the pressure off. Next, use your eyes to train your thoughts on sensations, as opposed to internal ideas: look down at the action or into your partner's eyes during sex; looking up into space will only encourage your mind to wander. Rather than analyzing what's (not) going on, participate in what's going on. Focus on what you're feeling in the moment—muscle tension, a change in your breathing, your desire to thrust or writhe—rather than where you're hoping to wind up (or what you're doing later that evening). Instead of interrogating your orgasm, interrogate your body. Keep asking yourself these questions: "What does it feel like when he does that?"; "Why does being in this position feel so different?"; "*Where* does it feel different?" and, "Do I like it?" But don't ever ask, "Why haven't I come yet?" If it helps you stay focused, you could even say your responses out loud. That way, your partner gets to benefit from the answers, too!

Different "Kinds" of Orgasms?

Describing the quintessential orgasm is tricky. Climaxing is different from person to person, and from day to day. Some orgasms are weak, some are intense, some are localized, some are full-body, some just scratch an itch, and some are religious experiences. There are nocturnal orgasms, multiple orgasms, extended orgasms, and simultaneous orgasms. Then, in women, there are more variations: you've got so-called clitoral orgasms versus vaginal orgasms versus uterine orgasms, even. We say a rose by any other name… Rather than categorizing and commodifying them into stupid human tricks that sell magazines (and potentially set you up for failure and disappointment), let's first make sure everyone can have an orgasm, period. Your first and foremost goal should be to get to know your own body, your own preferences, and your own methods of attaining orgasm (no matter what "kind" it is). The better you do all that, the better you can control and manipulate your sexual response alone or with a partner in order to achieve various results—whatever you call them.

Improving *Any* Orgasm

Lose the Routine—Once you've developed a tried and true method of climaxing, alone or with a partner, it's hard to muster the patience or willpower to give up that direct route from A to Oh for a less traveled, meandering path that may turn out to be a dead end. After all, having just one way to climax is far better than never having an orgasm at all. Plus, some people just have very specific arousal and orgasm patterns. So don't stress that you "should" be doing it differently—that may just have negative consequences on the orgasms you already do have. That said, if you believe there's only one way to climax, then you'll always climax that one way. And just like a strict diet of chocolate and red wine would eventually lose some of its appeal, so too can your orgasm. So experiment: go slowly, make sure you're fully aroused before you try something new, and add the kind of stimulation you want to learn to like to the kind that you already do. But don't put yourself on an orgasm diet just for the sake of learning a new trick: there's nothing wrong with ending in the same position every single time, so long as you don't always start in that position, too.

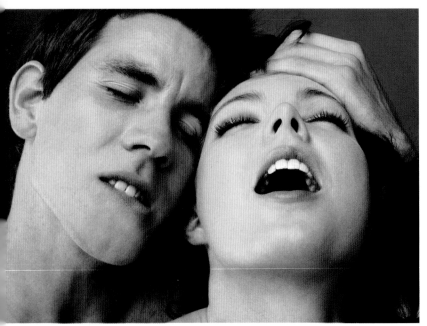
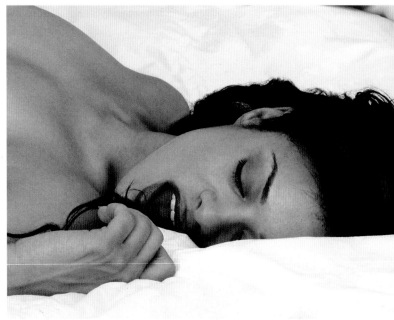

Delay Gratification—If James Joyce could make Molly Bloom wait 45 breathtaking pages for her orgasm in *Ulysses*, you can probably hold out for an extra minute or two, right? So the next time you're having fun on your own, don't go straight there. Bring yourself to the brink (or rather just before the brink), stop, take a breather, switch positions or techniques, resume and repeat. And then try this with a partner, too. Guys can experiment with slower and more shallow alternatives to pelvic thrusting (which she may actually prefer), alternating intercourse with offering oral sex, gently pulling the testicles away from the body, and perhaps even wearing a cock ring. (For info on premature ejaculation, see p.177.) Delaying gratification will not only ensure that she's fully aroused (i.e. prepared for orgasm), it will help build sexual tension in both of you, which can intensify eventual orgasms. Plus, when you know your body and have control over when you climax, you can try to sync up your orgasms.

Spread the Love—Just before, during, and just after your orgasm, you can draw that energy up through your body, rather than keeping it one place, simply by using concentration, focus, and the power of your mind. But if that's too Eastern for you, you can use a free hand or two (yours or your partner's) to help sweep waves of pleasure throughout your body, using long, smooth strokes up your belly or your back.

Just Breathe—Lots of people, especially women, hold their breath when they feel they're getting close to an orgasm. But that can sabotage your orgasm by throwing your body into self-preservation mode. So let your breathing reflect the intense feelings you're experiencing and you may find all that heavy huffing in turn makes those feelings even *more* intense.

Read the Rest of this Book—Relaxing (p.20) can be the first step in setting the stage for achieving successful orgasm. Accessorizing with a sex toy or even just lube (p.129) can introduce you to new or more intense sensations that you never knew existed. Getting your mind in the gutter with outside sexual stimuli, like erotica or porn, can be a great arousal trigger (p.144). And doing your Kegels (p.175 and p.177) can lead to stronger contractions during your climax.

The Pressures of Sex

Almost everyone has faked at least once in their lifetime. Yes, that includes men: their orgasms are expected to grow on trees, as we are guilty of suggesting ourselves, so imagine the kind of pressure that puts on them to perform! Your reasons may seem justified in the heat of the moment: you do it to spare your partner's ego, to give an impressive erotic performance, to fast-forward a particularly extended session in order to avoid love burn, or to keep from admitting you're just not sure how to come at all… But no matter how you break it down, faking is a fib. And that kind of dishonesty will only get in the way of you achieving genuine orgasms. The more often you fake, the harder your partner will find it to accurately tune into your body. Hence the vicious cycle of faking: the longer you do it, the easier it is to get away with, and the further you'll drift from each other in the bedroom—and eventually, in the relationship, too.

Sex doesn't always have to end in a climax (for either of you). If you're able to think of sex as being less goal-oriented, sometimes that makes it less intimidating to get things going. Think of it as just having dirty fun (and if you're not having fun, then you're doing it wrong). Because if you assume that every time you make out, it has to lead to "mind-blowing, God-finding, orgasmic sex!", then you're going to start avoiding making out if you're not in the mood for sex, and then no one ever gets in the mood.

That said, everyone has a right to sexual satisfaction in bed. And you and your partner should make it a priority to figure out how to attain that satisfaction together. With any luck, this book will help.

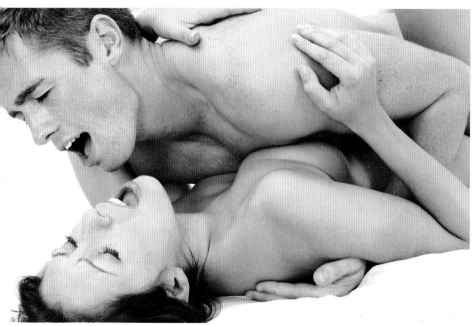
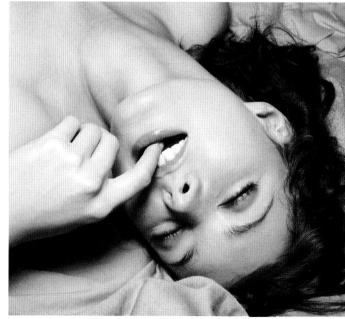

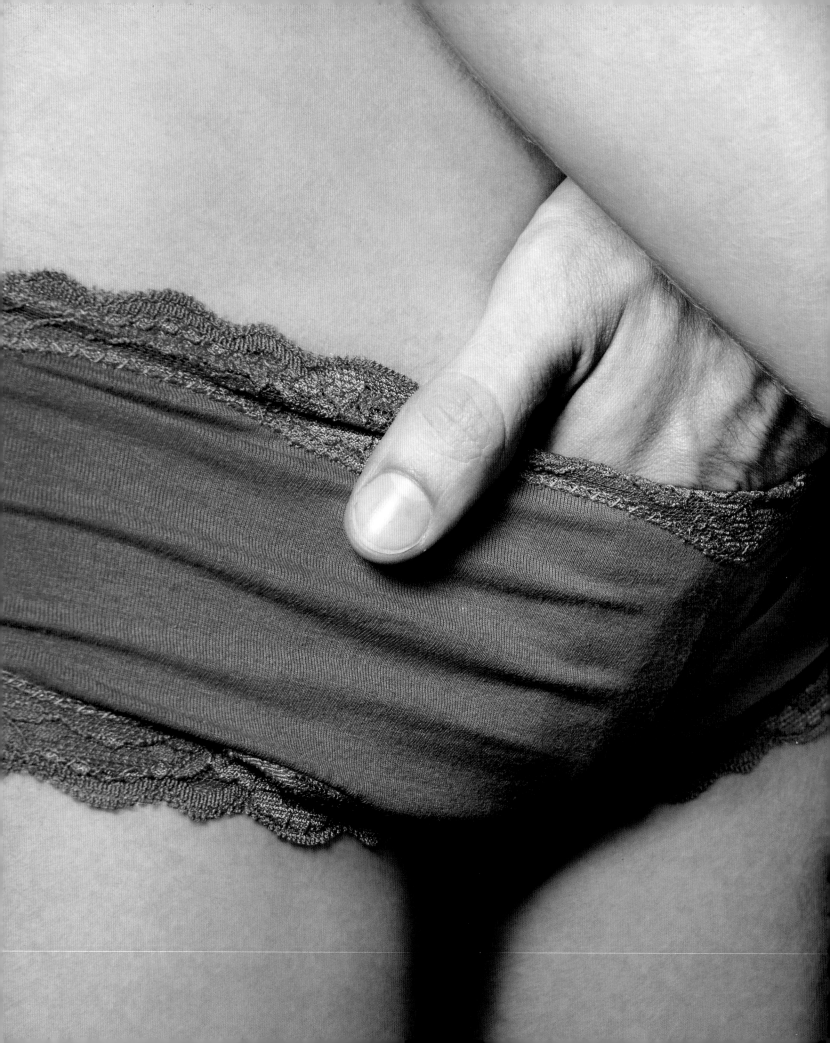

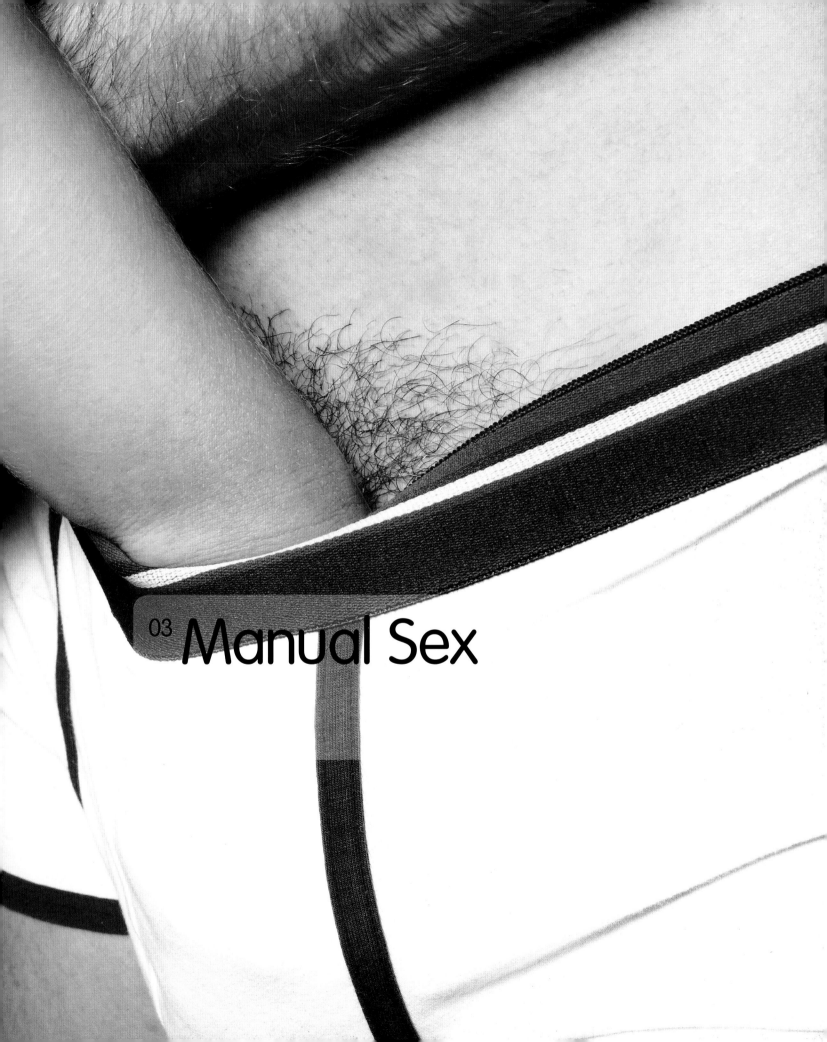

⁰³ Manual Sex

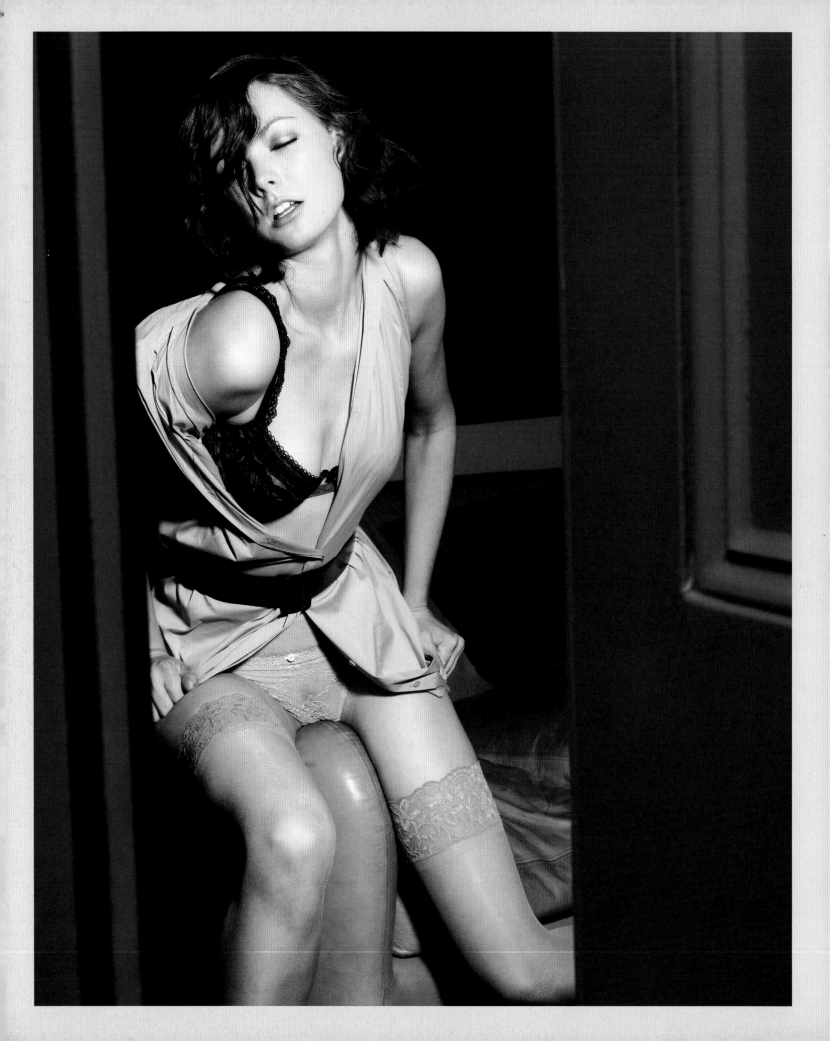

There's the Rub

Manual sex. No, it's not sex by the book. Nor is it hard labor. Manual sex is handwork: sex *without* genital-to-genital or oral-to-genital contact—basically, anything you can do with an appendage, whether on yourself or your partner. This includes masturbation, handjobs, and, for lack of a better word, fingering. In fact, that's why we say "manual sex"—it is a better term! After all, these three activities *are* sex. Purists tend to dismiss them as inferior to intercourse, something that only the inexperienced, freshly post-pubescent resort to. What a shame! Because dismissing all the wonderful things you can do with your hands results in unnecessary and unhealthy shame about masturbation, a self-imposed limitation on the kind of stimulation an adult couple can enjoy together, and often a failure for women to get the kind of stimulation they really need in order to orgasm when hooking up.

Learning how to diddle yourself or others doesn't always come naturally. Some people (okay, women mostly) think that masturbation is self-indulgent, juvenile, or plain old embarrassing—or else they just don't know where to start. Same thing with handwork: trying to pleasure your partner with your own two hands—the same set of tools that they themselves already have access to 24-7—can be incredibly intimidating. How can your inept, bumbling fingers possibly compete with their own digits, which have a direct line to the pleasure directives coming from their brain?!

Even if you're an avid masturbator (good for you!), you still run the risk of falling into a rut. Once you establish a pattern of physical stimulation and response, there's an understandable tendency not to stray from it: hey, it's the quickest route from point A to point Orgasm. But self love shouldn't be a routine any more than intercourse should. The more you vary your masturbation routine, the more options you'll have for climaxing when you've got a helper.

And as for handwork on your partner, admit it: you have a tendency to think of it as homework, something to wrap up before the "good stuff" of genital-to-genital contact. But that's a tad selfish, no? We realize the tips of your fingers aren't exactly hot erogenous zones, and that manual sex, like oral sex (pp.64–77), is usually a fairly one-sided endeavor in terms of physical pleasure. But that can be a good thing. Not being distracted by your own impending orgasm allows you to focus more on your partner's pleasure: what truly works for them and what doesn't. You can ask questions and learn about their sexual preferences and responses, rather than just conveniently assuming that what feels good to you during, say, intercourse, also feels good to them. Would that it were so easy.

So do your homework by doing your handwork. When working on yourself, don't rush to the finish line with your patented moves: make it last longer, bring yourself to the brink and pull back, try new positions and techniques, experiment. When working on your love object, take the opportunity to observe how their equipment works and responds. Read the rest of this chapter for more inspiration on hand-to-inner-thigh coordination. And revel in the knowledge that manual sex is one of the safest forms of sex there is.

Before you can be a good lover to anyone else, you've got to be one to yourself.

Why?

We once met a woman who claimed (quite proudly, we might add), "I've always had dick, so I don't need to masturbate." Our eyes bulged, our jaws dropped, our ears began to bleed a little. How could she utter such scandalous words? We tried desperately to explain that it's not about "need" but about "want." It's about taking responsibility for your own sexual pleasure and being your own sexual agent. It's about figuring out for yourself what you like instead of always leaving it up to somebody else. We begged her to see the light, and then we begged her to buy a vibrator (p.130).

There are myriad reasons why this particular lost soul might cling to such an antiquated notion. Maybe her mom caught her touching her "naughty place" when she was little, freaked out and told her to "Stop that right now!"—and from then on she always considered masturbation to be a social no-no, like stealing someone else's doll or picking her nose. Maybe no one ever taught her how to do it—most sex education is pretty inadequate when it comes to making women feel comfortable with and knowledgeable about their own bodies. (Lesson 1: the sexual equivalent of the penis is not the vagina, but the wonderful clitoris!) Or worse, maybe someone passed onto her some "wisdom" from the previous century—like the misconceptions that masturbation is beneath refined human beings; that clitoral stimulation is a poor woman's substitute for the "perfect" pleasure of a man's inserted penis; that "excessive" masturbation could damage the vagina, nerve endings, or even reproductive capabilities; that any kind of non-reproductive sexual act is a sin; that women don't have sexual needs or desires quite like men; or that masturbation is for lonely losers. The list of possible reasons for this woman not getting to know herself intimately goes on and on…

But still, there are so many more reasons why she, and all those like her, *should* get it on with themselves. First of all, it's just plain good for you. The World Congress of Sexology, an international gathering of sexuality scientists, states, "Sexual pleasure, including autoeroticism [masturbation], is a source of physical, psychological, intellectual, and spiritual well being." In fact, some studies suggest that denying yourself can do more harm than good. According to one study, women who do the electric boogaloo with sex toys achieve higher levels of sexual desire, higher levels of sexual satisfaction, and higher rates of success in achieving orgasm! Masturbation also releases endorphins, those chemicals that create an all-natural high and help fight the blues. And orgasms have been known to relieve menstrual cramps and PMS. Plus, the involuntary workout your pelvic floor gets from regular stimulation will only aid future genital health.

And the benefits of masturbation don't suddenly disappear once you're no longer single: you don't give up the morning paper, ladies' nights, or going to the gym when you're in a relationship, so why would you sacrifice self love? First of all, getting to your happy place solo is the first step toward orgasming with a partner: the better you know your body, the better directions you can give. Secondly, self-loving can be a booster shot to your libido, making you want partner-sex more. It develops your sexual sensitivity and trains your nerves to respond more efficiently. Finally, you may feel more comfortable indulging in your naughtier fantasies, especially those that don't include your current partner, and especially if you feel guilty about those fantasies (for the record, you shouldn't—but *acting* on them? Now that's a different story).

Every woman should know how to get herself off. It's an essential life skill that ranks right up there with boiling an egg, writing a résumé, and plucking your eyebrows. At the very least, it's the easiest way to get sex whenever you want it, however you want it.

Masturbation for Her

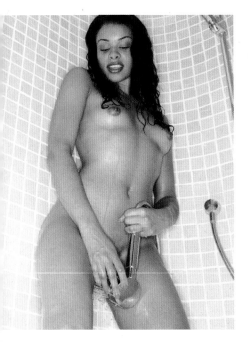
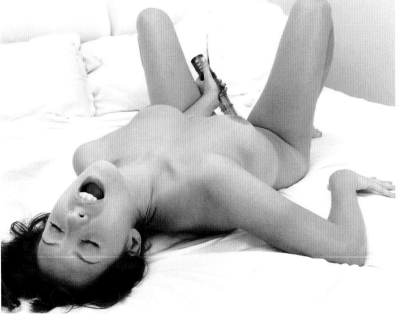
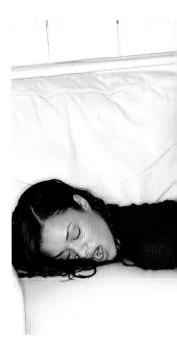

How?

Women don't always climax during intercourse, but they almost always do during masturbation, and often within minutes. Of course, it may take a bit of practice. And even if you're a record holder for fastest orgasm in the West, you should keep practicing just to keep things interesting. Here's how, drawing on other chapters for inspiration:

Female Anatomy—p.38 Study Chapter 2 to understand what you've got to work with. See how you compare, using a hand-held mirror and some exploratory probing. Remember your parts may not look exactly like the diagrams, nor will they all necessarily work in typical ways. Doesn't mean you're abnormal, just unique—like a snowflake. So learn and love what you've got: the look, the smell, the taste…

Getting in the Mood—p.16 Seduce yourself: you know you're a sure thing, but that's no reason not to pamper yourself. Turn down the lights, turn on some music, slip into something more comfortable. And make sure you're relaxed: give yourself 30 to 60 minutes of uninterrupted play time, starting with a bubble bath. You might find the faucet, whirlpool jet, or detachable showerhead is all you need (but never shoot a stream of water inside yourself—it's dangerous).

Massage—p.30 Give yourself a light, all-over body massage with your fingertips. Think of this endeavor not as sexual, but sensual: touch yourself everywhere without trying to turn yourself on, but just focusing on which kind of attention feels best. Use some oils or a mini-vibrator, start at your extremities, and slowly work toward your more erogenous zones.

Handwork for Her—p.56 Using your fingers is often the best way to achieve orgasm and show your partner how you like to have sex. Give yourself a hand with the techniques in this chapter. Once you find something that works, try to condition your body to respond to another sensation, so that you—and eventually your partner—will have more options.

Sex Toys—p.125 Most women employ handy props to help get them to their happy place. The intense stimulation from a vibrator can awaken a hibernating orgasm. Plus, once you know what your O feels like at the end of a vibrator, it's easier to get there by hand. The Toy chapter outlines a plethora of options, but perhaps none more important than lube, which can make any kind of stimulation—whether with your fingers, a vibrating phallus, or a flesh and blood one—feel much better for much longer. You can also go DIY with the props by squeezing a pillow between your legs, riding a couch arm, pressing up against the washing machine on spin cycle…

Kegels—p.175 Contract and relax your pelvic floor muscles, cross your legs, squeeze—all to help focus feeling in your genital area and unlock your orgasm: a fantasy and strong muscles may be all it takes for a hands-free, cross-legged O.

Playing and Posing—p.144 Let your mind wander to an erotic story—one you've read, seen, or made up in the dirty corners of your mind. For many women, imagining a sexy scenario with lots of details can put you in the right head-space to enjoy sexual stimulation when no one else is around.

Mutual Masturbation—p.54 Do it together. Turn the page for *why*. As for *how*: start pleasuring yourself when he's otherwise engaged (driving home from dinner, on a conference call…). The fact that he can't immediately join in may take the pressure off you. Plus, you might just discover that you like being watched. Hey, millions of fantasizing women can't be wrong! (See Exhibitionism, p.150)

Elements of Style—p.82 Use masturbation as part one of a two-part masturbation/intercourse session, to ensure that you're good and ready for penetration. In the middle of the night, masturbate to orgasm (or to the point just before), then wake up your man for an impromptu ride—you'll be raring to go. This also works right before he gets back from a grocery run, or even when he's just in the other room.

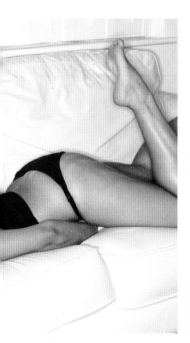
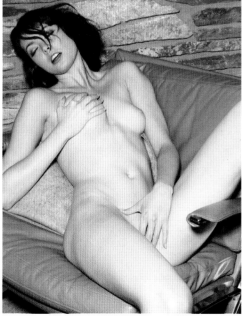
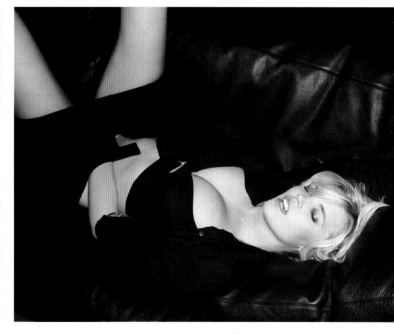

Most men don't need to be encouraged to masturbate—it's a given, as sure as the sun rising, as the tides ebbing, as a one-legged duck swimming in circles. And you already know the best reason for doing it: masturbation just feels good.

But maybe you don't know all the other reasons it's good *for* you. Studies suggest regularly flushing out your prostate gland can help prevent blockage, infections, and maybe even prostate cancer (scientists in white lab coats didn't make the Aneros "prostate massager" for nothing—p.136). Masturbation can ease tension and aid sleep. If you think you climax too soon with a partner, you can use masturbation to train yourself to recognize that point of no return and not pass it. Or if you have trouble climaxing with a condom, you can practice on your own, getting yourself used to the sensation and conditioning your body to love safer sex.

Or maybe you feel guilty about how often you like to "feel good" like this. Let's hope we're all enlightened enough to forgo addressing those ludicrous myths about masturbation that somehow still abound (it's a sin, it'll cause acne, it'll give you hairy palms…), and focus on more realistic concerns. Do you worry that you're addicted to masturbation? As long as it isn't keeping you from doing your job properly, attending to daily responsibilities, or having sex with your partner, then whack away (if not, consider counseling). Does the frequency with which you jerk off make you concerned about physically damaging an admittedly delicate organ? As long as masturbation isn't painful and you're not rubbing yourself raw or doing anything that results in blood in your ejaculate or urine, then keep diddling (if not, seek medical attention). Do you feel like you're betraying your partner? Individual people have individual sexual needs and desires, and very rarely do

two people's match up perfectly: as long as you have a healthy relationship based on communication and compromise, and aren't using masturbation as a way not to deal with intimacy problems, then feel free to polish your pole when the mood strikes (if not, try couples counseling).

Of course, it may be more a matter of making your partner feel okay with this self-love. If she's threatened by your masturbatory habits, reassure her that she's more than enough for you, that it's a physiological itch that needs scratching and that it's not indicative of any dissatisfaction with her. If her sex drive is lower, explain that masturbation helps even that playing field—but give her the option of joining in. We wouldn't recommend keeping self-love a secret (which only perpetuates feelings of shame and mistrust), but we also wouldn't recommend leaving your porn lying around or turning to the Internet when she's doing the bills in the next room and you've got thin walls, especially if she's not an avid fantasizer herself. For many women, it's the idea of you looking at and thinking about other women—rather than the physical act of touching yourself—that's most distressing. Remember, there's a big difference between being shamefully secretive and respectfully discreet. And definitely encourage her to masturbate on her own too. Try engaging in some mutual masturbation sessions, for a start (see below).

Finally, just as you probably don't need to be encouraged to masturbate, you probably don't need to be told how to do it. If you've made it through your teen years, then you've probably tried every trick in the book (remember wrapping your dick in banana skin?). But even if you've put away childish things, that doesn't mean you can't experiment: try some toys for boys (p.136); use lube (not short-lived lotion) even if you're uncircumcised (p.129); contract and relax your pelvic floor muscles during masturbation (p.177); forgo the porn, slow down, and concentrate on the physical sensations to get more "connected" to your body; and finally, employ the handwork techniques on the following pages.

Masturbation for Him

Mutual Masturbation

Definition 1—
Masturbating in front of each other simultaneously.
• The self-imposed obstacle of not being able to touch each other can add to the sexual tension.
• You can indulge any number of look-but-don't-touch fantasies: peepshow, bubble boy, prison visitation with glass divider, etc.
• It's voyeuristic and exhibitionistic at the same time—you're on an even playing-with-yourself field.
• Not only is seeing your partner masturbate arousing, it's educational: you can learn how they like to touch themselves and store that info for later bedroom use, all the while teaching *them* how *you* like it.
• It's great (we might even go so far as to say essential) practice for phone sex.
• If you're both avid, confident masturbators—and relish the exhibitionism of touching yourselves in front of each other—you're both practically guaranteed an orgasm.

• And so long as you don't do anything else, there's zero chance of giving each other an STD or accidentally ending up pregnant.

Definition 2—
Performing manual sex on each other simultaneously.
• It takes you back to a more innocent time, when fumbling for hours in the backseat of the car just to finally get the chance to touch each other's genitalia, was to fall in love, understand the nature of the universe, and find God.
• Putting your hand down each other's pants forces you to slow down, build up sexual tension, and tease more.
• Manual sex is often the best (if not only) way to give her an orgasm.
• It allows you to give hand-produced pleasure while you receive it, too—it's the manual equivalent of 69 (p.76).
• In terms of STDs, it's lower-risk than oral, anal, or vaginal sex (though not 100 percent safe, see pp.178–181).
• As long as all ejaculate stays away from her genitals, there's no chance of unplanned pregnancy.

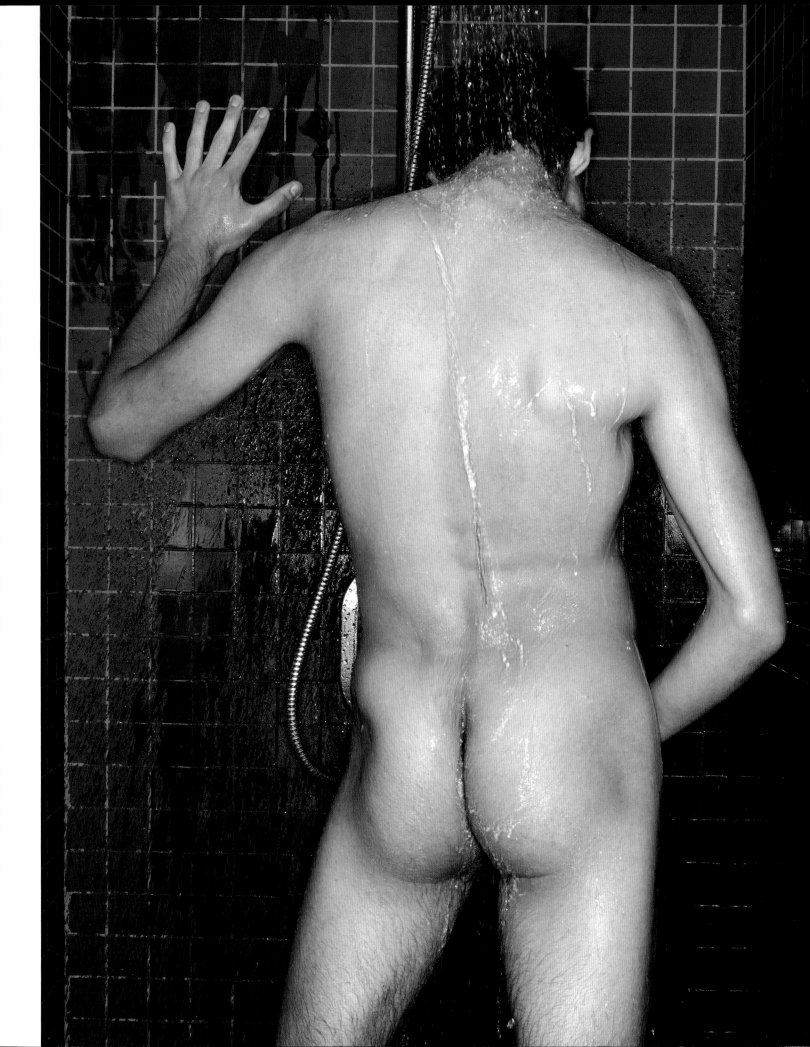

Perhaps more than any other technical area of sex, female manual sex is where most men (and women themselves!) need an attitude readjustment. Get your head straight here and now.

Mind Setting

Handwork on her should not be considered foreplay; it should be considered sex. In fact, it may often, if not always, be the main event for her. For many women, digital manipulation is far more effective than hands-free intercourse in eliciting orgasms: think about how much more control and range of motion you have with your fingers than your penis; then consider how crucial her clitoris and perhaps her G-spot are to her orgasms (way more so than her cervix at the end of your penis). So if you're holding onto any old-fashioned prejudices about orgasm via intercourse being sexual nirvana, throw them out the window! You should also get in the habit of insisting that her (first) orgasm come first. After all, her post-orgasmic vaginal state is ideally suited for further stimulation: she's aroused and erect and will probably continue to experience pleasure and perhaps even more orgasms (much more easily than you can after you come). You could even try holding off on intercourse until she's climaxed—that way you'll know for sure she's as physically ready as you are for penile penetration, and it'll probably feel better for her (and you). Another thing to burn into your brain: manual sex on her is not something that necessarily stops during other forms of sex, whether intercourse, oral, or anal. If manual's her thing, then continuing it during these other endeavors will ensure greater pleasure and a greater chance of orgasm for her. Finally, turn back and review her various hot spots—sometimes known as her orgasmic or arousal curve—in Anatomy & Orgasm (pp.38-41).

Prepping

Wash your hands, moisturize, and cut your nails. No need for regular metrosexual mani's, just make sure your fingers and tips will be soft and smooth against her sensitive parts. We highly recommend—actually, we insist—you use a high-quality water- or silicone-based lubricant (p.129) to add to any natural wetness: it lasts longer than her own natural lube, allows for more varied stimulation for longer everywhere, and basically just feels better. (Avoid anything oil-based, which can lead to vaginal infection).

Props

Manual sex with any kind vibrator is not cheating, it's enhancing. For some women, it may even be necessary for her orgasm, at least until she trains her body to respond to other similar, non-electronic stimuli (and you both should be working on that!). Don't think of a battery-powered prop as a replacement for your fingers or penis; think of it as an extension of them for all the moves outlined in this chapter. You're the one controlling the on/off button, the speed, the angle, and the pressure of the device. Revel in turning your sex tech-savvy. And remember that most women are fully aware of the fact that their vibrators make terrible cuddlers.

Encouraging Her Erection

Before you go in like gangbusters, you've got to make sure she's aroused, engorged, and, yes, erect (though not necessarily wet with natural lube, as that is not a reliable indicator of arousal). Just as with a male erection, blood should be flowing to her genitals and everything should be expanding and puffing up. Let her lie back and focus on the pleasure—and maybe even engage in her favorite fantasy—as you stimulate any outlying erogenous zones, slowly

Handwork On Her

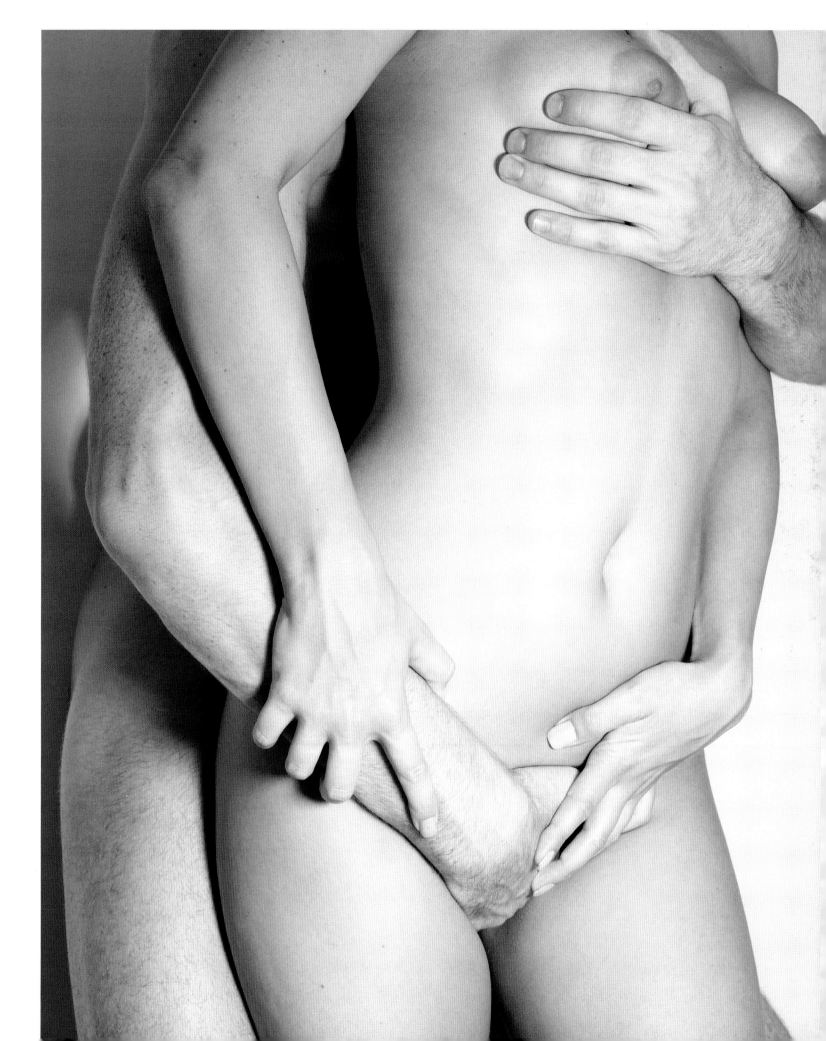

working your way in. For inspiration, reread the section on erotic massage (pp.30–33). Lightly run your fingers through her pubic hair (if she has any) and barely tickle the entire area. Place the whole of your palm over her, from pubic bone to perineum, and apply gentle pressure as you rub. Give focused finger attention to her outer labia first, then her inner labia and then follow the illustrations below.

Communicating

Don't ever be afraid to ask for some direction. We know, we know: guys hate asking for directions. Get over it already: every woman is different, and even your own partner's likes and dislikes may vary according to her mood, the time of the month, the weather, etc., so you can't go on auto-pilot. Pose quick and easy questions like "harder or softer?" or "more of this… or more of this?" That said, she's not your personal GPS, so don't expect her to give you instructions at every turn—especially if she needs to close her eyes and fantasize a little. Learn to read her moans and non-verbal cues, too, e.g., she pulls back ("go a bit softer, please" or "not directly on the clitoris, please") or her breathing gets heavier and her inner labia and clitoris look larger and/or darker ("I could get used to this"). A note to ladies: if you don't want to be interrupted with too many questions, then get talking and moaning!

Clittage

Clitoral massage, or "clittage" (a catchy term coined by the Douglass sisters in their fantastic book *Are We Having Fun Yet?*), is the one of the best ways to arouse her entire sexual network and eventually secure her an orgasm. Remember, the clitoral head is just the tip of her iceberg: when the clitoris is stimulated, its bulbs and legs—which extend around the urethra, urethral sponge (or G-spot), and vagina—become aroused, having a knock-on effect of pleasure (you'll move onto those other areas next). Depending on your partner, she may need lots of warm-up before you make direct contact with the clitoral head, or she may prefer you to stimulate it over its hood or even over a pair of pants or jeans, or she may even need you to pull up tightly on the mons to expose the clitoral head for some hard and fast stimulation. When in doubt, ask. A good rule of thumb is to start light and slow, and gradually build up pressure and pace, asking for feedback as you go. For specific techniques, see the illustrations below. And remember, once you find a pattern of stimulation she enjoys, clittage may be done with other body parts besides fingers: use your palm, knuckles, fist, wrist, leg, even penis in similar ways (if you can resist jumping into intercourse). And think of oral sex as just another method of clittage.

The U-Spot

Her urethral opening is just below her clitoral head. The area around it, known as the U-spot, which contains the paraurethral ducts and is analogous to the area right around the penis's urethra, is an often overlooked erogenous spot. But just as it is sensitive to touch on the penis, so is it on her. Often clittage and penetration indirectly stimulate the area (as rubbing can move it up and down quite a bit), but it may be helpful to visualize this as a potential pleasure point between her clitoral head and G-spot, especially since stimulating it can help arouse the urethral sponge (a.k.a. the G-spot).

Internal Affairs

Moving from the clitoral head past the U-spot, you'll get to her vaginal opening. Remember that the vagina is surrounded by the clitoral legs and bulbs, the pelvic floor muscles, and the urethral sponge (from the top side), and when she's aroused, all these structures will be engorged, causing a tightening effect on the vaginal opening. This is what makes penetration

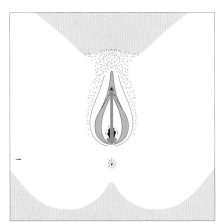

Warming Up—Move your finger from her clitoral head down to the perineum and back. Think of this as a warm-up move, grazing the area lightly, moving moisture around, then building up pressure. Never go all the way to the anus and then back to her vagina and urethra, as this can lead to infection.

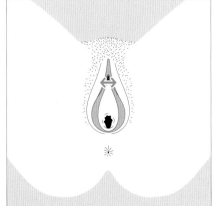

Crosstown Bus—Move your finger in a small, rapid side-to-side movement across her clitoral head. Ask what kind of pressure she likes: some like a light touch while others prefer you to really press down hard. Make sure you cover the entire clitoris. If hers is small or buried, it may be difficult to position your finger right on it, so don't be afraid to search it out visually and ask for direction.

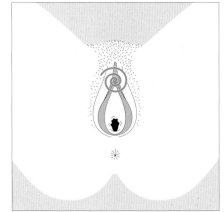

The Swirl—Move your fingertip in a small swirl-motion around (and closing in over) the clitoral head. The swirl should start out big enough to circle around the clitoris. In fact, you can repeat the outermost circles several times to build up tension. Or, if you're dealing with someone who doesn't like direct clitoral stimulation, keep the circling around the clitoral head the whole time.

feel nice for her—and this is why the girth of a penetrator is often more important than its length. It's also why shallow penetration is often preferable to deep, cervix-poking thrusting—at least for her. That said, women's equipment varies more than the soup of the day, so once inside, you should explore thoroughly to find exactly where she likes pressure, stroking, or poking. Cover all the walls of her vagina, as you may find that pressing in the opposite direction of her G-spot may help tighten the orgasmic network, stimulate her perineal sponge, and indirectly stimulate the nerves of her anus. Or she may be one of those women who does enjoy having the back of her vagina stimulated—this is where you'll find her A-spot and cul-de-sac (p.40). During arousal, the innermost area of the vagina around the cervix actually expands, creating a pocket between the cervix and the inner back vaginal wall that can be responsive to pressure from your fingers (though probably not to thrusting from your penis). For G-spot stimulation, see below.

The G-Spot & Female Ejaculation

Continuing along her arousal curve from the vaginal opening, you'll reach the G-spot. To make sure you hit it, have her lie on her back (she can pull her knees up or place a pillow under her bum for better access), and insert one or two fingers about two inches in and up, as if you were aiming behind her pubic bone. (See the illustration below.) You're feeling for a rough, ridged area on the front or upper wall of the vagina, about the size of a stretched-out coin. Remember, the G-spot actually sits behind this wall—it's the spongy tissue that surrounds her urethra and is known as the female prostate. Since you'll be pressing on the urethra (and in the vicinity of the bladder), it's only natural that she might feel like she has to pee when you do this. If she urinates beforehand, then she'll know she can ignore this feeling and you can keep on G-spotting. Once there, curve your fingers in a "come hither" gesture and massage firmly and steadily. Some women find

this sensation downright uncomfortable and can't get past the resulting "urge to purge." But others actually require this kind of stimulation for orgasm, or even ejaculate as a result of it.

If she should fall into this last category, here's what's happening (and it's a good thing, by the way): upon arousal, the glands and ducts embedded in the urethral sponge fill with fluid (not urine) which may be expelled through the urethra and the paraurethral ducts during stimulation or orgasm or when she contracts her pelvic floor muscles—in other words, ejaculation could occur before, during, or after orgasm. Some women may spurt, some may release a flood of fluid, and some may emit just a few drops of ejaculate, making it almost impossible to detect. This is another kind of pleasure for her, but not one that should be pursued like the holy grail. The fountain-like squirting you see in porn is not universally attainable—and in some cases, may not even be real.

The Backdoor

Considering that her pelvic floor muscles wrap around her nerve-rich anus too, perineal and anal stimulation can be another carriage on her genital train. To avoid infection, keep any fingers, appendages, or toys that have stimulated her anal area (either externally or internally) away from her vagina, urethra, and clitoris. Read Anal Play (pp.112–123).

The Happy Ending

Now we've reviewed all the parts, you can pull them together to create one orgasmic whole. She may not like all of the above areas stimulated, but some combination will usually do the trick. When it comes to the home stretch, remember: continual, steady stimulation. With your new attitude and approach, her elusive orgasm should run out of places to hide.

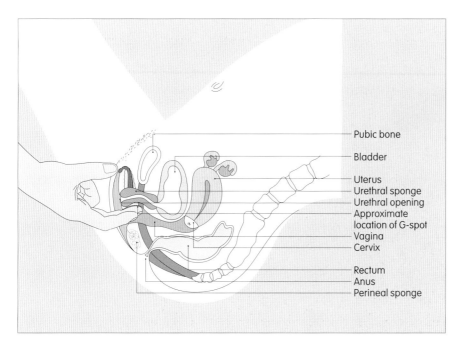

Pubic bone

Bladder

Uterus
Urethral sponge
Urethral opening
Approximate
location of G-spot
Vagina
Cervix

Rectum
Anus
Perineal sponge

Stimulating the G-spot—Insert your index and/ or middle fingers, palm up, into her vagina and stimulate her G-spot by curving your fingers in a "come hither" gesture in the direction of her urethral sponge.

Sure, he's been doing it himself since he was 14 and knows what he likes better than anyone, but that's no excuse not to bother. Besides, we're guessing that if he had to choose between a self-administered handjob and one from you, he'd choose your helping hand every time. Handwork is a useful skill in your sexual repertoire—if you're not in the mood to get all worked up and naked, handwork on him can be a quick, easy, and neat way to satisfy him. Chances are, though, once you see him grow in your hands, you'll soon get in the mood too.

Mind Setting

Don't let his masturbatory adroitness intimidate you. And don't worry that your rusty techniques have been gathering dust in the closet of novelty moves since high school. You can learn to give a great handjob again, or for the first time. Consider it the sexual equivalent of pottery making: you're working with a somewhat malleable, albeit delicate, piece of flesh to create something of kinky beauty (sure, he'll soon be reduced to a soft lump of silly, blissed-out putty again, but all great art is fleeting). All it takes is following the steps outlined below. If, after reading them, you're still not confident enough in your manual sex skills to attempt to elicit an orgasm, then practice by employing handwork as foreplay; as a beginning to, a part of, or a temporary break from a blowjob; or just in between intercourse-position switching.

Prepping

Your hands should be clean and soft and your nails should be well manicured and not too long—we're not talking weekly visits to the salon, just no rough edges or hangnails. Remove any rings. While he's likely to emit some pre-ejaculate during stimulation, it's rarely enough to be useful for an entire manual sex session, so we highly recommend you use a manmade lubricant, even if he's uncircumcised. Keeping things slick will help ensure your touch doesn't get too tacky or dry, which can make things uncomfortable for him. Plus, it'll help you run with that whole pottery-making analogy. Use a pump dispenser for easy, one-handed reapplication. If there's a chance of intercourse afterwards, then your best bet is a water-based lube (you can certainly use a nice silicone-based lube, though you might find that, while long-lasting, it gets a little too thick and sticky). If there's no chance of intercourse, then you can go with a really slippery oil-based lube—some products are actually specially made for handjobs for him. Just remember that oils can break latex condoms and cause vaginal infections. Whatever you do, make sure the lube isn't chilly: run the bottle under warm water or rub it in your palms first. And be sure you've got something handy to clean up with should his geyser blow: tissues, a hand towel, an old T-shirt that's less important to you than erotic ecstasy (i.e., not one with nostalgic value).

Taking a Stance

Sticking your hand down his pants feels naughty and is a playful foreplay move (would that be "foreplayful"?), but you won't be able to get much range of motion. So if you'd like to work his shaft seriously, make sure it's freed from the confines of any clothing. If you're approaching from one side—for example, lying beside him in bed—it will be difficult, if not impossible, to use both hands, so try to position yourself so you can use your dominant arm. That way you'll have more

Handwork On Him

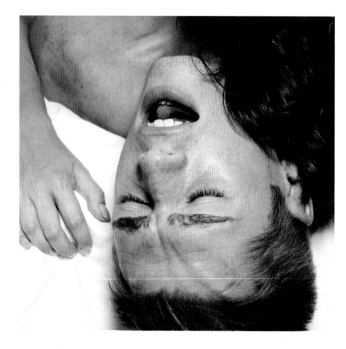

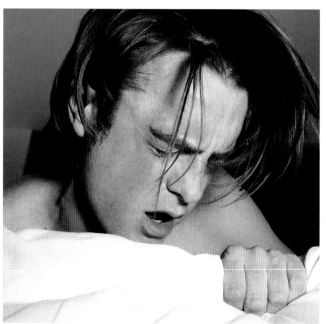

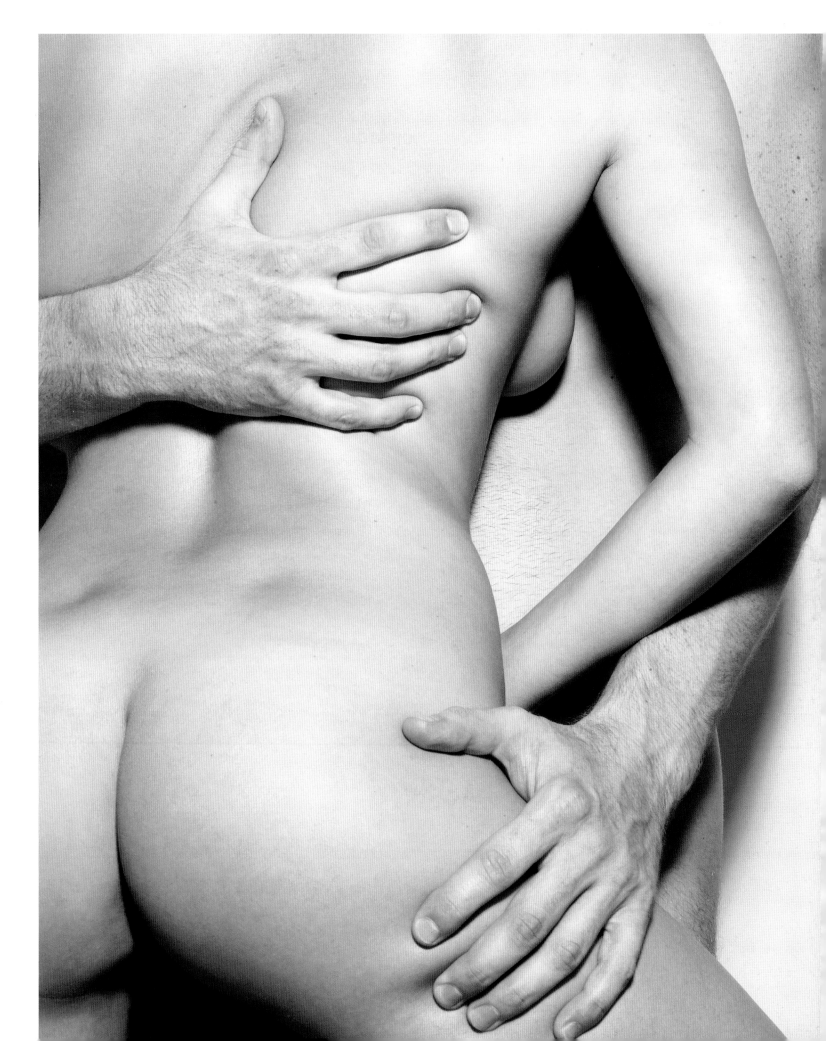

pumping endurance. Reaching around from behind him with one hand can replicate the sensation of masturbation—which could make him salivate like a Pavlovian dog and act as a shortcut to his orgasm. You don't want to get an arm cramp at a crucial moment, so don't be afraid to set up shop between his legs—that way you'll have a lot of freedom to use both hands in a variety of positions. Plus you get the scenic view, which includes his unit (you can watch what you're doing and look for any tell-tale impending O signs like his balls rising up toward his body) and his face (great for reading facial expressions and making *très sexy* eye contact). You can also kneel beside him, though access to the sensitive underside ridge will be limited. If you want another angle of approach, it's better—and dirtier—to kneel over his chest, especially if he's a "butt man."

Communicating

Reading body language is all fine and dandy, but as with any sexual endeavor, you can learn a great deal by asking questions, too. Guys can be very particular about their handjobs, so ask him exactly how he likes it to be done. You can even have him give you a personal demonstration with his own hand. And encourage him to give you feedback and guidance as you go—tell him you like to hear him talk dirty.

Turtlenecks

If you're working with an uncircumcised specimen, you'll want to use the foreskin as a sort of natural masturbatory sleeve that moves with your hand motions. Lubricant will not be essential here, but it's often welcome. Keep in mind that pulling the skin out of the way and directly addressing the über-sensitive glans may be more touch than he can handle.

Skimming the Surface

Before his boxers come off, run your fingers inside the waistband, run your hands up his thighs, caress under his butt cheeks, finger-comb his pubic hair (if he has any). Touch everywhere but his penis with your fingers. Once you make contact with his genitals, keep the touch light and slow at first: do not jump into rapid-fire pumping right away. Start with your fingertips, rather than a full, firm grip. Cover all penile, testicular, and perineal areas—not just his shaft. If at this point he is still soft or growing, use the fingers of one hand in an upward-only stroke along the shaft, as if you were David Blaine trying to magically elevate a wand. You could then switch to a soft, full-handed grip, still working with just an upward stroke. Try squeezing and pulsating gently, too, like you're pumping up a blood pressure cuff (though your grip shouldn't be nearly as tight as those cuffs!).

The Essential Up-and-Down

The foundation of manual sex for him is the essential up-and-down: think of it as creating a virtual vagina with your hand. Grip his erect shaft in your dominant, well-lubed hand. You can use your other hand at the base to stabilize or position his penis. He need not be at a perfect 90-degree angle to the rest of his body: his shaft may be naturally inclined to lean in either direction. (Pulling it toward his lower body will probably only weaken his erection or maybe even hurt him.) Move your dominant hand up and down the shaft in a fluid motion, never losing contact with it completely, and closing your grip as your top fingers pass the head. At first, work the entire length fairly slowly; closer to orgasm he may prefer you to focus just on the top half while picking up speed (when in doubt, just ask). Start off with a light grip, then slowly increase firmness. Never increase to what might be called a "death grip." Always keep the movement steady rather than jerky. When you feel comfortably dexterous, you can add a slight back-and-forth

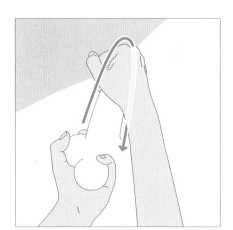

Over the Hill—One hand cups the balls from underneath. The other hand starts with an inverted grip at the base of the shaft (so your thumb and index finger are up against his body). Move up the shaft. When you get to the top, roll your palm over his head. Then fluidly move into a traditional down-stroke without losing contact. Keep doing this U-shaped movement.

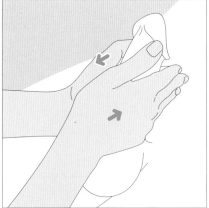

Warm-up Act—Imagine that you're rubbing your flat palms together to warm up. Now put an erect penis between those palms, so the palms are midway up the shaft. One hand should move in one direction while the other hand moves in the opposite direction—they don't move a great distance before they both switch directions (the object is not to twist his dick off or start a fire).

twisting motion as you go up and down—you shouldn't be pulling the skin with you, just letting your light grip move smoothly over the skin.

Tricky Techniques

You can build upon an up-and-down foundation with some simple techniques, like those outlined in the illustrations below. Or try these moves, too:
• Get your other hand in on the action by alternating moves with each hand. For example, if you're just using an upstroke, start with your right hand at the base (in either a traditional full-hand grip, a finger-and-thumb "okay" sign, or an inverted grip), move up, then when it reaches the head, place your left hand in a similar grip at the base and follow your right; as the right hand loses contact and the left hand moves up the shaft, the right hand returns to the base. Do the same with just a downstroke.
• Focus on the underside ridge of his shaft (it's called the raphe, in case you were wondering) by massaging it firmly with the pads of your thumbs (while resting the topside of the penis against your interlocked fingers). Position them side-by-side and slide them straight up and down, or inch them up the shaft in alternating half circles, like a penis massage.
• Take a break from the up-and-down: grip the shaft with an open fist and cup the head in the palm of your other hand and move it as as if you were polishing the silver bulbous top of a walking stick. Sensitive penises, especially the uncircumcised, may not be able to take much of this attention.

The Outer Limits

When not using both hands (on or at the base of the shaft), let your free hand roam. Play with his balls: tickle, caress… you can even pull them gently away from his body using an "okay" grip where they meet the base of the shaft in order to help delay ejaculation. Don't ever squeeze or pinch his testicles. If you're in a position where you can reach, stimulate his nipples (but only if you know he likes that). Indirectly stimulate the prostate by massaging his perineum (i.e., press up into him), especially when he's about to come. Or stimulate his anus externally or internally (but only if you really know he likes that, or you've given him warning that you're going to try).

Props

The only prop you really need for a stellar handjob is lube. But if you'd like to mix things up: use your cleavage as a new set of hands; wrap his unit in a soft silk scarf during foreplay and initial stimulation (before you've added any wet lube); add a butt plug down below for backdoor stimulation that doesn't take one hand away from your work up top; try one of your mini-vibrators (set on low) at the base of his shaft or on his perineum.

The Happy Ending

As you approach his orgasm, most men like firm, steady, uninterrupted strokes that are a bit faster and more furious than what you started with. Remember not to violently yank and bend it like a video arcade joystick, but know that you can probably treat it with a little more fervor than your own mini penile head (a.k.a. the clitoral glans). It's nice to ask him beforehand what he prefers you do once his first ejaculatory spurt erupts: keep pumping until the last or hold still and squeeze through the orgasm? Once he's spent, loosen your grip and resist the urge to keep playing, even lightly. You can certainly cuddle him in your still hand, but any movement (for example, when taking your hand away), should be slow and almost undetectable, as if you're trying not to disturb a sleeping grizzly. Finally, it's always a nice touch to help him clean up.

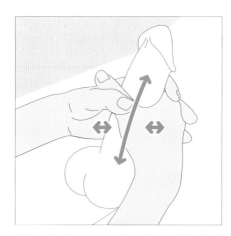

Giving Thanks—Put your hands around the shaft with your fingers interlocked and your thumbs overlapping on the opposite side (to replicate the feeling of the vagina). Move up and down with firm pressure, closing in on the head when your fingers pass it (don't lose contact with the shaft entirely). You can add a slight squeezing and releasing around the shaft as you go.

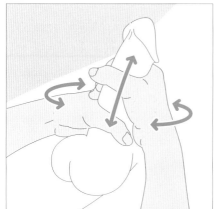

Let's Twist Again—With each hand, form an okay signal with your thumb and index finger (you can add the middle finger, too, if you like). Place your hands one on top of the other, starting at the base of the penile shaft. Twist each hand back-and-forth in opposite directions as they move in unison up and down the shaft.

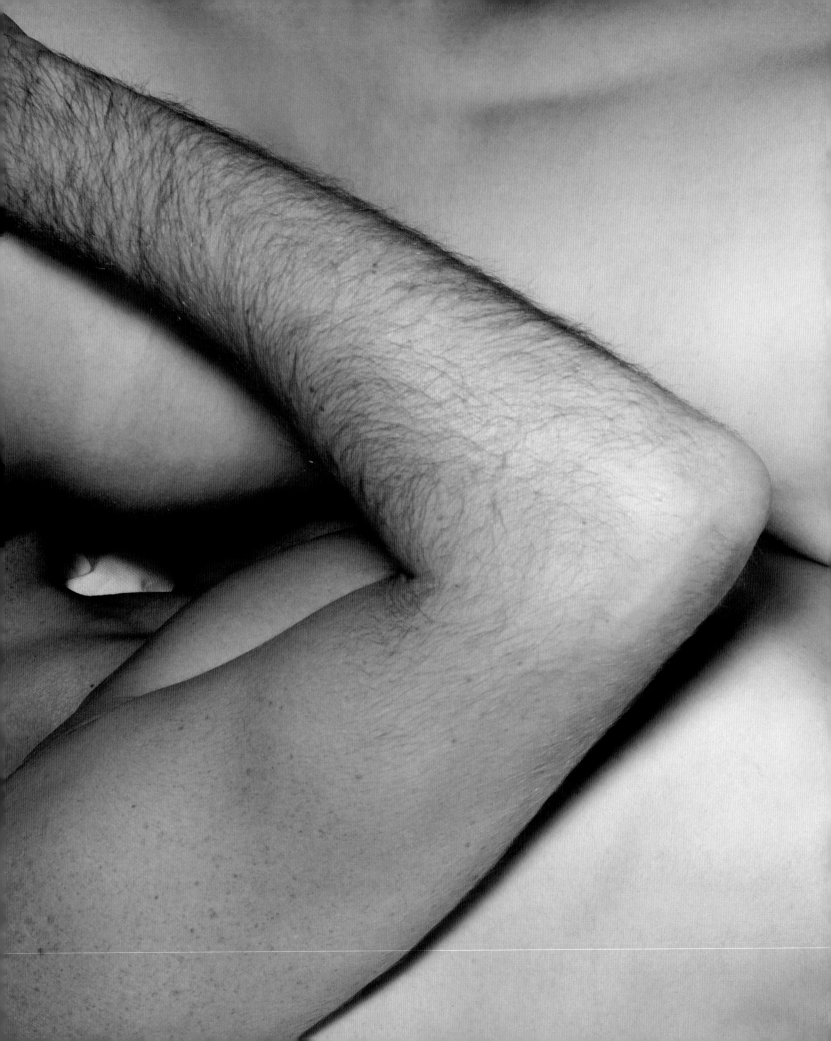

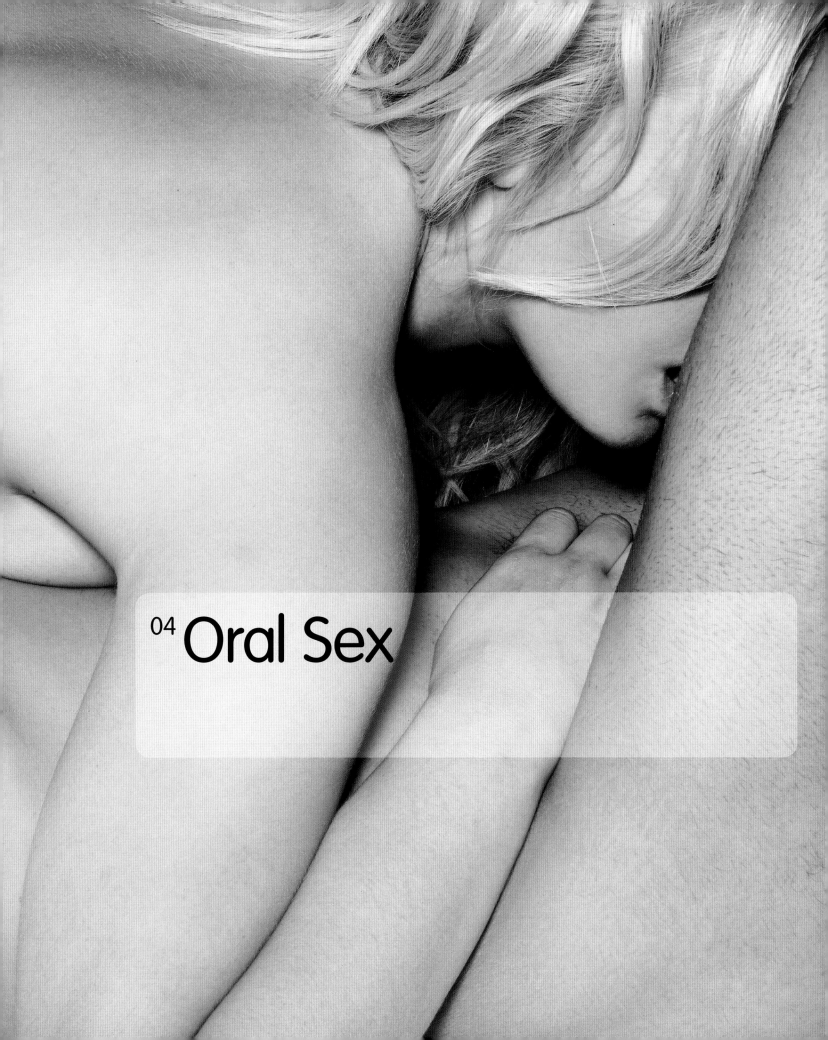

04 Oral Sex

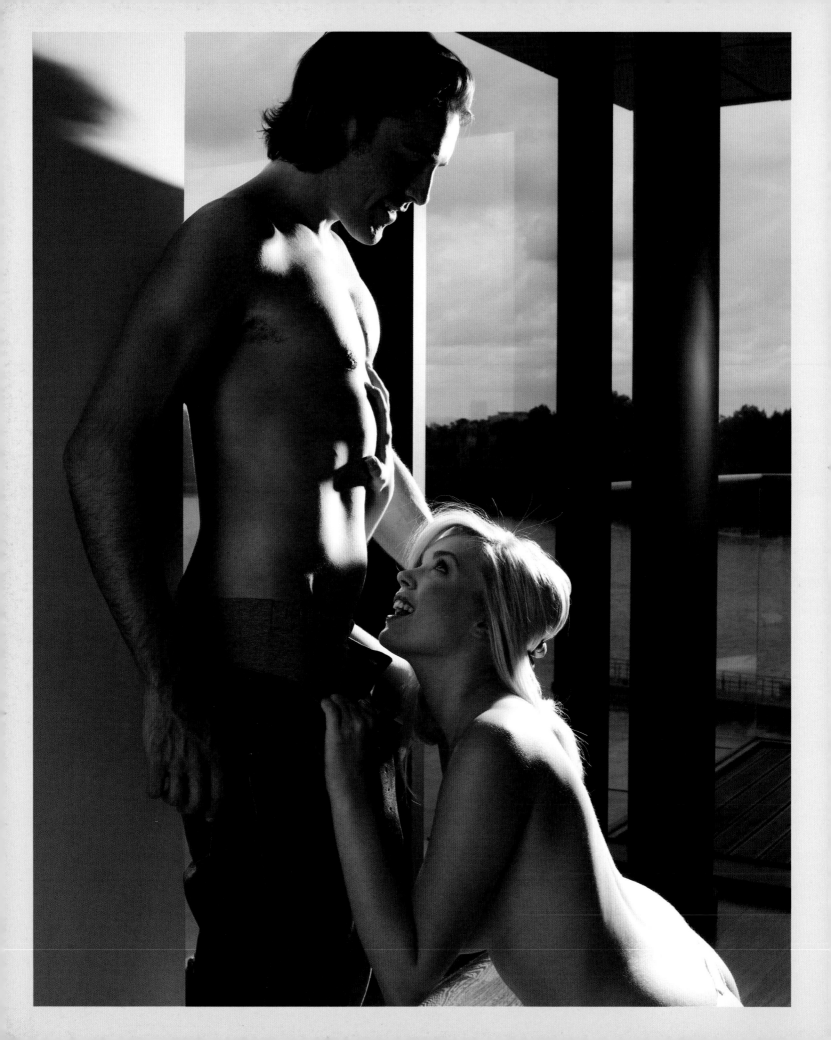

Paying Lip Service

Not counting Japanese rope bondage, going down is about as complicated as sex gets. For some people—especially adult women—it feels more intimate than intercourse and belongs somewhere between going steady and saying "I love you." And yet for others—especially teens, adulterers, and people saving themselves for marriage—it barely even "counts." For some, oral conjures flowery terms like "worship" and "devotion," while for others it's more likely to inspire feelings of duty or dread. For some, oral sex is an afterthought and for others it's an orgasm essential…

Can't we all just get along?

Of course we can! When it comes to oral, everyone's right every now and then (or, at least, most of us are). Sometimes oral sex feels so intimate, you'd swear you just melded souls. Other times, it's the kind of get-the-job done act that's tailor-made for a booty call. Sometimes going down is a selfless gift—and other times it's a heady thrill. And, yes, sometimes it's just about returning the favor.

You've got to learn to overcome any prejudices, bad habits, or self-defeating mantras that are holding you back from enjoying giving and/or receiving. After all— unlike with Japanese rope bondage—a lack of southerly attention, in either direction, might just be a relationship deal-breaker.

Does oral administration feel like a job— and you're the underling? Then don't wait to be asked: initiating has been scientifically proven to make you feel 57 percent more in charge (also, who says you have to kneel?). Fantasize about who you are down there (p.144). Or just use bondage (p.158): their hands bound, your mouth on their genitals… now who's the underling?

Are you a wallflower, shying away from any one-sided, put-upon-a-pedestal attention? Are you always bickering over whose turn it is? Do you tend to be a chronic giver in the bedroom? Then try a 69 (p.76) to level the playing field!

Does your other half not like the sensation? Well, reciprocation doesn't have to mean a begrudging "10 minutes for me, 10 for you". If she hates cunnilingus and he'd be happy to accept blowjobs for every birthday, national holiday, and weekday from here to the retirement home, he can find another way to return the favor… extended handwork, her favorite position, a 20-minute massage, etc. And remember: reciprocation doesn't have to be immediate—unless it's a one-night stand.

Squeamish? Then shower first—or go down in the shower. That said, aficionados will recommend a shower that's recent (an hour or two) but not too recent (mere minutes) if you'd rather taste your partner than their shower gel. You could also try cutting down on coffee, cigarettes, beer, asparagus, red meat, spicy foods, and junk food in favor of kiwi, pineapple, strawberries, cinnamon, and lots of water—the science is flimsy, but it's a great excuse to experiment!

Is your partner lost down there? Then make some more noise: moans of pleasure and positive reinforcement ("that feels so good, don't stop!") will help clue them in to what you like—not to mention serve as their own personal cheering section. Or are you the lost soul? Then keep reading.

Cunnilingus is one of the most daunting sexual tasks for a man. It's an unfair fact of life but there's more variation among gals than guys, so there's no set moves that guarantee her orgasm. This doesn't mean you should consider her orgasm high maintenance; we prefer the word *individual*.

Getting Started

In recent decades there's been a much-welcomed focus on oral sex as the key to a woman's orgasm, but that's put a hell of a lot of pressure on the men. And frankly, there are plenty of women out there who could take or leave the cunnilingus. So lower your expectations, cut yourself some slack, and just enjoy yourself. This is one of those sex acts that's more about the journey than the destination.

Mind-Setting—First, you've got to get in the right frame of mind: remove selfishness from your vocabulary, cover all the clocks, and become a rainy-day New-Age sensualist (no ponytail necessary). Now you need to make sure her head is in the game, too, otherwise all your efforts will be for naught. If she tends to stress out about reciprocation, try heading south when there's no time for her to respond in kind (like, right before a movie). Or tell her that for the next half hour you are her love slave. Make sure there is no possibility of interruption. And if she still can't stop worrying about your penis, then tie her up so she's got no choice (with her consent, of course).

Prepping—If you think she's worried about hygiene (or you are), then shower together or run her a relaxing bath. If you've got a pubic hair preference, don't heighten her insecurities with demands. Instead, phrase everything in positives ("It

would be so hot if…"), offer to do any trimming yourself as a sex game, and be willing to sport the same hairstyle yourself. (And remember, contrary to widespread belief, the French and 70's porno styles can be sexy, too.) Speaking of trimming, you might want to check on your beard situation: a few-days-old soft growth might feel kind of good, but a mean 5 o'clock shadow might end up sandpapering her labia.

Taking a Stance—If you're attempting an orally-induced orgasm, then chances are you're going to be here for a while, so get comfortable. Encourage her to lie back on a bed or comfy chair with a pillow under her hips. You can kneel between her legs or on the floor (put a pillow under your knees). But if control (rather than relaxation) is what gets her to her happy place, then she might want to straddle your face or even stand over you. For something a little novel, try approaching her from behind (ask first!): she can still relax and moan into a pillow and you'll have an all-areas access pass—though you'll probably need to bring in your fingers or a toy to properly address the clitoral head.

Fluffing Her Up—Nuzzle, kiss, nibble, lick, and suck the outlying areas—her mouth, breasts, stomach, inner thighs, mons—gradually closing in on your ultimate target. Gently spread her legs as your fingers get closer. Lightly run your hands over her vulva and through her pubic hair (if she has any). Cup your arms under her thighs or bum to pull her in close to you. Breathe over her entire vulva (but never blow into her orifices—it's dangerous).

Communicating—Besides telling her how good she tastes and smells, ask for feedback, at least until you learn what she loves. And as with manual sex, tune into her non-verbal cues: she pushes into you ("nice job!"); she really pushes into you ("harder!"); she grips the sheets or arches her back ("brilliant job!"); she grips her head in your thighs ("don't change a thing"); she squeezes her thighs *and* holds your head in her hands ("I'm coming"). Assuming she's not a faker.

Cunnilingus

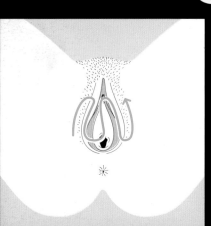

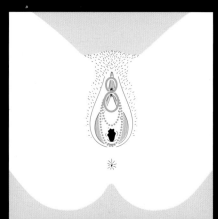

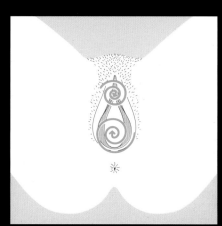

The Rollercoaster—Starting on the left, take your tongue up the outer lip and down between the outer and inner lip, then up and down over the vaginal opening, crossing the clitoris, then down between the opposite set of lips and up again.

The Lazy Eight—For the upper half of the "8", swirl your tongue over the clitoral hood, stimulating the shaft; for the lower half, alternate between short loops that cross the urethral or vaginal opening and longer loops that cross the perineum. The intersection between the upper and lower loops is always over the clitoral head.

The Double Swirl—Move your tongue in ever decreasing circles, first around (and closing in on) the vaginal opening and then around (and closing in on) the clitoral head.

Getting Finished

The closer you get to the clitoris, the more women are going to vary in terms of the kind of stimulation they enjoy and how long they'll enjoy it—so the more techniques you've got to try out, the better. That's what we're here for!

Lollipopping—When it's time for tongue, start by French kissing her vulva. Bury your face. Use your nose as a stimulation tool (this move is also a good one to return to later, when your tongue may need a break). Then get everything really wet with a wide, flat, soft tongue. Keep your jaw relaxed and lick slowly from her vaginal entrance up to her clitoris—or even longer, from her perineum up to her pubic bone. Lick up the center then down again, lick up and down either side, and go side to side, too. Spread her labia with your lips or tongue. Hold each set of her lips between your lips and run your tongue between the inner and outer labia, first one side then the other. Or pull her lips into your mouth and suck on them. You may graze the clitoral head with these broad strokes, but don't pause just yet: she'll probably need to be much more aroused for that.

Going In—You're not painting a wall here, so you'll probably need a little more in your arsenal than a soft, wide tongue, no matter how well the two of you "communicate." But wait until she's pushing into you, physically begging you, before you go any deeper with your tongue. During your long, slow tongue strokes, start dipping your tongue inside as you pass over the vaginal opening. Remember, it's the outer third of the vagina that is most likely to respond to friction and pressure, so there's no need to pull a muscle trying to get all the way in there: just circle your tongue around the opening and move it in and out. If she seems to want a little more in terms of penetration (there we go again with that communication), bring in a finger or three while your tongue continues on the outside: move your fingers in and out using short but firm strokes, or keep them inside, rubbing against her G-spot—basically, try anything you learned in the Manual Sex chapter. Move your tongue and fingers in sync if you can.

Coming to a Head—As you get closer to the clitoral head, keep in mind what a sensitive little thing it is and be gentle, at least at first: some women never want direct stimulation of the clitoris, while others can't seem to get enough of it. Remember that the more you tease and the more turned on she is, the more stimulation she'll be able to take. Keep your licking very light until she pushes into you for more. Some women prefer to have their clitorises attended to over the hood, so ask first if she'd like you to try pulling it back a bit for more exposure. Experiment with what feels best to her over and around her clitoral head: a soft, wider tongue technique or a stiff, pointy one. Never let the area get dry. Feel free to roam, but keep coming back to this focal point, taking cues from her all along the way—ultimately, she'll probably want you to stay put once you've found something that works. For some tongue-specific moves that address the clitoris, see the the illustrations on the opposite page. Then try these, too:
• Lick around it in circles, up and down either side, then up and down over it, or from left to right.
• Try tracing the alphabet over her clitoris with your tongue if it helps keep you focused.
• As with the labia, you can suck on her clitoris, too: pull it into your mouth and suck and lick gently, maybe flicking your tongue over and around it while you hold it.
• Place the tip of your tongue on the hood and move your tongue in circles without moving off the clitoral head.
• Apply a firm, pulsating pressure with a wide tongue.

Tricky Techniques—Whether you're covering the entire vulva or honing in on the clitoris, anything you tried with your hand in chapter three can be tried with your tongue here (especially the moves in the illustrations on page 58). You can also:
• Shake your head back and forth with a slightly stiff tongue.
• Nibble with caution—and if she loves it, then nibble with slightly less caution: the inner thighs, the labia, the mons, even, eventually, the clitoral head (gently).
• Try some deep, guttural moans—the vibration may have a pleasing effect. Plus, she'll know you're happy to be there.
• And don't forget that your fingers can do more than just penetrate: dip them into her mouth, play with her labia while your tongue is elsewhere, gently tug on her labia and pubic hair, pull up on her mons or rub it in a circular motion, let your hands stray to her nipples, her perineum, or her anus (but never before the fingers-in-the-mouth move).
• Three sensitive spots not to overlook: where the inner labia meet, just under the clitoral head; the area around the urethral opening; and her perineum.

Props—Cunnilingus can be a hard day's night, and there's no shame in turning to props. You can help things along with edible lube, either flavored or, if you don't have a sweet tooth, tasteless. A hint of strawberry or pineapple may help her relax about how she tastes. (Choose a glycerin-free product if she's prone to infection, see p.129.) A vibrator can give your tongue a break—try bullet vibes, finger vibes, a vibrating dildo, or a G-spot vibe if that's her thing (look at chapter seven). You can even try a gimmicky oral vibrator in your mouth, though the teeth-rattling effect may not be worth it (to say nothing of the choking hazard!). If she likes a little backdoor action during oral sex and you don't want to "reserve" a lubed finger for that purpose, insert a small, lubed butt plug instead. For novelty, try a mint in your mouth or a sip of hot tea or ice water before starting or during the session.

Rhythm Is Going to Get Her—The key to good cunnilingus is patience and a steady stroke. In general (though we hate to generalize, especially in this chapter), women tend to like firm pressure and a repetitive motion. You can build up speed and pressure slightly as she gets more turned on—but if she pulls back, then so should you. Chances are, quick, sporadic tongue flicking is not going to push her over the edge. And when she moans, that's not necessarily a cue to speed up—no matter what it means when you do it yourself during a blowjob. If you've figured out the rhythmic key that unlocks her orgasm, then during build-up you can sometimes even go in the opposite direction: get her almost there, then back off, then repeat, so that when she does finally climax, it's really *&$#!**. If her orgasms are more elusive, keep doing exactly what you're doing until she's yelling *&$#!**.

The Happy Ending—With any luck, all this oral attention will lead somewhere very good. But if it doesn't, don't feel down—while some women like you to go all the way with it, others prefer cunnilingus as foreplay. At this close range, you should have a pretty good idea when she's coming. Remember, her orgasms may last longer than yours, so don't stop until she releases you. She may want you to keep up the exact same motion all the way through her final shudder—or she may just want you to pull her in tight and provide firm pressure. If you forget to ask how she likes it, don't worry: we're pretty sure she'll grab you with her hands and guide you. If she doesn't, ask her for next time. And if you can't seem to achieve the desired effect, be prepared to throw in the towel when she suggests it. Because if you've applied all the above advice, then—no matter the orgasmic result—you'll have secured your place in the Boyfriend Hall of Fame.

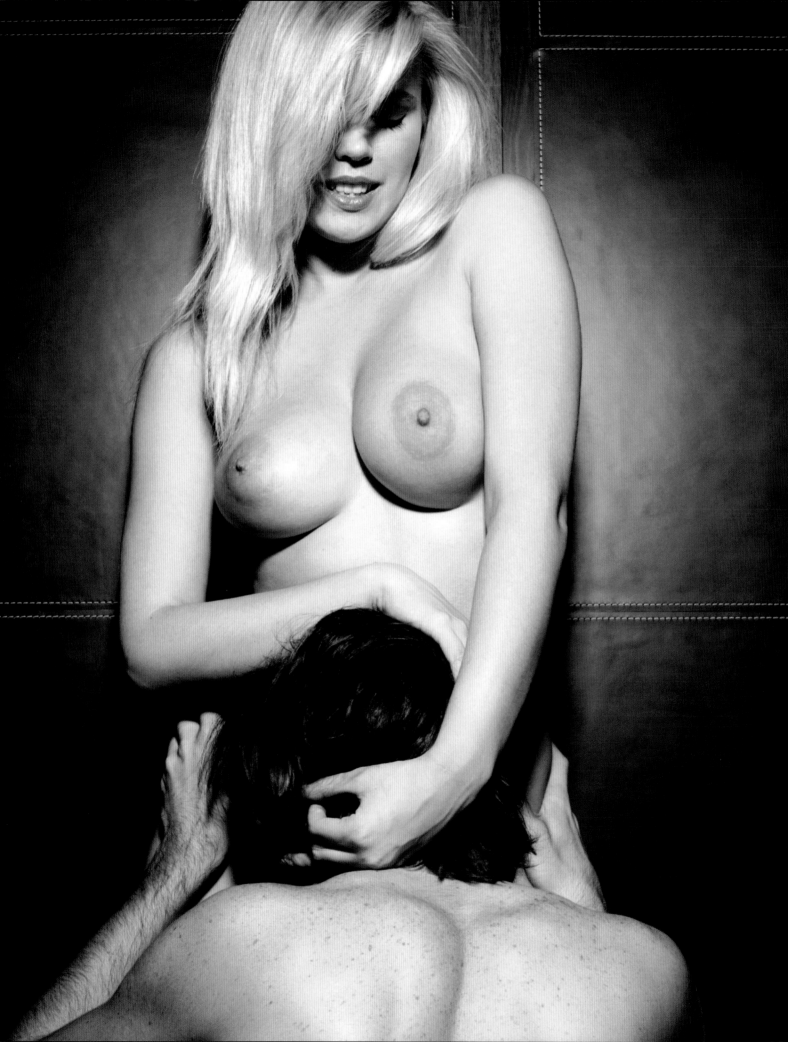

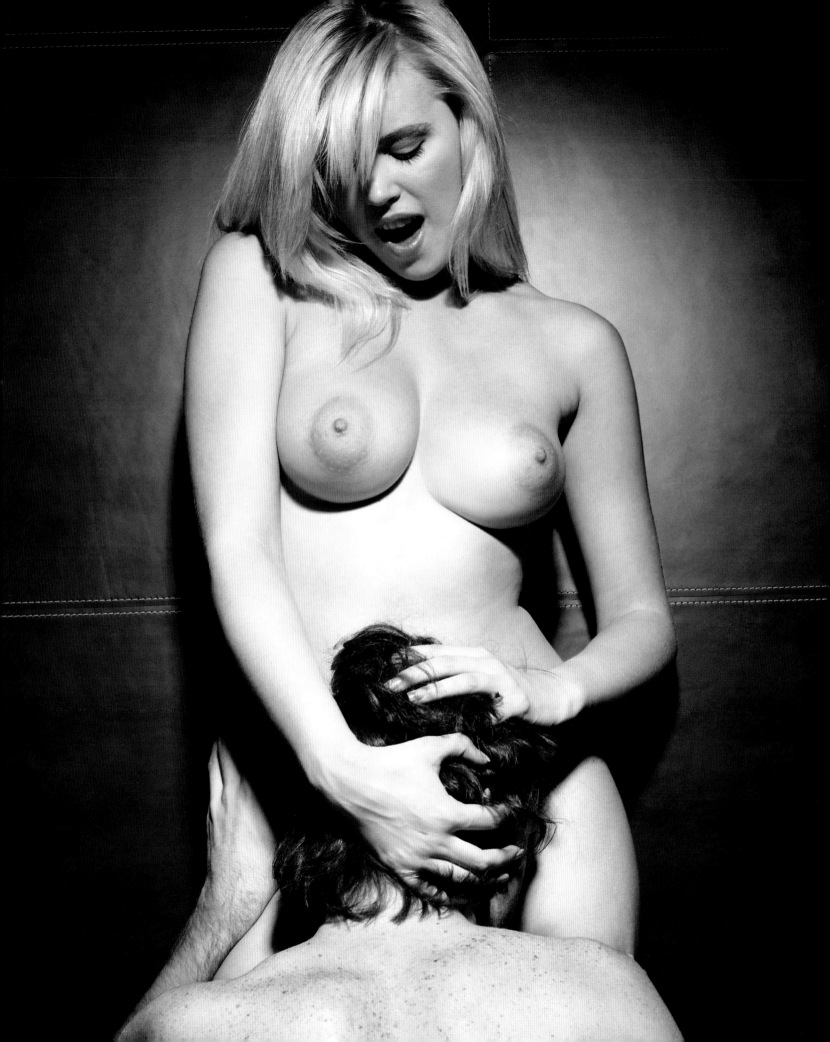

Plenty of women dread going down, whether because they're insecure about their skills or they just don't enjoy it. But many, many guys would give their non-dominant arm for a regular dose of oral—a lot of them would even choose it over intercourse. So the tips on the next few pages are designed to improve your skill set and your enjoyment level. Soon, you'll like giving bjs as much as he likes receiving them! (Okay, almost as much.)

Getting Started

The best oral sex comes out of the blue: a blowjob that is offered up rather than requested, begged for, or traded for a favor always feels better. As a bonus, initiating makes you feel like the boss—and the more confident you feel, the more fun everyone will have. Think of making the first move as a way to gain instant points in the skill department—it beats trying to master impossible techniques that may result in lockjaw.

Mind-Setting—You may feel vulnerable down there, but remember, when his balls are in your mouth, who's really in charge? It's all about getting into the right headspace, because a timid blowjob isn't a good time for anyone—and besides, the more you get into it, the faster he'll probably come. So learn to love his penis at least a little. Fake it at first, if you must—with any luck, you'll eventually start to believe in your own enthusiasm. Assuming you enjoy sex with this person, surely there are lingering feelings of affection for the guy downstairs? Let those feelings flow!

Prepping—Think fellatio is dirty, and not in a good way? Don't like the way he tastes? Hop in the shower together first—or stay there. (Pretty soon "Why don't you take a shower?" will sound as sexy as "I want to suck your cock.") Make sure you're hydrated so you don't get cotton mouth (keep a glass of water handy). And brush your teeth beforehand, too: when you're dealing with that much of your own saliva, fresh breath makes things more pleasant for you (and potentially tingly for him!).

Taking a Stance—For high comfort and control, have him lie back on the bed while you kneel or lie down between his legs (kneeling offers more maneuverability). If you're feeling lazy, both lie on your sides and place a pillow under your head. If you'd like him to do some of the work, you trust him not to get carried away, and it doesn't make you panic or gag, then he can kneel or hover over you, supporting his weight on his arms, as you lie on your back, maybe with a pillow or two under your head: you'll get great access to his balls and ass, not to mention your own naughty bits. If you're going for a worship-the-penis vibe, he can sit on a chair or stand and you can kneel on a pillow at his feet. Remember, so long as he respects you, there's nothing demeaning about getting on your knees—and if he doesn't respect you, then what are you doing down there in the first place? In a happy, loving relationship, kneeling for oral is just a bit of fun roleplaying (p.146). Plus, if you're inexperienced, the naughty factor of this position may compensate for any lack of artistry. Start off standing and move to the bed when his legs or your knees start to ache. In fact, it's always acceptable to adjust positions to stay comfy. And if he's been very good or he's had a very bad day, push him against the wall the moment he walks through the door and pull down his trousers. A note to gentlemen: if you even think of pushing a woman's head down as a "hint," karma will ensure that these sorts of good deeds never ever come your way!

Charming the Snake—Assuming this isn't a quickie in an airplane toilet, tease him first. Follow all the instructions for

Fellatio

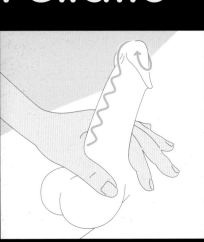

The Scenic Route—Use one or two hands to steady the base of the penis and run your tongue from the base to the top along the raphe in a back and forth motion, following the squiggly line. Try this early on to warm things up, or later if your jaw needs a break.

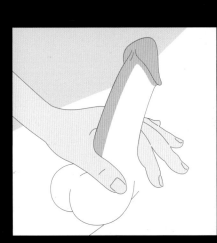

The Harmonica—Again, one or two hands steady the base. Turn your head to the side, create a mini suction cup with your mouth, and run it along the raphe, from the base to the head, enveloping the entire head with your mouth when you get to the top. Then return to the base and repeat—the shaded area indicates mouth-to-penis contact.

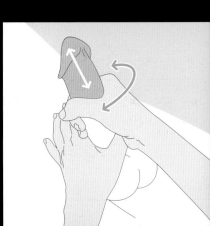

The Twist—One hand at the base, the other hand is an extension of your mouth, as in the basic up-and-down. This time, though, your wrist twists back and forth as you go up and down. Try twisting your head in an opposite back-and-forth motion to your hand as you go. You can even use your other hand to lengthen the tube of sensation and add more opposing twisting sensation.

"Skimming the Surface" during a handjob (p.62). Once he's naked, graze everywhere but his penis with your lips: thighs, bum, stomach, chest, pubic hair, balls, back of his knees, behind his ears. Or just breathe on him. And don't forget that guys like to be complimented, too: profess your ardor for his love unit and tell him you love the way he tastes. All this teasing says you don't care if this takes a while, even though it's okay to want the serious, energetic up-and-down work to last less than 10 minutes. Plus, building up tension now will shave minutes off your up-and-down time later.

Communicating—If at any point you don't know how he likes it or what to do next, just ask. As long as you're not in the crucial homestretch and orgasm is imminent, it won't spoil the mood—in fact, it proves you're not on auto-pilot.

Lollipopping—Now you can start kissing and licking his penis all over—refraining from any oral envelopment just yet. Keep your tongue flat and soft like you're licking a you-know-what (don't make us say the bj cliché). Or use the pointy tip of your tongue in a paisley pattern. Keep your tongue in constant motion, mixing moves. Lick all the way from the base to the head, either in one long smooth stroke, or in lots of little upward licks. Dry friction is the blowjob's worst enemy, so you want to get the shaft good and wet before you start any fancy moves. If neither of you are neat freaks, feel free to slick up the balls and perineum too. Though keep in mind that wet balls get chilly fast—so warm them with your hand, the sheet, or a soft towel. And if you're truly dirty birds, you can even spit on the general area. If you find the sloppy wet sounds off-putting, you could always put on some tunes—though chances are, he finds those sloppy wet sounds a turn-on. Kiss, lick, suck on the balls—don't bite. Play grownup Operation and see if you can get his shaft in without touching the sides. Finally, save the sensitive head and frenulum until last: take just the head in your mouth and swirl your tongue around the rim, lick and press your tongue into the frenulum and U-spot. Repeat as necessary until he's raring to go.

Blowing It—The following is a fairly provocative and controversial move: once everything's wet, blow gently on him from the testicles all the way up to the head. Resume contact soon thereafter, otherwise all that wet surface will start to chill in your breeze. We wouldn't recommend this as your first warm-up move on a new partner, lest he think you're taking the term literally. And be warned: he might just find it so gimmicky that it's more humorous than hot.

Getting Finished

Once he's completely hard, you can start to get a bit fancy. There are two schools of thought here: some people say, always go down in one fell swoop to announce your presence dramatically, while others think you should tease him by going down a little bit further on each downward stroke until you make it to the bottom. We say, why choose?

The Essential Up-and-Down—At its most pared down, the blowjob is just moving up and down on the shaft with your mouth, and this is where you should start (and finish). Place one or both hands at the base of his penis so your thumb and first finger form a C that holds him steady. Some people like to stretch their lips over their teeth to avoid scraping sensitive flesh at all costs, but holding this facial expression for long is quite difficult, not to mention a little funny looking. As long as you're careful, then soft, slightly puckered lips against the shaft will be fine—in fact, ideal. Try to keep your lips in constant contact with the penis. You might find loose on the way down and slightly firmer on the way up works well. Gradually get into a rhythm—go slowly for now and keep the suction at a minimum, breathing through your nose if possible. Inhale at the top, exhale on your way down. The sucking action isn't nearly as important as the steady up and down movement, especially at the beginning—and besides, too much suction makes it hard to get into a groove and keep your teeth out of the way. At some point, bring your tongue into play, stimulating the shaft and head as you bob up and down. Take the penis out every now and then to lick the top and sides.

Mouth Extensions—Deep throating is by no means a prerequisite for an excellent blowjob. It's a gimmick. And one that most women can't master for purely physiological reasons: there's that inescapable, naturally-occurring gag reflex about three inches inside your mouth—much shorter than your fella's penis (we hope!)… so do the math. Stop dreaming the impossible sword-swallowing dream and instead work with what you've got. Add one hand around the shaft as an extension of your mouth, while the other supports the base. This will increase sensation for him and give you more control over his thrusting. At first, you can delicately hold the shaft with light fingertips (the way Celine Dion might hold a microphone). Then, you can move on to a loose grip that glides up and down in sync with your oral up-and-down. Eventually, you'll use a firmer grip and keep your hand connected to your lips as you move up and down. On the upward stroke, you can take your mouth off the penis entirely, closing your lips as you do, followed by your hand gently squeezing his head. You can even continue the upward motion until your closed fist is just resting against the very tip, but don't lose contact completely or linger there: initiate the downward motion—hand then mouth—immediately. You can even get your other stabilizing hand in on the motion, creating one, seemingly never-ending orifice. And if he's the kind of guy who enjoys deep throating because of the sensation of his penis hitting a dead end, then try making him hit the roof of your mouth or the inside of your cheek instead while using this grip.

More Handwork—When you have a free hand or hands (usually during the earlier stages of a blowjob or once you've mastered the above mouth extension with just one hand), let your fingers wander to his thighs, balls, butt, nipples. Use your hand(s) in a sweeping motion across his abdomen toward his penis, as if you're drawing in all bodily energy to the center of his universe. Give him your fingers to suck on. Switch to a full-on handjob to give your jaw a break. Rub or press firmly on his perineum with a fingertip or two, a knuckle, or a thumb. Circle the surface of his anus with a well-lubed finger, and if he's amenable, slip it inside for stimulation at both ends of his shaft (i.e., internally with your finger at one far end and externally with your mouth at the other). Stating the obvious: do not give him your fingers to suck on after this move.

Turtlenecks—If he's uncircumcised, you can put your mouth on his foreskin and move it up and down—though once you get into the swing of things, you'll want to pull it back to expose the sensitive head. Once he's really hard, it should just stay out of the way on its own.

Tricky Techniques—The key to an excellent blowjob is variation: you don't want him to be able to predict exactly what you're going to do next, except, of course, when he's "coming to a head" (see below). Anything you learned to do with your hands in the previous chapter is worth trying to do

illustrations on p.72. Then mix things up as follows:

• As you reach the head during the basic up-and-down with one hand, remove your mouth, glide your palm over the head, twist it like you're screwing and unscrewing a lid (but oh-so gently!) then glide it back down the shaft, followed by your mouth.

• Never stop moving your tongue. Run it up and down along the raphe. With the head in your mouth, take the underside of your tongue back and forth across the frenulum. While you're going up and down, trace your tongue around the head on each upstroke. Or take a break from the up-down and concentrate on just the head with little flicks of your tongue or concentrated sucking.

• Try getting tactile with your teeth. No, seriously: some guys actually like a hint of tooth as you go up and down the shaft. Go very slow and be prepared to back off if he hates it. If he loves it, try delicate nibbling, too: underside of the shaft, the foreskin, the head, inner thigh, scrotum (not the actual balls).

Kinking Up Your BJ—Nothing wrong with employing tried and tested porno techniques, especially if your partner is a porn enthusiast. Hump his leg while you're down there—not only to prove this turns you on, but also to give yourself a little more physical satisfaction. Rub or smack his penis against your cheek or breasts. If you can bring yourself to moan or just say "mmm" while you're down there, he'll feel special and he'll enjoy the vibrations (hey, it's better than humming). Remember, anything that can be licked can be sucked, too: perineum, just the head, balls (one at a time or two if you're feeling heroic). And though you might find the pube-mustache effect of eye contact during cunnilingus somewhat laughable, most guys love it when they're on the receiving end: the occasional dirty look reminds him you're there for him, you're not just getting on with a job. You could even tell him you want him to watch you.

Props—No need to go it alone: edible lube (plain or flavored) can help keep things wet and even tasty if you run out of spit. Or DIY food-lube on him is fine, too: whipped cream, heavy cream, olive oil, your favorite liqueur… Just be sure he pees afterward to flush out his urethra, and showers before intercourse, because such leftovers can lead to vaginal infection. Sucking on mints or sipping hot tea or ice water are tricks that'll work on him, too. And if he's a fan of backdoor play (you'd be surprised what a little Pavlovian conditioning can accomplish during a blowjob), then try a small butt plug or anal beads instead of your finger. Finally, he might like a vibrating ring or a mini vibe held against his balls or shaft, or one of those novelty oral vibes you hold in your mouth—then again, this may just annoy him or rattle your teeth.

Coming to a Head—He'll almost definitely want more speed as he nears the finish line. And he'll probably enjoy or even need a bit more suction and a firmer hand grip, too—though again, you'll have to ask (unless you're the penis whisperer). Definitely don't slow down or suddenly change anything at this point, unless you want to tease him and drag things out. If you've both got the time and the stamina, this may only increase the intensity of his eventual orgasm; but you may also risk losing his orgasm for good, due to frustration and rawness. Don't worry about what you look or sound like as you go harder and faster—he'll probably be too busy making his own funny noises to notice (it's safe to say he's in a pretty self-focused place right now). If he does notice, the most coherent thought he's likely to muster is a scatterbrained, Hilton-esque, "That's hot".

The Happy Ending—Sometimes a blowjob is just a prelude to intercourse—especially if you're still learning his likes and dislikes. But if you decide to make this the main (or at least final) course, you'll need to decide between swallowing, spitting, or handworking. Each has its pros and cons: swallowing is neat, tidy, very intimate, and very dirty, but many women find ejaculate tastes worse than castor oil and is just as hard to get down. Spitting allows you to complete the bj without interrupting the all-important, orgasm-inducing sensation and without having to force ejaculate past your gag reflex, but you end up holding it in your mouth three times longer and guys may feel rejected by your spit-take. Switching to manual sex right at the end allows both parties to enjoy the visual without any aftertaste, but the dramatic change in physical sensation may be jarring, disappointing, or even orgasm-defeating to him (though if you're already using your hands like you should, the climactic finale should be in your grasp, literally). As with dildo selection (p.137), the one with the receptive orifice has final say: how you end things is entirely up to you, as long as you keep applying sensation all the way through his orgasm and then stop as soon as he does. And as long as you do it all with love.

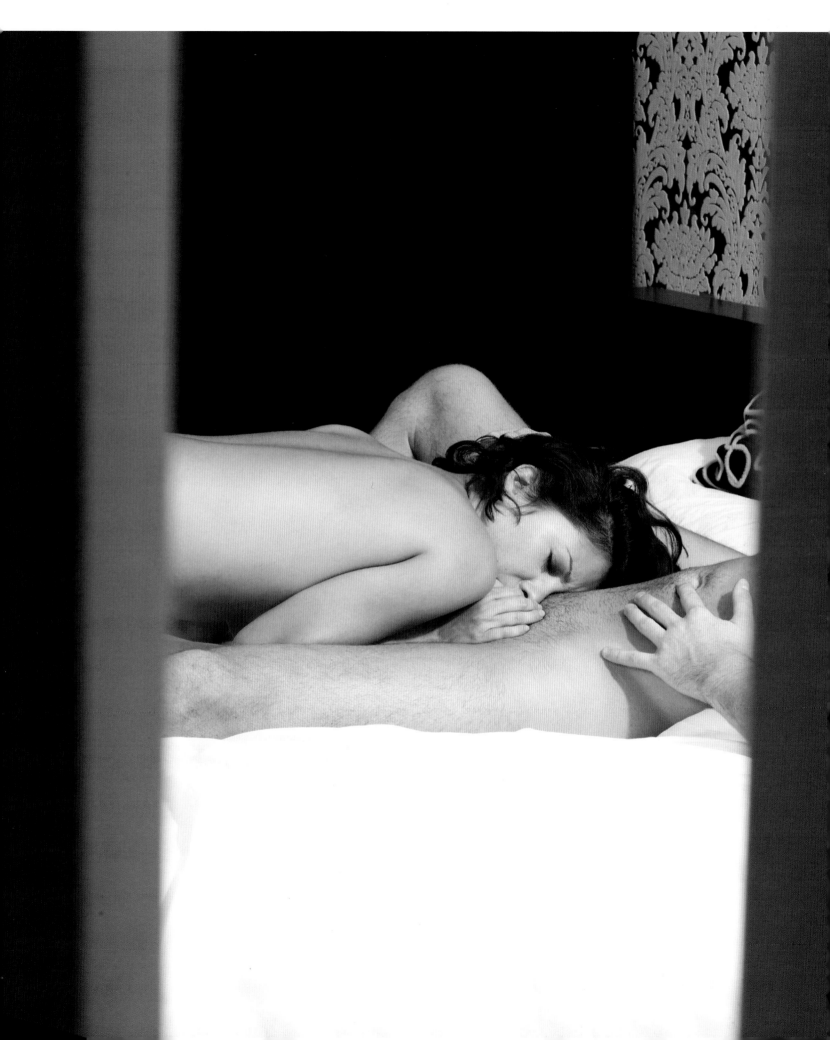

The 69 position is kind of like communism: brilliant in theory, but rarely as equitably satisfying in practice. Theoretically, what could be better than simultaneously providing each other with the kind of stimulation that is almost guaranteed to lead to orgasm for most people? (Sure, we know oral isn't for everyone, but the odds are way higher than with intercourse.) But in practice, well, if 69s lead to simultaneous orgasms every single time, don't you think we'd have a harder time getting people to breed? Still, its merits keep some people coming back for more, so to speak. We've assembled the various positions, pros, and cons of this ancient art so that you can make up your own mind.

Positions

Woman on Top—He lies on his back and she gets on top of him, her tush pointed toward his face. She can rest her weight on her elbows or his chest, and he can bend his knees to bring his penis into a better position.

Man on Top—The reverse of the above. Less common, because most women prefer to be in charge of the pace. Plus, if he's a lot bigger, she might get smothered (there's so much going on during a 69, it's easy to forget your partner needs to breathe).

Side by Side—Both lie on your sides, head to toe, usually with each of your top legs bent and up for easier access. Add pillows under your heads for comfort—or use each other's thighs as pillows, assuming you're both cushy enough. This position is the most popular because it frees up your hands to get in on the action (very important, given the odds of mutual satisfaction) and is easier to adjust if you're not the same height.

69-Inspired—If your genitals simply don't align in a 69, no matter the position, you could get side by side and head to toe and just stimulate each other manually instead. Or perhaps one of you provides oral while the other goes manual (if one of you is a hands fan, you may prefer this anyway).

The Standing 69—One person stands while supporting their upside-down partner, whose arms and legs are wrapped around the stander. Hilarious, but 100 percent ineffective. On this, there is no debate.

The Case For and Against 69

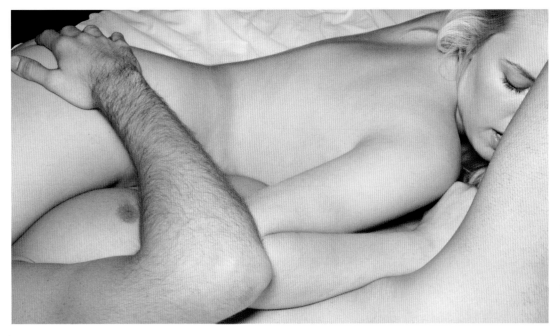
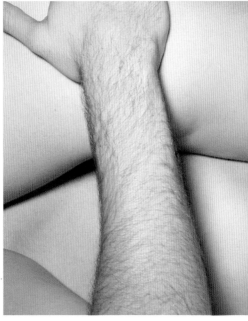

Pros

For devotees of the 69, the number one benefit—mutual oral-genital stimulation—outweighs any drawback in the book. It's an intimately bonding experience no matter the outcome. But that's not the only reason to give this position a whirl. Engaging in such gimmicky sex can make you feel young again—it can take you back to a time when experimenting, no matter how silly, was wholly erotic simply because it was new. Physically speaking, the genitals are approached in the opposite direction from typical oral sex, which could make for an intriguing new sensation. If either of you is shy about either giving or receiving head, then a 69 dims the spotlight. Which is not to say that it's any less intense—in fact, when you're this up close and personal with each other's naughty bits, you'll probably feel pretty darn adventurous (and pleased with yourselves). You couldn't be any more exposed to each other, which is perfect if you're in a full-service kind of mood: perineum, bum, *everything*. And at such close quarters, it's easy to get caught up in each other's sexual excitement. Sure, the timing isn't always perfect, but it still makes for excellent foreplay, especially for women: she can tease and slow down the pace on him, which in turn means his stimulation of her will last longer. So she gets the extra foreplay she needs without worrying that he's feeling disengaged, bored, or in a rush to get to the intercourse. And you can always take turns taking breaks if you start to feel overwhelmed by the level of concentration required. Or perhaps one of you works with your mouth while the other works with your hands, and then you switch off. In the 69 position, this kind of back and forth is practically seamless. And it's also a great way to learn about each other's oral preferences: since the penis head and the clitoral head are homologous organs, you can demonstrate exactly how you like you to be licked, using each other's genitals as the display model. Genius.

Cons

First of all, mutual oral-genital stimulation does not necessarily mean mutual satisfaction. If you're the type who likes to lie back and drift off to your happy place while you're being orally pleasured, then a 69 will be a total buzzkill—this is especially true for women, who are more likely to need to lose themselves in the moment. "Multi-tasking" is incredibly efficient at the office, but since when does efficiency = explosive orgasms? Going down on a partner can take a fairly high level of concentration —maintaining a rhythm, watching the teeth, paying attention to your partner's responses—which can make it all but impossible to relax enough to enjoy the attention you're receiving. And if you do start to relax into the receiving, you're liable to get a little lackluster in the giving department. The closer you get to your own climax, the more likely you are to lose track of what you were doing—or even to bite down accidentally in the throes of passion! That's why some people prefer the spotlight effect of first-me-then-you oral sex. Plus, in a 69, where's the view? For many people, watching their partner is the hottest thing about oral. And instead, you get within millimeters of their asshole—which is not for everyone, especially if the shower is a distant memory or you're just not ready for that sort of introduction yet. Also, the much ballyhooed "approach from the opposite direction" can actually be disappointing, especially for him: his sensitive frenulum will most likely be against the roof of her mouth, making it harder to access with her tongue. And if there's a massive height differential, you might well miss each other's genitals altogether! (Or else end up with a serious neck cramp.) With odds like this, it's a wonder anyone ever gets off in a 69. As for simultaneous orgasms in the position? They're at the end of the rainbow, along with all the unicorns and pots of gold.

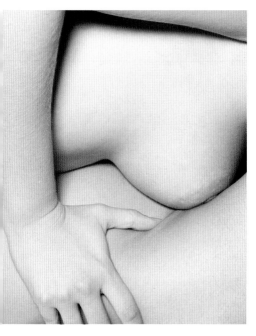

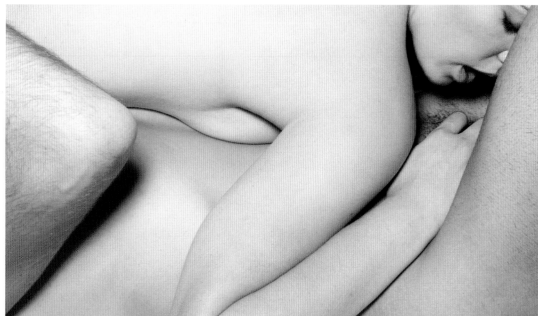

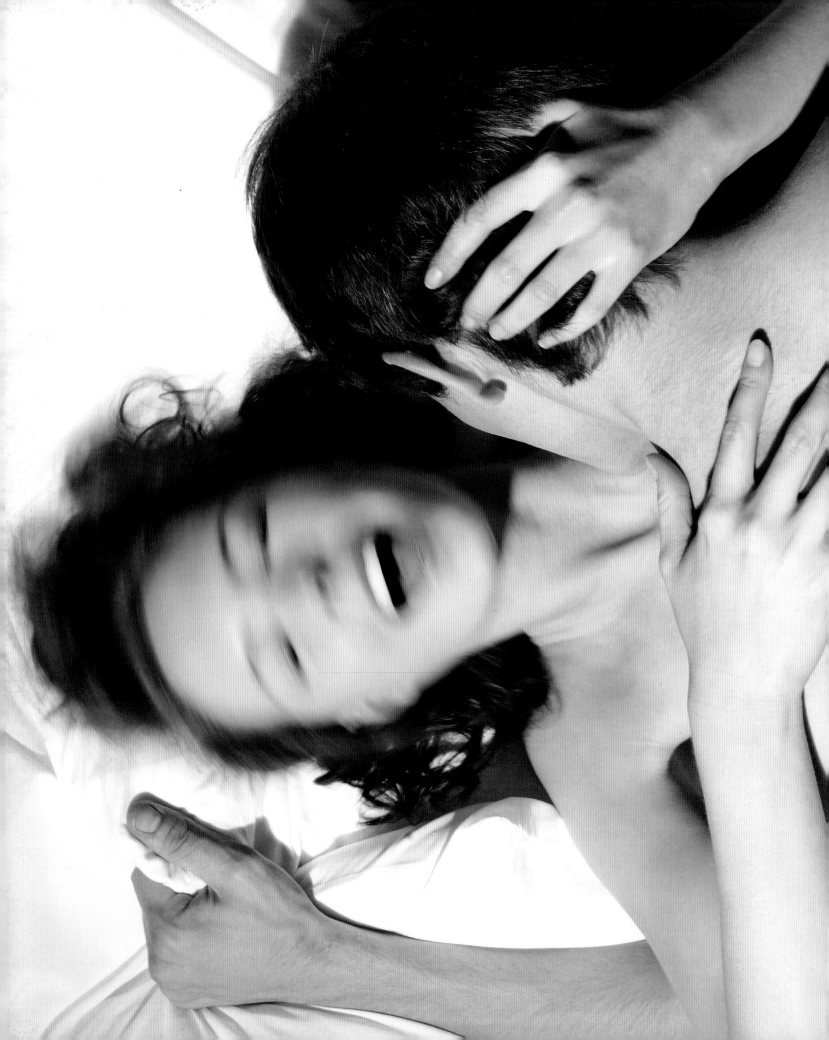

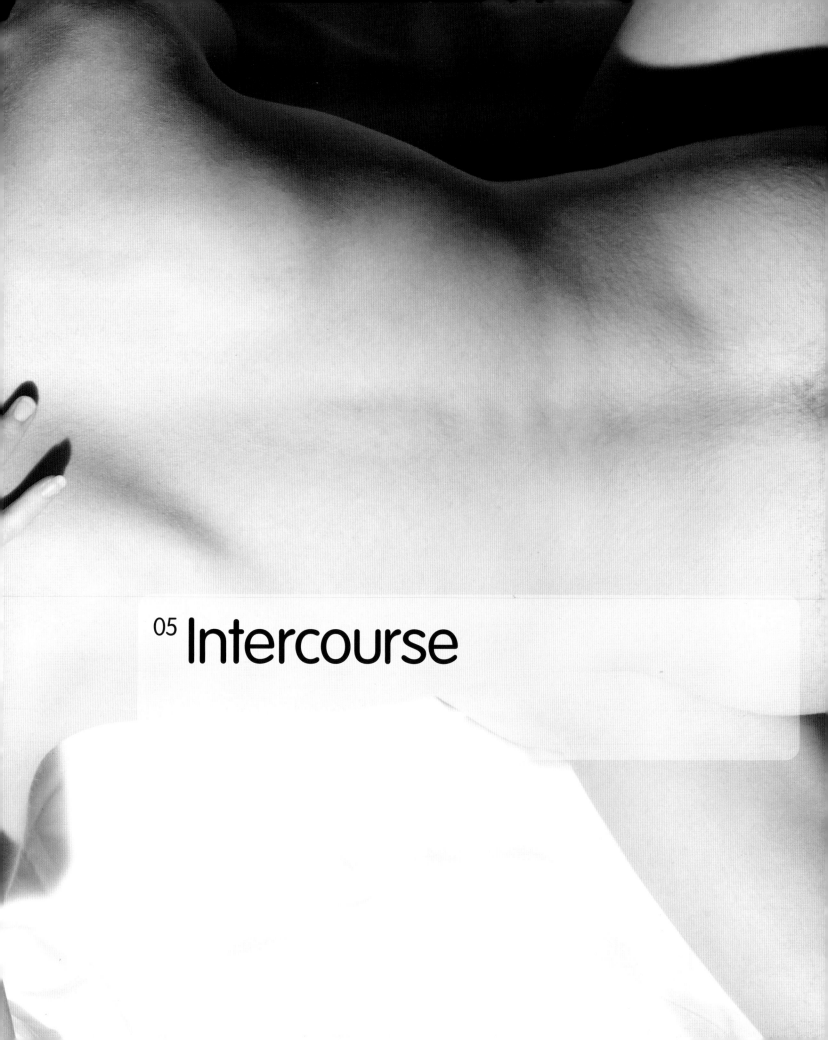

05 Intercourse

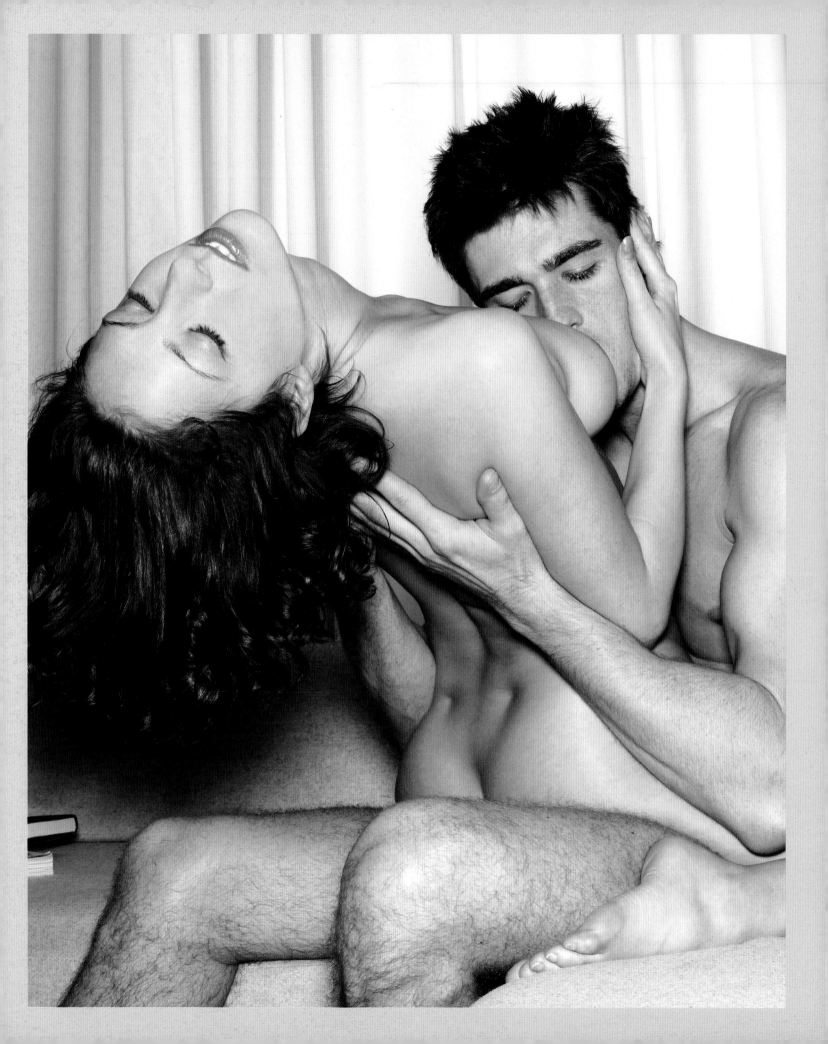

Beyond the Old In-Out

The definition of sex is not "intercourse." If you skipped the previous four chapters to get to the "good stuff," then stop, turn back, and read them (not just the pictures!) before you even *think* about joining us here.

Ready? Good. You won't find terms like "going all the way" in this chapter, because intercourse is not the last lap you complete to win a medal—in fact, it's not even a *requirement* for "winning" at sex. No, intercourse is one of *many* ways to engage in sexual pleasure—sometimes it's on the agenda, and sometimes it's not.

Intercourse is also more than a series of steps: insert tab A into slot B, thrust, repeat as necessary. At least, mutually satisfying intercourse is. Mastering the technical skills of the various positions outlined on the following pages is the easy part. The hard part, as it were, is making style, flow, grace, and equality a sexual priority when it comes to intercourse. It's what separates us from the animals.

Which is not to say that sex shouldn't be animalistic: some of the best sessions are rough-and-tumble romps driven by instinct and punctuated with lots of back-of-the-neck biting. But as anyone who's ever watched a nature show can tell you, sex in the wild often lacks creativity, stamina, romance, birth control, and, perhaps most importantly, orgasms for the female of the species (less than 30 percent of women orgasm from hands-free intercourse).

While many a poo-poo-er will claim that sex should come naturally (and not from a manual), we would suggest that anything (or anyone) worth doing is worth doing *well.* The difference between just getting by and excelling—at anything, but especially sex—is a willingness to learn, to open your mind, to try new things. And the most frequent victim of just "getting by" is intercourse.

There are more ways to move than the scenes in Hollywood blockbusters and skin flicks would suggest. The fast-paced, ass-clenched, two-dimensional humping of four-legged creatures is not the all-around winner these movies make it out to be. What looks normal and what feels good are often two very different things—and the next pages outline a few sexual philosophies and elements of style that will help you tell the difference.

Reinventing intercourse isn't just about trying new positions. In fact, that's the least important step. First you've got to change how you do it. Women, study closely: it's time to welcome your clitoris to the intercourse party! And men, study even closer: it's time to find out just how good intercourse can be when your partner enjoys it as much as you do.

Not the Be-All End-All—MYTH: *Simultaneous orgasm during intercourse is the highest sexual ideal you can attain.* This is an old-fashioned fairy tale, a 20th-century (sub)urban legend. Sure, it's nice work if you can get it (and yes, some couples can), but for many women, the intercourse-centric view goes against their very biological nature (have you noticed how far away the clitoral head is from the vaginal opening?). It sets up unreasonable expectations for both men and women (she thinks, "What's wrong with me that I can't come from his dick?" and he just thinks, "What's wrong with my dick?"). And more often than not it leads to serious—but often unspoken—sexual disappointment and frustration for her. How many men do you know who'd put up with an orgasm-free sexual relationship?

For women who don't get off on intercourse alone, intercourse is a dish best served *after* they've enjoyed at least one orgasm of their own by whatever means necessary: penetration just goes over better with a fully satisfied vagina. And, let's be honest here, most men find it, shall we say, challenging to sustain interest once they've been satisfied (which is not to say that they shouldn't try, but "ladies first" tends to put everyone in a better mood).

Safety First—If intercourse is on the menu, then barrier protection and birth control should be too. The majority of STDs can be spread with minimal genital-to-genital contact (i.e., no penetration necessary!). And pre-ejaculate can include enough sperm from a previous ejaculation to result in pregnancy. So if you're planning on bumping beauties with someone with whom you haven't a) been tested, b) jointly agreed to be monogamous, and c) established a birth-control plan, then at the very least, wrap up his cookie with a condom before going anywhere near her cookie jar—because the five-second rule that applies to candy dropped on the floor does not apply here. (See pp.178–185 for more very important info.)

Willing and Able Doesn't Always Mean Ready—You wouldn't think of attempting intercourse in the absence of a man's erection. So don't try it without a woman's either: her genitals should be engorged with blood, aroused, and just as "ready" as his. The best way to achieve this is to give her the kind of genital attention she likes best: manual sex (p.56), clittage (p.58), G-spotting (p.59), or oral sex (p.68). Or perhaps she prefers more teasing attention, like being being tied up, tickled with feathers, or titillated with naughty words (p.20). By the way, willing, able, *and* ready won't necessarily mean wet—arousal is no guarantee of lubrication. In this case, a liberal dose of a store-bought lubricant isn't a *replacement* for her arousal but rather a happy accompaniment to it (p.129). Even if she is slick herself, adding a dab of the man-made stuff can extend her staying power. Oh, and it feels pretty excellent for him, too.

Must-Have Accessories—After condoms, lubricant is the next most important bedside accessory for intercourse. But don't close your nightstand drawer just yet! There are now wonderful, high-quality, beautifully designed, ergonomic vibrators and love rings and vibrating love-ring combos made specifically for heterosexual intercourse. They can enhance sensation for both partners and help keep the clitoral head

Elements of Style

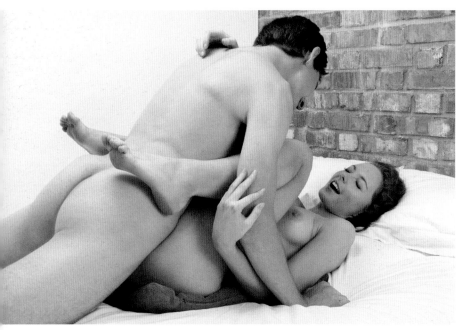

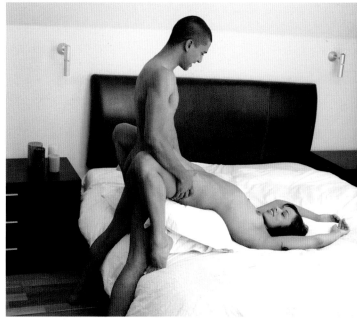

from feeling left out (p.38). Wearing cute little butt plugs can spice intercourse up for both of you, too (p.135). And don't forget strategically placed pillows or even made-for-sex bed wedges that can help support your neck, back, ass, and legs to make trickier positions more comfortable for you two.

Going Deep?—Don't always have tunnel vision, so to speak. Penetration can be more than a means to an end—it can be its own independent sexual activity. Build up to it. Draw it out. Vaginal pressure feels especially good in the outer third, thanks to the surrounding clitoral and other sexual structures—so don't go racing to the cervix: hang out in the shallow end, too. In fact, shallow penetration is great for targeting her G-spot with the penis—try missionary positions like The Squeeze (p.85) and The Aerobix (p.87); woman-on-top positions, such as The Backward Lean (p.90) and The Comfy Seat (p.92); any of the sideways positions (pp.96–97); the Cookie Twist (p.102); and the CAT (p.106) or the Reverse CAT (p.107). Which is not to say that deep penetration doesn't have its own rewards: he'll most likely enjoy the lengthening of any in-out motion and, once fully aroused, she may enjoy having her cul-de-sac stimulated (p.41).

The Motion of the Ocean—Continuing with this theme of "out with the old, in with the new," we'd like you to throw out the old in-out move as *the* intercourse standard. Jack-hammering, piston-thrusting, old-fashioned screwing, whatever you want to call it—let's try something different for a change, shall we? Swivel your hips, rock side to side, slide up along each other's bodies and back down, squeeze and pulse your pelvic floor muscles (see p.41), use your pubic bone to create more overall genital pressure... (And, ladies, don't make him do all the movement work.) Basically, find a cadence and a motion that might not *look* like stereotypical intercourse, but that feels right to both of you. And if one of you likes leisurely pelvic squeezing while the other prefers it fast and furious? Take turns, people: a bit of what she likes, a bit of what he likes, and everyone goes home happy.

Not a Hands-Free Zone—The majority of women enjoy—and often require—clitoral stimulation to gain and maintain arousal. Unfortunately, too many of these women don't ask for it during intercourse (or at all). Ladies, speak up! Guys, step up! Don't hesitate to keep attention on the clitoris with a finger, hand, or sex toy should the clitoris in question want it and the position engaged in logistically allow for it. (For example, clittage ain't gonna happen with "The Wheelbarrow" on p.108, which is just another reason why that position is kind of useless for most of the population.) And don't forget about all the other fun outlying areas that can be manually handled during intercourse on either partner: probe the mouth, tweak the nipples, massage the perineum, circle the anus, rub the tummy, scratch the back, squeeze the bum, lick the earlobes, nibble the neck, and, of course, kiss.

The Tortoise or the Hare?—Sadly, there's a lot of pressure on men to break stamina records during intercourse. We're here to relieve that pressure, because an extra 15 minutes of fast, deep pumping rarely translates into orgasmic bliss for her. So don't worry about that sort of perseverance—you're off the hook, gentlemen. Instead, earn your stamina points early in the game (remember those chapters you were going to go back and read...?). Take your time during slower, subtler, more rocking and repetitive intercourse—conveniently, you should find that this approach naturally extends your endurance anyway. Or try pulling out and offering some oral or manual sex before going back in. Ultimately, when it comes to timing, you just want to make sure you're dedicating equal time to the techniques that work for each of you, whether they fall under the category of "intercourse" or "other."

Now we're ready to assume the positions.

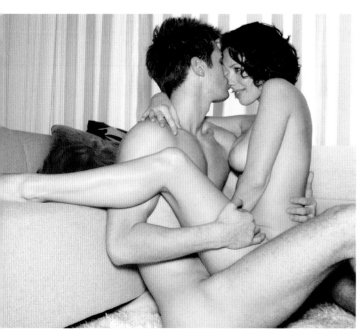

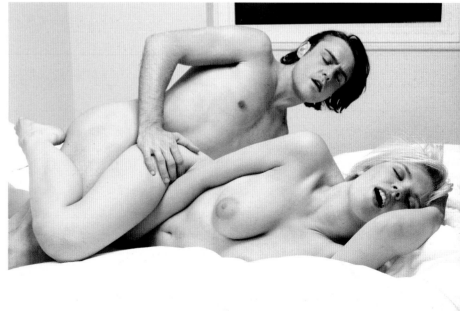

We all know we're supposed to take sex out of the bedroom to keep things hot. Variety is, after all, the spice of your sex life. But there's a reason we devoted 24 pages of this book to intercourse in your bed and only two to intercourse in the rest of your house: beds and sex go together like beanbags and movie-watching… like brownies and nuts… like beds and sex! Once you've got the right partner and the right attitude about intercourse (see Elements of Style on the previous pages), it doesn't really matter where you have sex. But we can't help but ask: why not be comfortable when you do it?

The Missionary Position

Many people assume that engaging in the missionary position is kind of like talking about the weather: you resort to it because you've got nothing more interesting to offer. But just as there are weather freaks and weather porn, so there are missionary fanatics—and for good reason, too. Men and women alike enjoy this bread-and-butter position for the intense eye and skin contact it provides. Women who feel overwhelmed by the responsibility of setting the pace or inhibited by performance anxiety while on top prefer the me-time they get on the bottom. And who doesn't like the freedom to get swept up in the screwing without fretting over whether the much-loved penis is going to break at some crazy angle? It's not lazy to love a position low on theatrics and high on physical pleasure. And let's be clear here: this is *sex*, not small talk, so it's really nothing at all like chatting about the weather. Lovers of the world, unite and take back the missionary position!

Basics for the Bed

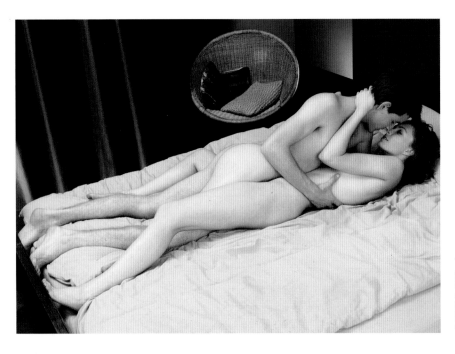

The Standard—This is as basic as the missionary gets—her legs are straight, right outside his— and is excellent for soul-melding sessions. She can use her hands on his hips to have a bit of say in the motion and pace. Or she can just grab a butt cheek in each hand and hold on, as if to say, "Don't even *think* of answering that phone."

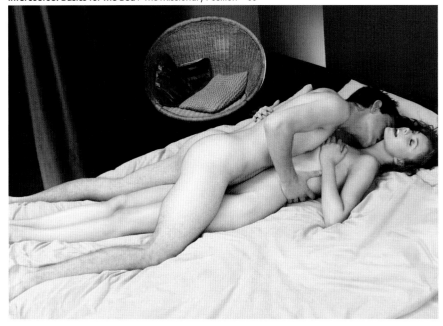

The Squeeze—The closer together and straighter her legs are, the tighter everything's going to fit, especially during slower, closer thrusting… which may well lead to labial and even clitoral stimulation for her. A little external lube (p.129) on her may make the frottage feel even nicer. To tighten the fit further still, she can squeeze her pelvic floor muscles (p.41)—there's nothing like a friendly penis to inspire a good Kegel workout!

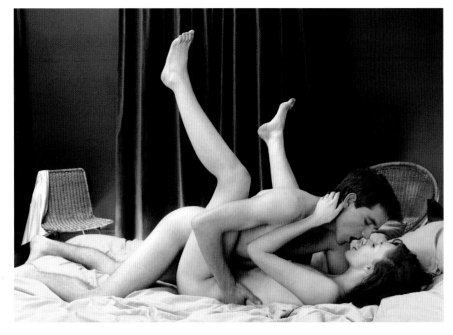

Legs of Victory—For a nice mid-intercourse stretch and deeper penetration, she can extend her legs straight up and out in the air, under his arms. However, this is not the kind of position she can maintain for very long unless she's got thighs of steel.

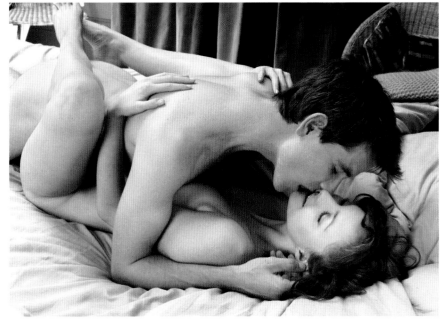

The Vice—For the woman who worries that the missionary position is too submissive: wrap your legs around his waist and you'll be the new pacemaker. This is another good position for pelvic squeezing.

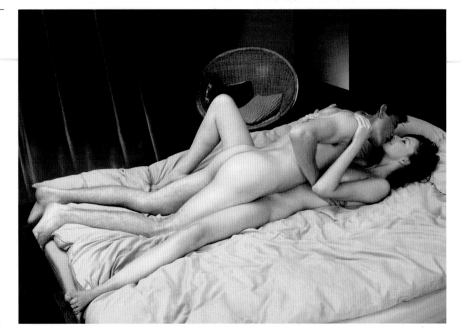

One Leg Up—Let's hear it for compromise! For the less limber woman, one leg bent at the knee and one straight is infinitely more comfortable (and sustainable) than bending both legs. Plus, it increases the depth of penetration without her losing clitoral contact altogether (which typically happens when she bends both legs at the knee).

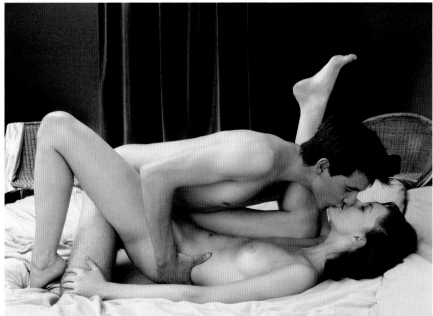

Over the Shoulder I—She rests one leg on his shoulder, for a *Kama Sutra*-esque twist on One Leg Up. She may find this position slightly harder to maintain, but the smug satisfaction you'll both get over how very *imaginative* your missionary is may make it worthwhile. She may also experience diminished clitoral contact, so he should feel free to pick up the slack with some clittage. (And massage her thigh later if she gets a cramp.)

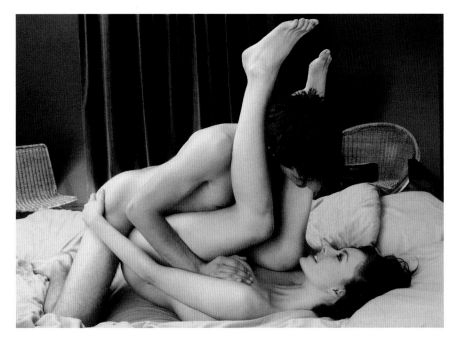

The Full-Court Press—Proof that even the missionary position can draw on your yoga skills! (We're serious: this is not a position for couch potatoes.) When she puts a leg over each of his shoulders, penetration is as deep as it gets for missionary sex, though the corollary is less overall movement and zero clitoral stimulation (unless she supplements with her own hand).

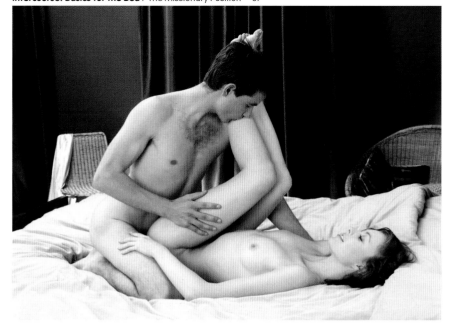

Over the Shoulder II—As we mentioned in The Squeeze, women often like their legs together during intercourse: they can Kegel and they can increase the pressure on their labia. Well, getting both her legs over one of his shoulders isn't the easiest to pull off (no lying back and thinking of England), but if you manage it, you'll get deep penetration *and* all the legs-together good stuff.

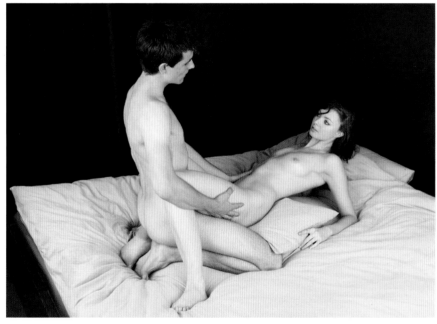

The Laptop—Want to experiment with a new angle of penetration? He kneels, resting on his feet, and pulls her toward him so her bum is resting on his thighs—or on a pillow if that's more comfortable. He can also support her with his hands.

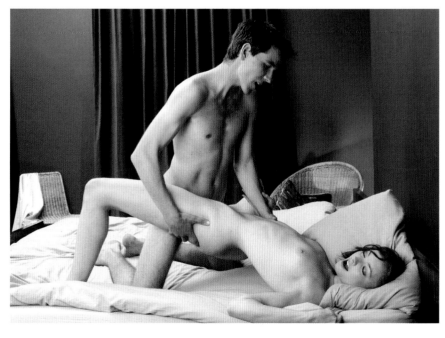

The Aerobix—Yet another cool angle (you'll find that G-spot eventually!): he's in a more upright kneel; she keeps her shoulders on the bed and then arches her back so her pelvis meets his—if he's a nice guy, he'll place a hand at each of her hips for added support.

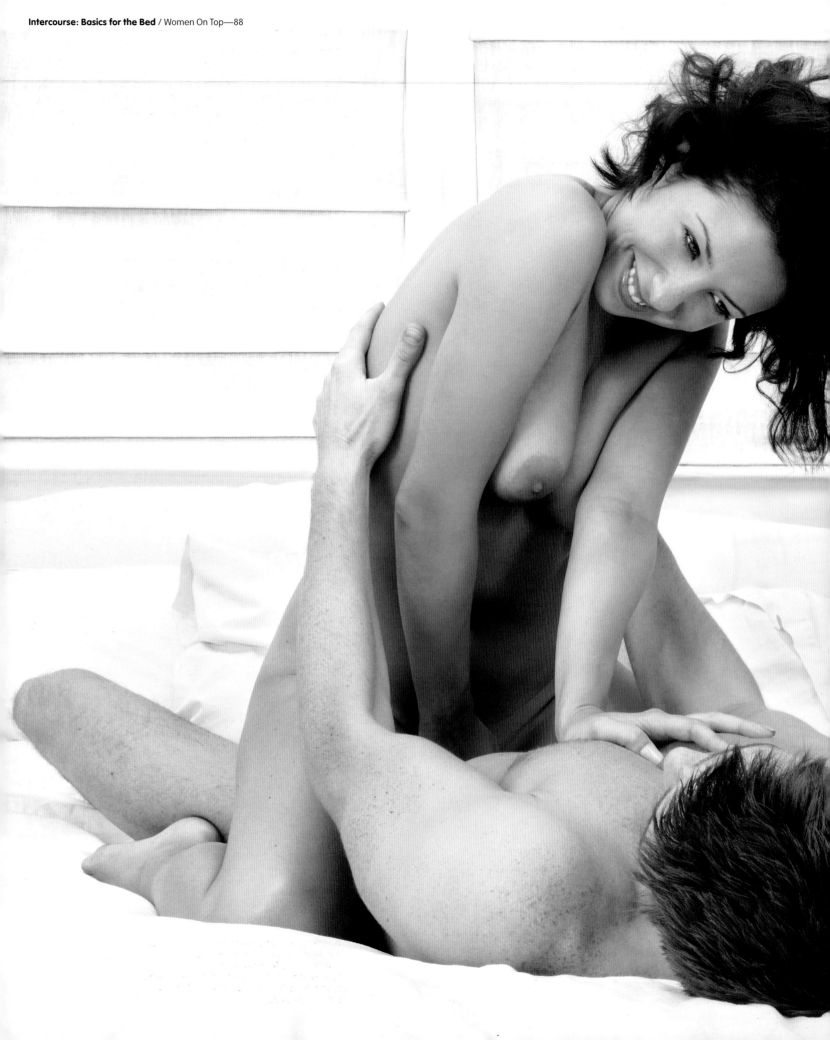

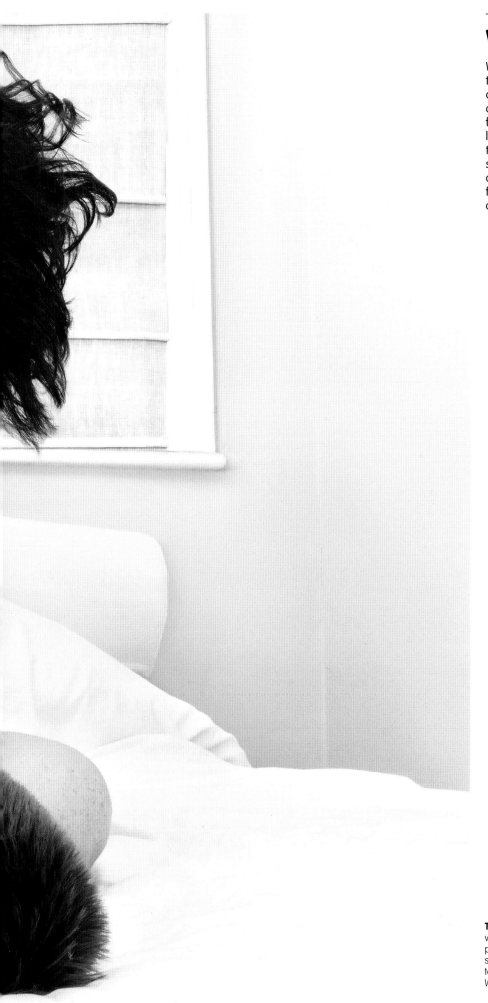

Women On Top

Women like to be on top for a simple reason: it feels good up there. It not only rates highly in terms of clitoral stimulation— all four hands on deck!—it also lets her control how much of his penis goes in, at what angle, and how fast. For G-spot fans, that's a big advantage. Plus she can move how she likes: sensual undulations of her pelvis, quick flicks of her hips, teasing shifts of pace, or fast bobs along the length of his shaft (and lots of other variations too). It's no wonder woman-on-top has a reputation for being the most female-orgasm-friendly position there is. And the men? They get to lie back and enjoy the view. Don't forget to tell her how great she looks!

The Cowgirl—This position is the most common woman-on-top pose, with great access for either partner to her clitoral head. It requires more stamina on her part than some of the woman-on-top variations, but it also provides the best "I Am Woman" power rush.

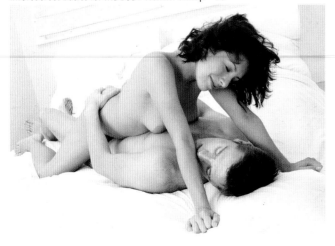

The Forward Lean—If she leans forward on her arms—resting on his chest or, if he's a fragile thing, the bed—she'll gain more leverage to lift her hips up and down or slide them front to back. Many women prefer this all-in-the-hips swiveling to the more bouncy action of The Cowgirl. Using her arms will take some of the pressure off her knees. A back and forth grinding motion will mean more labial and clit stimulation for her. Plus, as she leans into him, he gets to look *and* touch.

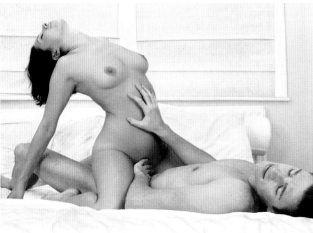

The Backward Lean—This time she leans back and arches her back, supporting herself on her hands, which are placed behind her. This pushes his penis to the front wall of her vagina, which means it may just hit her G-spot, thank you very much. Unfortunately, he may find his penis slipping out quite easily or, worse, hyper-extended in this position; therefore, slower, smoother movement is recommended. But a great close-up view for him may make it worth the risks: he gets to see *everything* as she moves in and out.

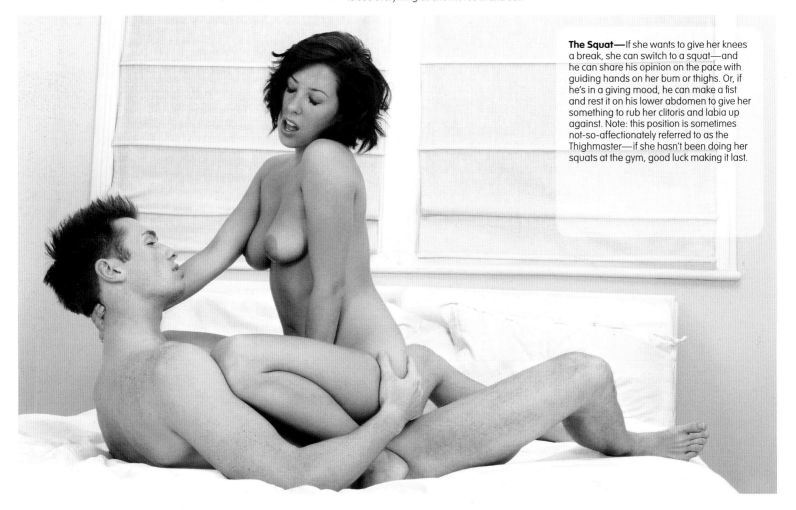

The Squat—If she wants to give her knees a break, she can switch to a squat—and he can share his opinion on the pace with guiding hands on her bum or thighs. Or, if he's in a giving mood, he can make a fist and rest it on his lower abdomen to give her something to rub her clitoris and labia up against. Note: this position is sometimes not-so-affectionately referred to as the Thighmaster—if she hasn't been doing her squats at the gym, good luck making it last.

Up Close and Personal—It gets lonely at the top sometimes, but if she leans all the way forward, so his and her torsos are touching, woman-on-top can feel a whole lot more intimate. And she can give her leg muscles a break by relaxing them into a frog-like pose. She may not have quite as much leverage as she does in The Forward Lean, but the friction is excellent.

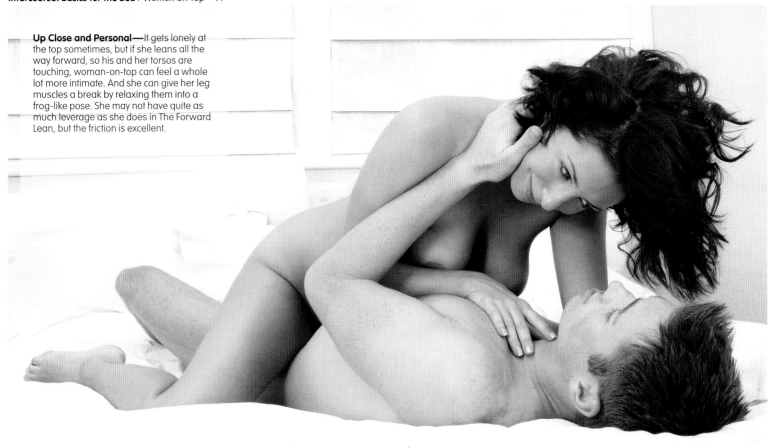

The Reverse CAT—If you *really* miss each other, she can hook her arms under his pits and cup her hands on his shoulders. Let's hear it for full-body contact! You won't get a lot of big thrusting in this position, which may be fine by her, as she's perfectly positioned to squeeze her pelvic muscles while rocking or grinding: there's much more opportunity for clitoral and labial, and potential G-spot stimulation. And he gets to lie back and enjoy a penis massage. For more on movement tips in this position, see The Reverse CAT on p.107.

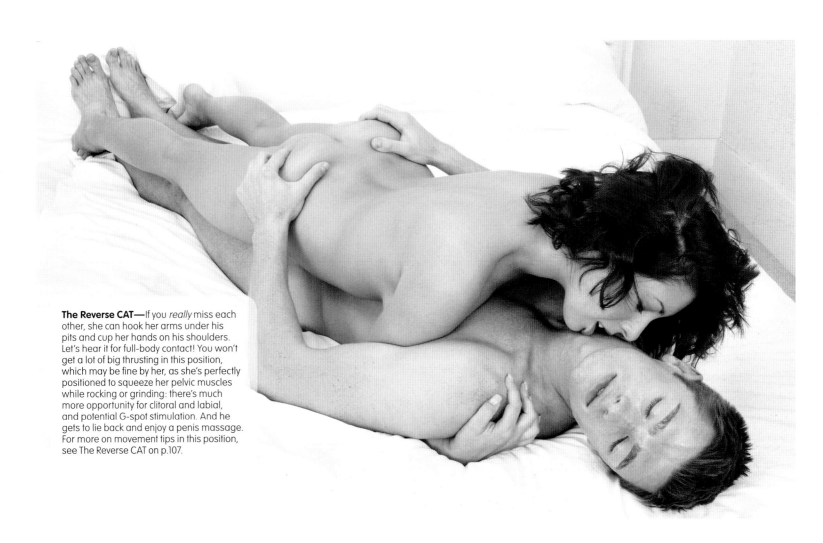

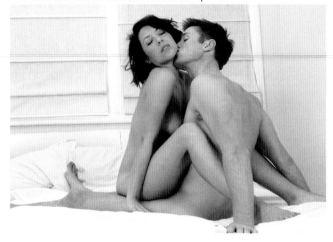

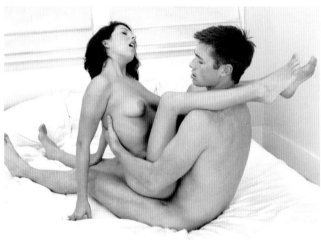

The Comfy Seat—This is like the cozy armchair of woman-on-top sex! He sits upright with his arms behind him and she sits on his upper thighs, with her arms supporting her and her knees in a relaxed bend, her feet flat on the bed. For variety, she can lean back slightly and put her arms behind her, but there's no dramatic arching— this position should be easy like Sunday morning, assuming his penis has got some give. If it does, chances are he'll hit her G-spot as she leans back. The only downside is that if one of you attempts to raise a hand for some clittage, the whole thing may come tumbling down.

The Neck Warmer—Feeling a little daring? She raises her legs over his shoulders, which shifts the angle of penetration and may offer another chance to target her G-spot. If her legs or arms get tired, or you find it too difficult to balance, she can shift easily back into The Comfy Seat or The Hug.

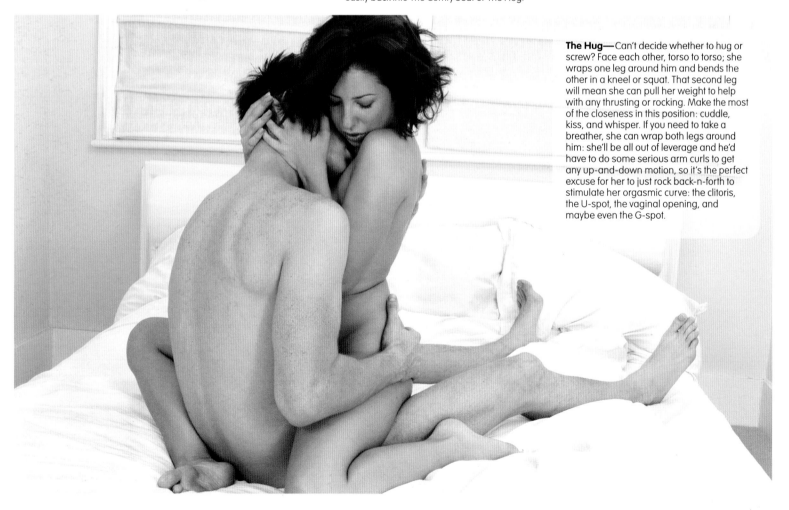

The Hug—Can't decide whether to hug or screw? Face each other, torso to torso; she wraps one leg around him and bends the other in a kneel or squat. That second leg will mean she can pull her weight to help with any thrusting or rocking. Make the most of the closeness in this position: cuddle, kiss, and whisper. If you need to take a breather, she can wrap both legs around him: she'll be all out of leverage and he'd have to do some serious arm curls to get any up-and-down motion, so it's the perfect excuse for her to just rock back-n-forth to stimulate her orgasmic curve: the clitoris, the U-spot, the vaginal opening, and maybe even the G-spot.

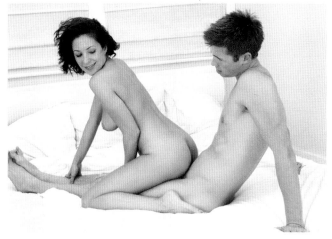

The Reverse Cowgirl—She kneels astride him with her back to him. She can lean either forward or back to find the angle that's best for both of them, though she'll probably have most leverage for thrusting if she leans slightly forward on straight arms. Plus, he'll have better access to offer an anal, perineal, or butt cheek massage. Just remember that his penis won't be able to bend as far in this direction and may slip out fairly easily. But if he likes to look at her backdoor (and she likes to show it off), what's the big deal about an occasional accidental disengagement? Re-engaging is just another sensation to enjoy!

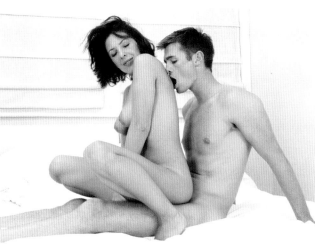

The Reverse Cowgirl Squat—Same as The Reverse Cowgirl, but she shifts into a squat. As in The Squat (p.90), it can take some pressure off her knees and he can offer support with his hands on her tush or thighs while he either lies back or sits up.

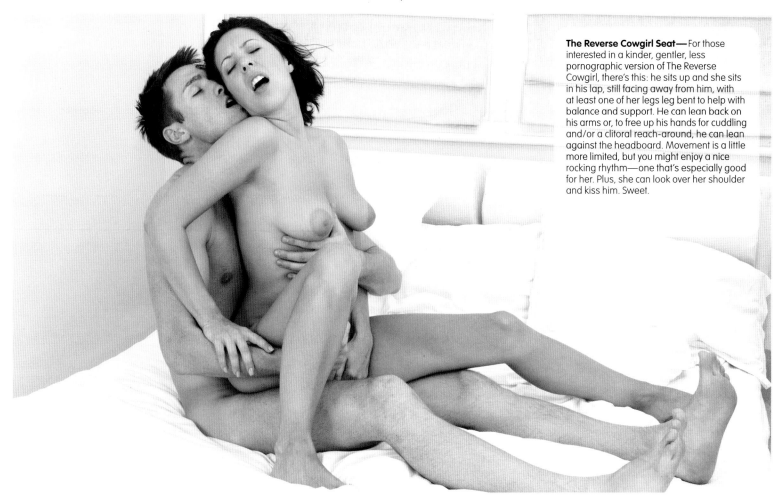

The Reverse Cowgirl Seat—For those interested in a kinder, gentler, less pornographic version of The Reverse Cowgirl, there's this: he sits up and she sits in his lap, still facing away from him, with at least one of her legs leg bent to help with balance and support. He can lean back on his arms or, to free up his hands for cuddling and/or a clitoral reach-around, he can lean against the headboard. Movement is a little more limited, but you might enjoy a nice rocking rhythm—one that's especially good for her. Plus, she can look over her shoulder and kiss him. Sweet.

From Behind

Rear-entry is unfairly maligned as being the favored position of cheaters, one-night standers, and commitment-phobes—after all, it's literally faceless sex. But why should the bad boys and girls have all the dirty fun? Loving, taxpaying couples in long-term commitments can reap this position's many benefits, too! Penetration is incredibly deep, which is always great for him (and *may* be good her). If you keep the penetration more shallow and aim downward with the penis—there's her G-spot. Both partners can easily reach her clitoris, labia, and/or breasts. And the faceless nature of rear entry means you can entertain your naughtiest grocery clerk fantasies. Ladies might like the raw, animalistic vulnerability and the sense of "being taken." Gentlemen often like *doing* the taking: the unencumbered thrusting, the feeling that his dick is the center of the universe, and, of course, the view (especially if he's what's known in clinical terms as an "ass man"). It's also a great standard "quickie" position. For an even easier position from behind, see Spoons on p.97; for a more challenging one, see The Wheelbarrow on p.108.

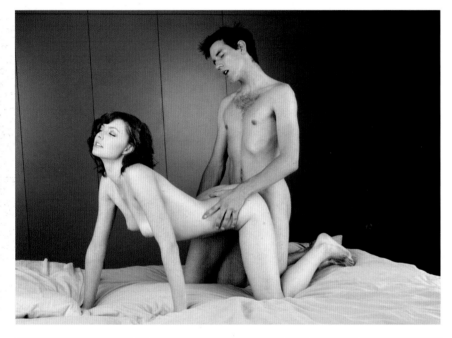

Doggie Style—This is your classic doggie style, which is probably why it feels the dirtiest: she kneels on all fours and he kneels behind her. Make sure you're on a soft surface, otherwise your knees may take a beating. He can hold or grab her hips, sides, shoulders, neck, or hair, or just give her a well-timed love-spank. She can wrap her calves around his thighs to help set the pace, rub her feet against his butt cheeks, or, if one leg is between his, use her heel to (*carefully*!) massage his crack. Up the kink factor by doing it near a mirror, so long as you don't find the reflected eye contact too funny-feeling.

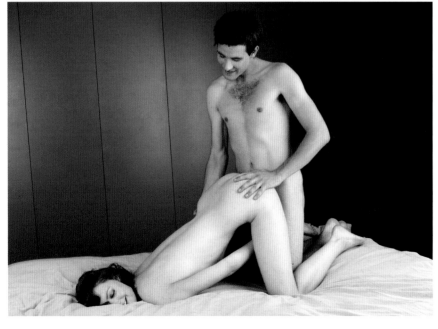

Half Doggie—She's still on her knees, but she leans down on her head and shoulders, raising her bum in the air to greet him. This position elongates her vaginal canal and provides the greatest depth, which often encourages jackhammering on his part (there is such a thing as going too deep—her internal organs can feel penis-punched). But if he can resist thrusting, she may enjoy having her A-spot and cul-de-sac (p.40 and p.41) stimulated by the head of his penis while he or she attends to her clitoral head (she's stable enough to give herself the constant stimulation that might get her off). Plus, he can stimulate her anal area with a finger or toy (as usual, he should keep anything that's been in or near her tush away from her vagina).

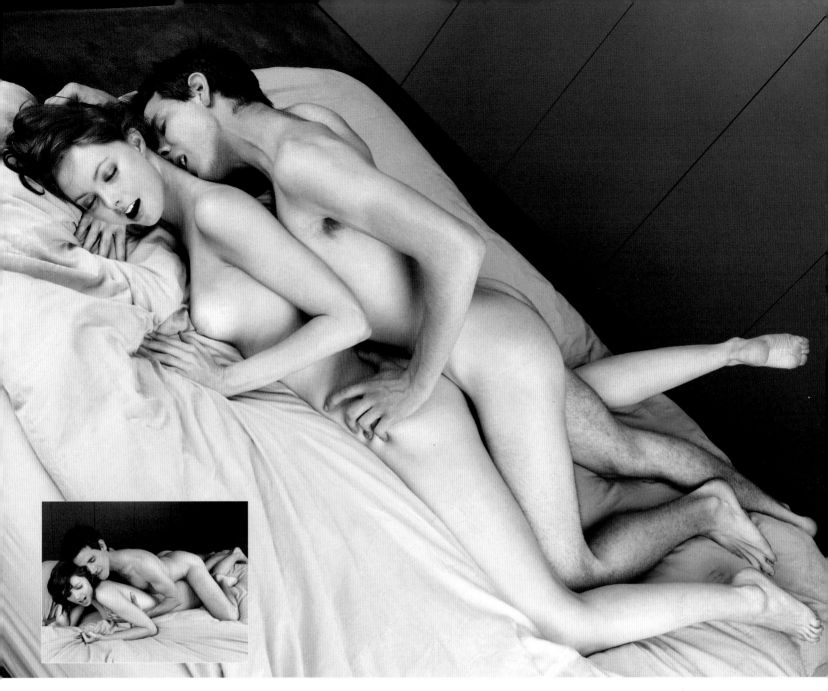

Human Blanket—She lies flat on her stomach and he enters from the rear (you might find it easier to start in a half-doggie and then slide down into this position). With the increased body-contact, this rear-entry position feels a lot more intimate and civilized, save for the lion-like back-of-the-neck biting that can occur. (The more reserved among you may also appreciate the fact that you no longer have to refer to the position you're in as "doggie"-anything.) Many women particularly enjoy the sensation of lying on something in this position—a hand, a wrist, a thumb, a body-contoured vibrator (see p.130),

a pillow, or even just some bunched-up sheets—it's how a lot of them first learned to masturbate. And she can vary the sensation in this position by bringing her legs together. As we've mentioned before, when a woman closes her legs during intercourse, it tightens things up for everybody. This means she may get more clitoral and labial stimulation, and she can squeeze her pelvis muscles around his penis, especially during slow thrusts where he stays close to her body (as opposed to during acrobatic piston-action, where she'll find it hard to get a grip).

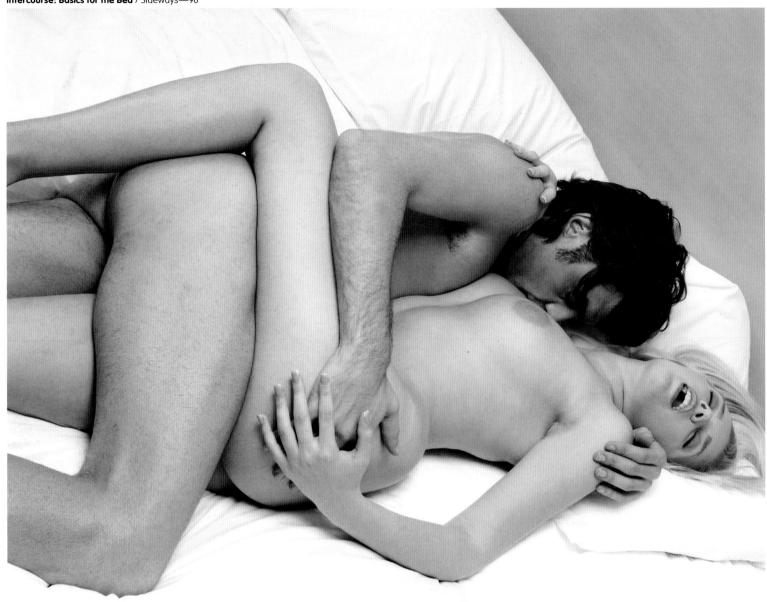

Sideways

Sideways sex is just as sweet as missionary but without the stodgy reputation. You won't get as much range of motion or depth of penetration when you're lying this way, but that can be a good thing: it'll force you to come up with a new way to move together (which might be just what she needs if she's the type of gal for whom traditional thrusting doesn't do it). Try rocking back and forth, or grinding against each other repeatedly like you've got all day. Sideways sex is great for taking your time, especially if you're a little tired and can't face anything more aerobic or if you just want to delay his climax. Whatever the case, don't forget to let those hands roam. And hey, if you get bored, most other positions are only a roll away!

Full-Frontal Sideways—This über-basic position is pretty much just the missionary or woman-on-top (depending on your perspective) turned on its side: you face each other and she props one leg over his leg or hip for better penetration. There should be lots of kissing, face-holding, and all-over caressing. Works great for sessions that might fall under the category "makin' sweet love": you've never done it with each other before, you told each other "I love you" for the first time, you just got engaged, you're trying to make a baby, it's Tuesday morning.

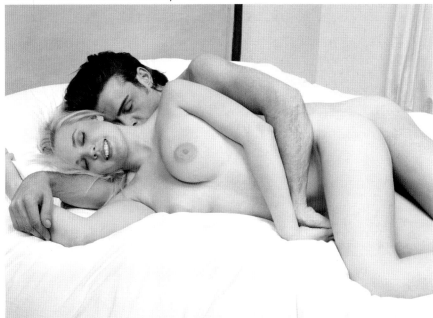

Spoons—This is basically rear-entry-lite: yes, he's entering her from behind, but you can just call it "being the outside spoon." As with sex from behind (pp.94–95), this position is good for her G, but unlike all those doggie positions, he gains his leverage here from hugging her close. And as with basic sideways sex, penetration and motion are somewhat limited—which means it's great for slow, easy, possibly hungover sex.

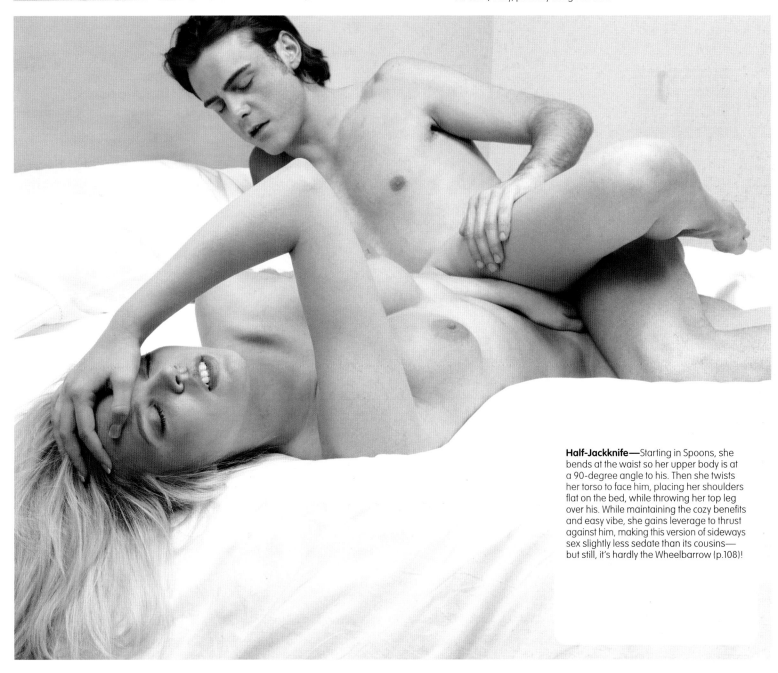

Half-Jackknife—Starting in Spoons, she bends at the waist so her upper body is at a 90-degree angle to his. Then she twists her torso to face him, placing her shoulders flat on the bed, while throwing her top leg over his. While maintaining the cozy benefits and easy vibe, she gains leverage to thrust against him, making this version of sideways sex slightly less sedate than its cousins— but still, it's hardly the Wheelbarrow (p.108)!

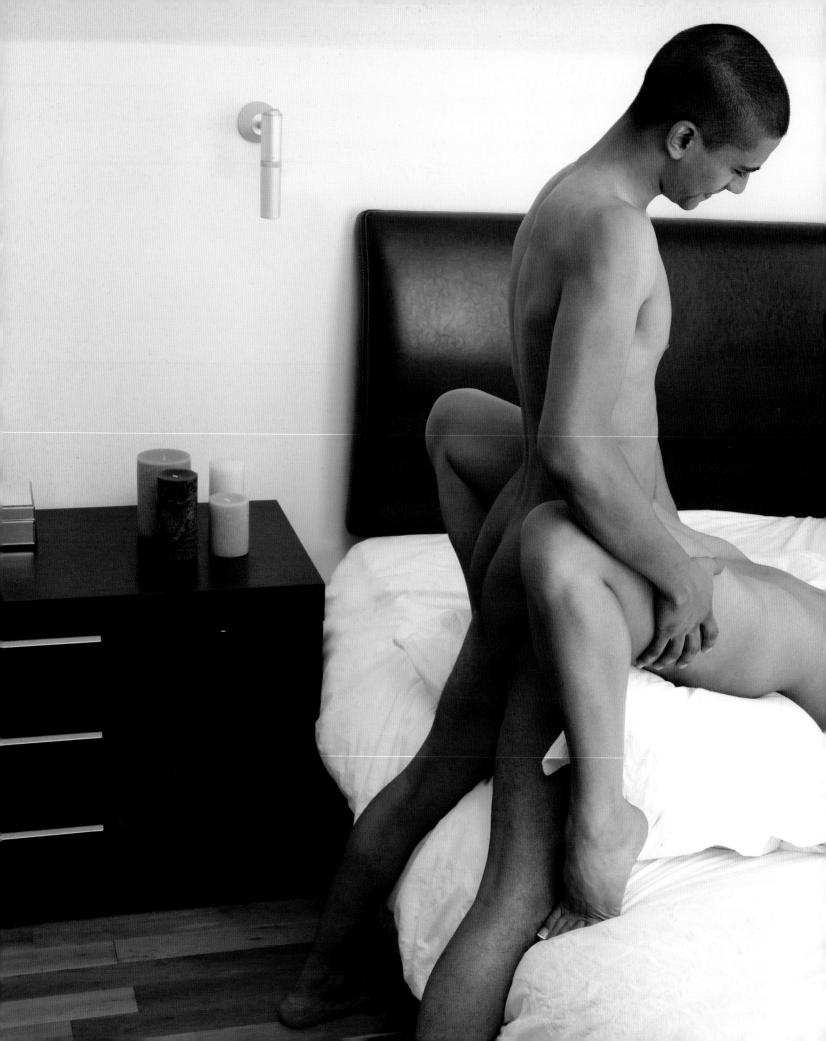

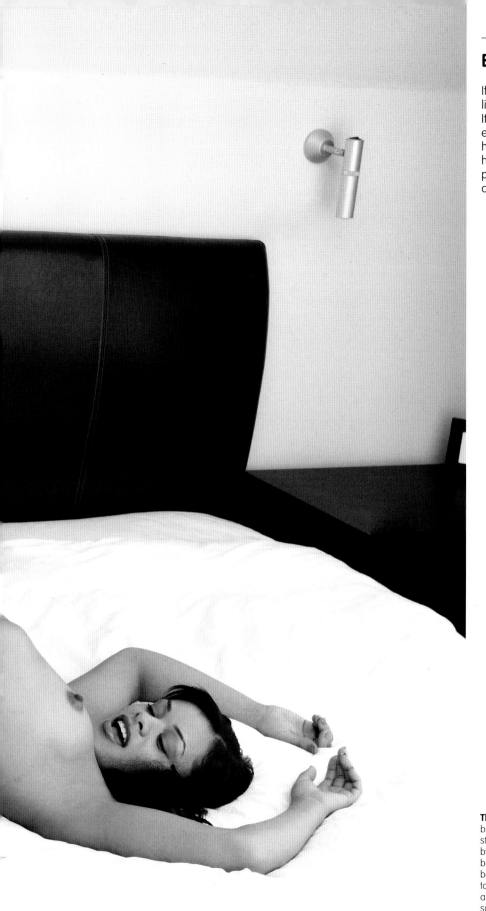

Edge of the Bed

If you want to feel adventurous but don't like the look of your linoleum kitchen floor, just move over to the edge of the bed. It's an easy way to try out different angles of penetration, especially with the help of a pillow or two. Plus, everyone's hands have more freedom to roam. And for couples whose height differential or low-risk personalities make high-gimmick positions like standing or shower sex disagreeable, it's the closest to loco they'll get. So go ahead, live on the edge a little.

The T-Bar—She lies on her back with her legs bent and her feet at the edge of the bed; he stands, and adjusts his height (for example, by widening his stance or standing on a phone book) in order to align his pelvis with hers. If the bed is a little low, she can lift her hips up off the bed to help their pelvises synch up (but unless she's a professional gymnast, he'll eventually need to support her with two helping hands or a few pillows placed under her tush). If you're working with a really low futon, he can kneel on a few pillows on the floor. These positions all provide him with pleasing leverage—both physical (freedom to thrust) and, perhaps, psychological (if power play is on the menu tonight, see p.154). Keep in mind that this position and almost all of its variations on the next two pages are practically made for clittage (p.58).

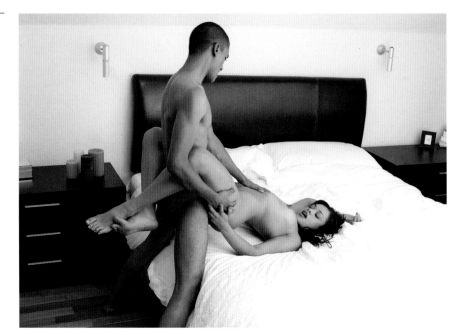

The Lift—Starting in The T-Bar (on the previous page), she then wraps one or both legs around his waist, giving her more control over the pace and depth of penetration. She may also find it easier to squeeze her pelvic muscles if she's wrapped around him.

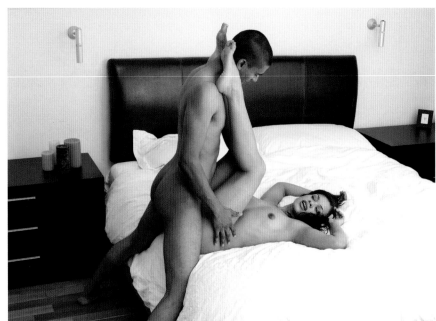

The Right Angle—She places a foot over each of his shoulders. This position will work best if your pelvises align when a) he's standing in a comfortable position and b) her back is flat on the bed from head to bum. Of course, this all depends on the height of the bed and the man, so don't force it.

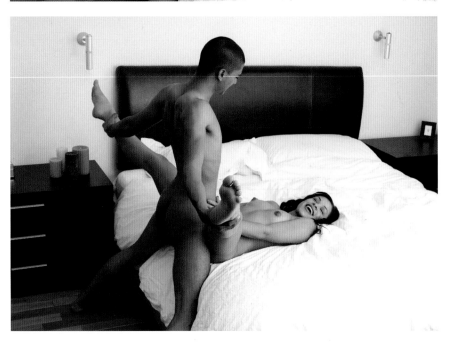

Legs of Victory—He takes each of her straight legs in a hand and spreads them out to either side. Rates high in porno-chic factor.

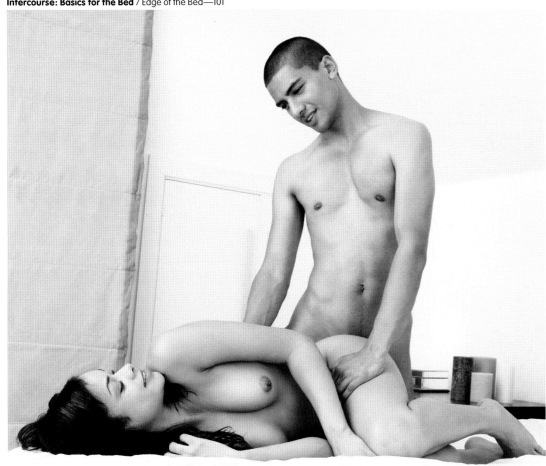

Sideboard—She lies on her side in a relaxed fetal position (i.e. *not* like her dog just got run over and she's rocking herself to sleep) with her ass at the edge of the bed. He stands and aligns his genitals with hers, for a sort-of sideways/rear-entry combo. This position sets up a "rotated penetration angle," as it's known in the biz, which is a fancy way of saying it'll give you a new and unusual sensation you may or may not like. Don't let the multi-syllabic terminology fool you: it's incredibly easy to pull off!

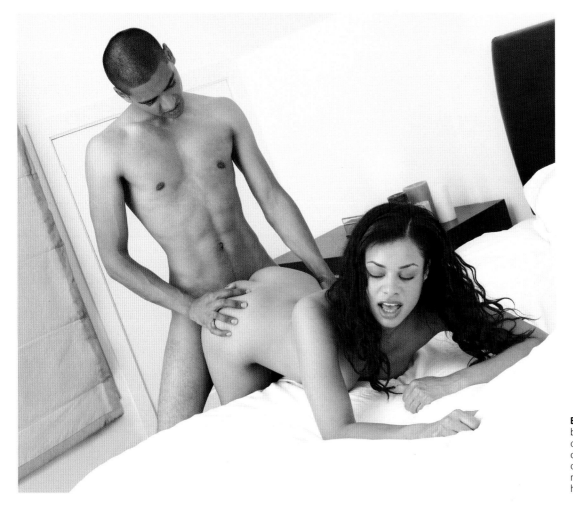

Bent Over—She folds herself over the edge of the bed with her legs spread and the balls of her feet on the ground, while he stands behind her. It's doggie-style for comfort queens! Plus, bending over *anything* has undertones of "you've been naughty"—think of it as instant roleplay, without having to come up with any dialog.

If you get bored of the basics, then you might want to add some more complicated moves to your repertoire (though if you adopt our elements of style on pp.82–83, we doubt you'll get bored of the basics). A few trickier positions can enhance pleasure, while some just provide a change of scenery, and others are made purely for kicks. Whichever flourishes you decide on, be sure to stretch first. And though we certainly wouldn't suggest it's a requirement for good sex, there's something to be said for the sense of accomplishment you might get from achieving a position with a difficulty rating of 9.8, or the fun you might have high-fiving your partner after nailing a tricky dismount.

Doing the Twists

There is no rule in the bible of sex (or this good book for that matter) that states you may not disengage genitals in order to switch positions—in fact, doing so may help stave off his ejaculation (if that's what you're hoping for). But sometimes it's nice to not break the seal—to stay connected. A blind dedication to not interrupting coitus, even when physics would recommend otherwise, expresses a mutual belief that this sensation of being united is just too good to stop. If you're both feeling this way or you'd like a new penetrative angle, then do a Twist. First-time twisters might want to start out on the floor—it'll give you more stability than a bed. You should be using lubricant to improve any position, but it is absolutely essential for making Twist positions as smooth as possible. As you twist, if something along the way feels good, then by all means stop and enjoy it. And if something along the way feels bad, then by all means stop, period.

Getting Fancy

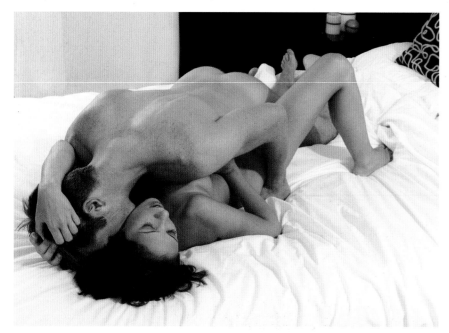

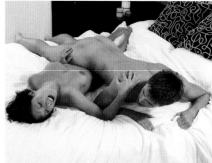

Cookie Twist

Step 1—Start off in a straight-legged stacked pancake position (with either him or her on top).

Step 2—Then, imagining your united genitals as an axle, the person on top *gently* rotates either clockwise or counterclockwise about 45 degrees, or however far feels good. The depth of penetration will be limited, which may well be a good thing. And if she's on the bottom, she may gain better access to her clitoris with her hands.

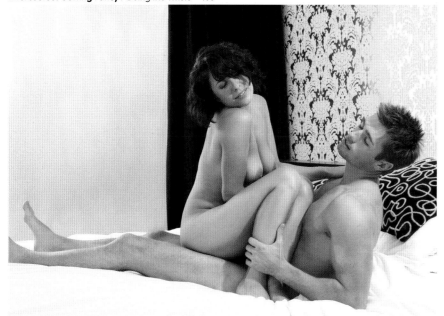

Sit & Spin

Step 1—From any woman-on-top position, she sits straight up, bringing her knees up close and putting her feet flat on the bed or floor. She takes one leg and crosses it over his torso to meet her other leg, using her hands on his body or the bed for support. He should help her balance and maneuver.

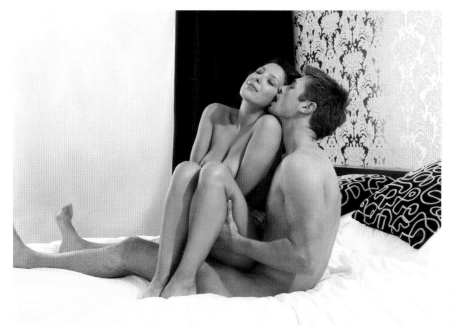

Step 2—Ever so *slowly* she starts swinging around to face the opposite direction, using his penis as an axle on which to rotate. Please remember, his penis is not actually sturdy, static machinery, so she should rotate with the utmost of care and the least amount of side-to-side movement. He should continue to help her twist around. If he sits upright, he might be better able to stabilize her.

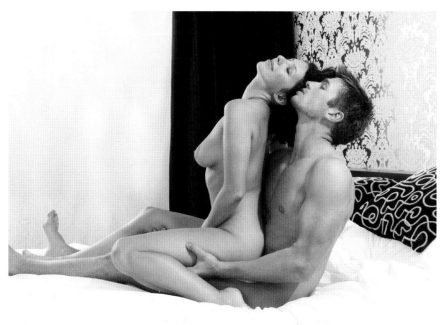

Step 3—She swings one leg over both of his and adjusts into her favorite reverse woman-on-top position (p.93).

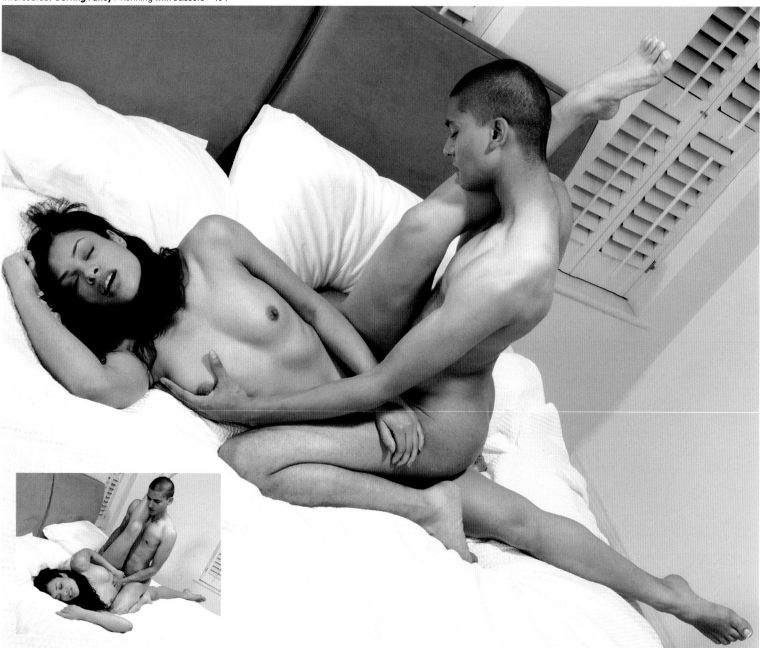

Running with Scissors

We'll be honest: scissor positions don't exactly rate high in the comfort factor, but it might be worth persevering for the unusual angle of penetration. Plus, you each have easy manual access to the other's genitals, should "unusual" not translate to "orgasmic" for either of you. And who knows, just being able to figure out how to get into these positions may be all the reward you need. Think of it as a naked version of Twister, without the colorful dots.

In Your Corner—She lies on her side with her upper leg straight up in the air. He kneels and straddles her lower leg and then she lets her upper leg rest on his shoulder or torso (unless she's looking for a simultaneous aerobic workout—though either way, this position is hardly a walk in the park).

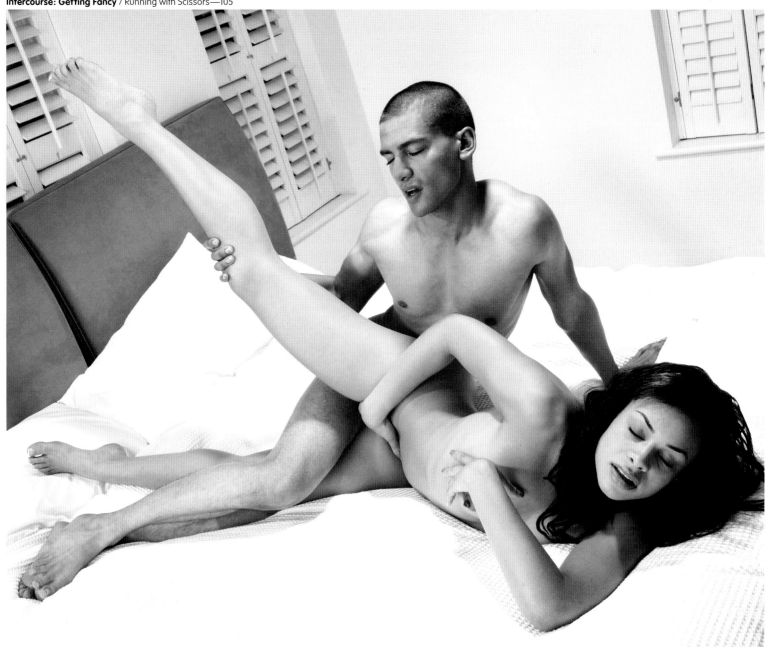

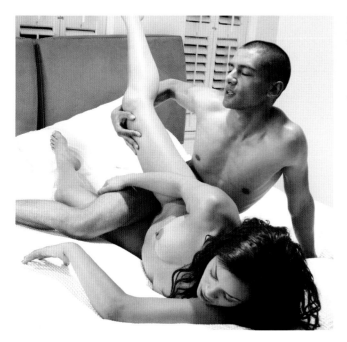

Interlocken—Both lie on your sides; if she's lying on her left side, then he should be too (and vice versa). Basically, this is what you want to achieve: his lower leg is the bottom layer, then her lower leg, then his upper leg, and finally her upper leg is the top layer—with penetration somehow occurring at the center of it all! If you get sick of trying, just roll over to rear-entry instead.

Letting the CAT Out of the Bag

By now, you've no doubt heard all about the Coital Alignment Technique (CAT). But have you ever actually tried it? It takes patience. It takes practice. And it goes against everything you've seen in pornos. But since when did pornos cater to what women want? Beyond following the specific steps below, mastering the CAT requires a *philosophical* readjustment. Abandon your assumptions that intercourse automatically means a piston-like motion, lots of flailing around, and a rush to climax. For the CAT, you've got to take what some might call a more "feminine" approach to sex: think small subtle movements, full-body contact with a focus on the clitoris and the pelvic mounds, and a Buddhist-like repetition of steps that may very well get her closer to Zen (i.e., orgasm) than any other hands-free intercourse position out there.

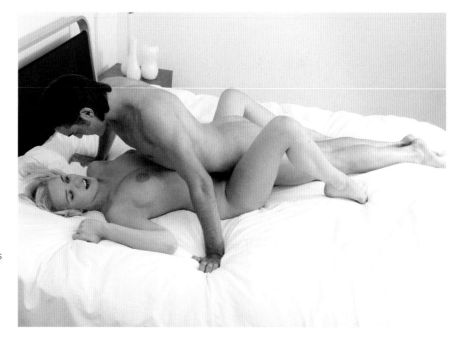

Step 1—Start off in the basic missionary: she's lying on her back with her legs just outside his; he's inside her with his legs very close together. In order to initiate penetration most easily, you'll notice his upper body is raised a bit and his pelvis may be a bit lower than hers (i.e. a bit further down her body) and between her legs. This is a great position for the typical in-out, but once penetration has occurred, you must kiss this movement goodbye if you want to successfully achieve the CAT.

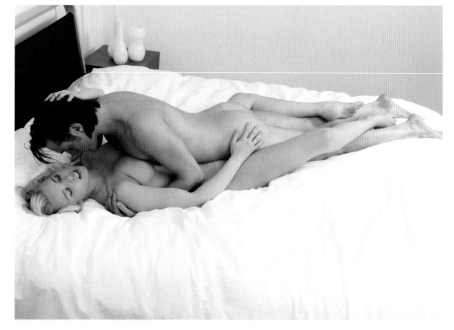

Step 2— Here's where the crucial alignment takes place: he cups her shoulders with his arms under her armpits so that he's resting on her (some of his weight can be on his forearms, but he should maintain as much body contact and pressure as is comfortable for her). While keeping his penis inside her, he pulls his body up along hers, toward her head, so that their pelvises are aligned (his directly on top of hers). His legs are straight and together, and her ankles are resting on his calves (her legs should be as straight and elongated as possible while wrapped around his lower legs; if it feels better she can try laying them straight on the bed right up against his legs). In this position, his head (the one on his shoulders) is beside her head (to one side of her face). His *penile* head should still be inserted, though much of the shaft will now be outside of the vaginal canal, pressing up against the top half of her external genitalia. Both spines should be as straight as possible. His upper body should be relaxed.

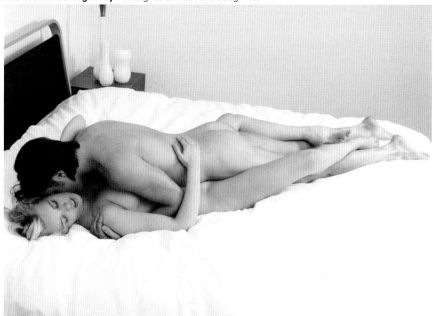

Step 3—As he's pushing up along her body (see step 2), she tips her pelvis away from him (down into the bed) so his penis comes almost all the way out and she can feel its base pressing against her clitoris. It's a very small, subtle movement—you don't want the penis to fully withdraw from the vagina.

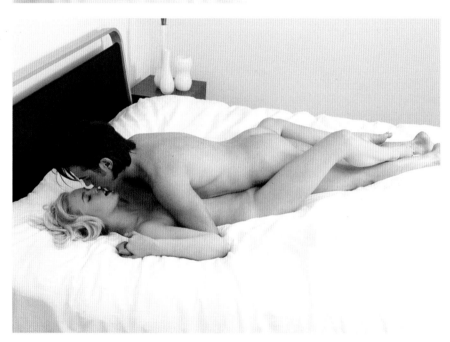

Step 4—Next, he pushes down with his pelvis so his whole body moves lower down her body and his penis enters her fully, while she tilts her hips up to envelop him. He's still lying on her, and both of your legs are in the same position as the previous steps—as straight as they can be with hers wrapped around his as low as possible. Her aim is to keep her thighs and knees close together rather than bent open (as in more traditional positions). The difference in his pelvis position between step 3 and step 4 is only about four inches (so in step 3, his pelvis is directly above hers; in step 4 it's about four inches lower down her body *and* his pelvis is closer to the bed, tipped at an angle and between her legs). Still with us? Now, just keep up this hip-rocking (alternating between step 3 and step 4): he moves up as she tips down, he moves down as she tilts up, and so on. Do not speed up. The goal is to maintain a constant pressure and rubbing against the area from her pubic bone down to her vaginal opening (the clitoral head and U-spot in between) with his penile shaft, his pubic bone, and the weight of his body. If you get it right and get into a groove, you might not be able to tell where one of you ends and the other begins.

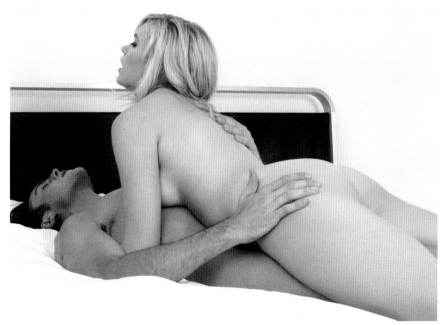

The Reverse CAT—He's on his back, she lies on top of him face down. His legs are together, hers are just outside his on the bed, but as close together and straight as possible (she could also try balancing her legs *on* his). Your pelvises are aligned (hers on top of his), and her arms under his, cupping his shoulders as he does to her in the basic CAT. She shifts down his body a few inches by pressing her pelvis down, so his penis shifts out of her a bit and its base stimulates her clitoris. Repeat the above, over and over. The difference between basic CAT and Reverse CAT is that fuller penetration occurs when your pelvises are aligned in reverse CAT; she gets the shallow penetration and genital stimulation from the base of his penis when she shifts downward. In Reverse CAT, she may feel like she has more control over the speed and range of motion, which may better suit her physical needs. But if she's light as a feather, he may need to help add some downward pelvic pressure by pushing down on her butt cheeks with his hands—not necessarily a drawback. (See also p.91).

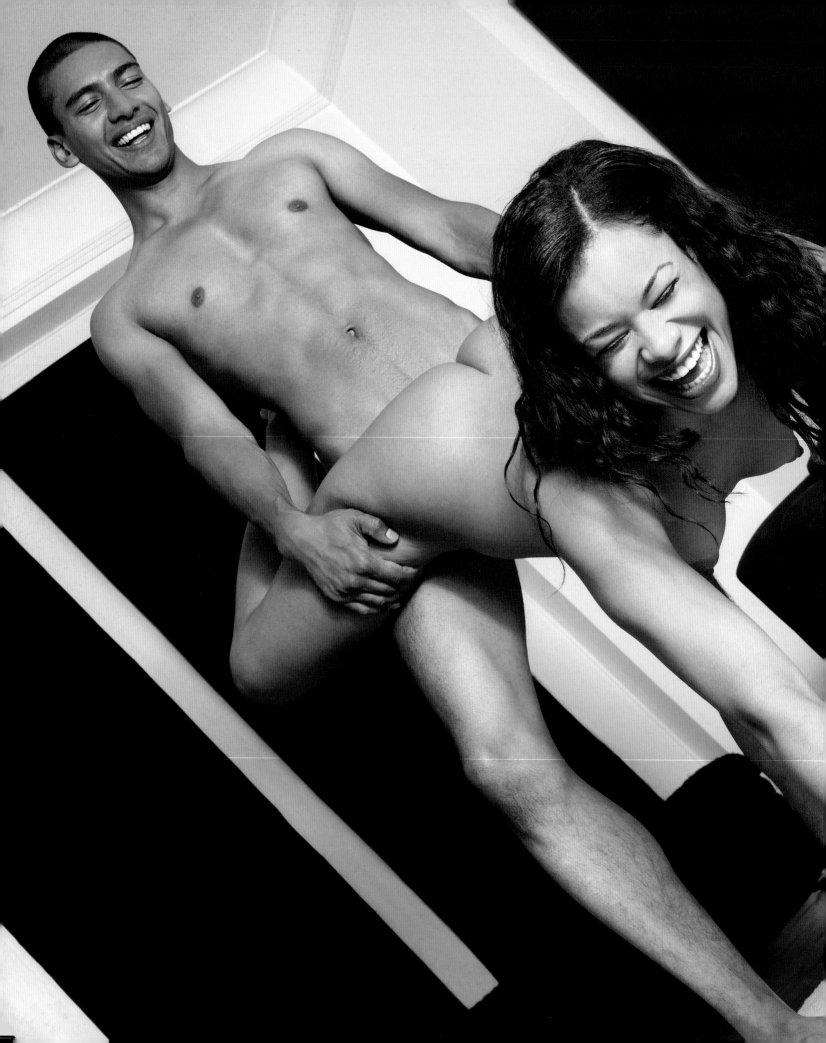

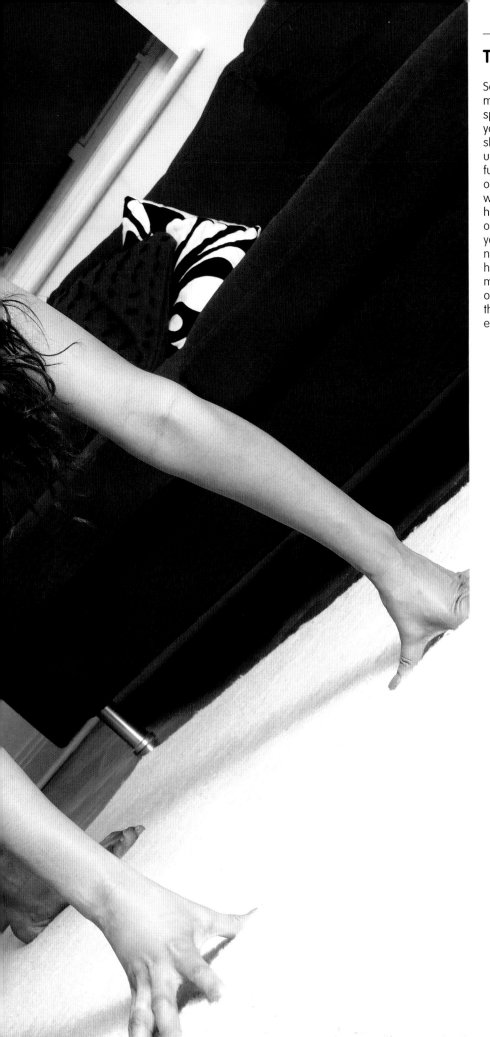

The Wheelbarrow & Co.

Some positions require a contortionist's flexibility, an iron man's strength and endurance, and an architect's grasp of spatial relationships. Before you put any undue pressure on yourself or, worse, throw out your back, remember this: sex should not be a checklist of stupid human tricks. You might be up to position 462 in the *Kama Sutra*, but if you're not having fun, or things don't actually feel good, what's the point? The only real benefit of a crazy position like The Wheelbarrow—where the standing man holds the woman's thighs like the handles of a gardening cart as she supports herself with outstretched hands on the floor—is the case of the giggles you'll get as you realize how silly you look and feel. Which is nothing to sneeze at: naked laughter is sexier than any handstand sex you can imagine. But if you're looking for multiple orgasms, simultaneous orgasms, plain old orgasms, or mere physical pleasure, don't expect it from positions like this or its ilk—"The Standing 69," "The Piledriver" (don't ask), etc. Don't say we didn't warn you.

Sex outside the bedroom: if the very idea makes you weary, *we get it*. But it's our professional responsibility to speak up on behalf of other venues. Doing it elsewhere is a way of saying that sex isn't compartmentalized, and it isn't any less exciting than what the Joneses are doing (not that we condone keeping up with the Joneses in bed, but a little healthy competition never hurt anyone's libido). Plus, how often are you just too freakin' exhausted to do it when you hit the sack? So think outside the bedroom and occasionally drop trou before you get there. Just remember to draw the living room shades. Or, you know, don't.

The Kitchen—We know it's terribly clichéd, but there's just something about sweeping aside the dishes to screw on the kitchen table or counter, even if it's not the most comfortable (or hygienic) sexual experience of your life.

The Hallway—Standing sex is really, really hard—especially if you're not one of those cute same-height couples who can share each other's jeans. Help yourself out with a handy phonebook or small footstool. By the way, door jambs are sometimes easier to get leverage against than a flat wall.

The Bath—Bathtub sex is not only guaranteed to flood your bathroom, it's notoriously orgasm-free for many women. So if you're going to be brave and do it, may we suggest keeping the water level low and adding a vibrating rubber duckie (p.139) for her? Also, water can wash away natural sexual slickness, so use silicone-based lubricant (the water-based kind will rinse right off)—it'll also come in handy for manual sex if you get too frustrated with the water-logged kind.

The Shower—Considering how slippery showers can get, engage in standing shower intercourse *at your own risk*. But maybe tempting fate and living dangerously turns you on. Just make sure you put down a no-slip rubber bath mat first. If you have a bathtub-shower combo, she can bend over and brace herself on the edge of the tub while he stands behind her. If yours is a stall shower, she should stand and brace herself with her back to one wall and one leg propped up on the opposite wall. If all this sounds too much like hard work (we're with you!), just take turns going down on each other. Your chance of orgasm skyrockets while your risk of soap-related injury plummets.

The Living Room—Though most sitting positions can be easily transported to the edge of the bed (see pp.99–101), they're often better on a couch that's a little lower to the ground: you both get more maneuverability when you can place a foot or two *flat* on the ground. A few things to remember: if she sits on his lap, facing away from him, she must respect the penis—an erect penis will bend only so far. And unless your couch is covered in tacky clear plastic already, you may want to put down a towel lest your next house guest find an unusual stain upon the upholstery.

The Dining Room—An arm-free dining room chair puts *all four feet* flat on the ground—which means that, with a bit of teamwork, you'll get great horizontal and vertical movement.

The Backyard—Just beware of mosquitos, poison ivy, nosy neighbors, frostbite in the winter, and sunburn in the summer (especially on your pasty butt!).

Marking Your Territory

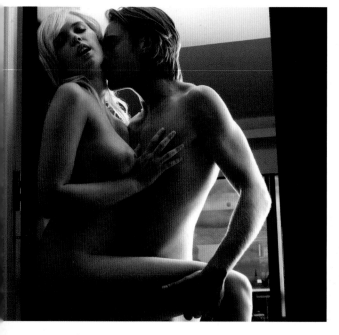

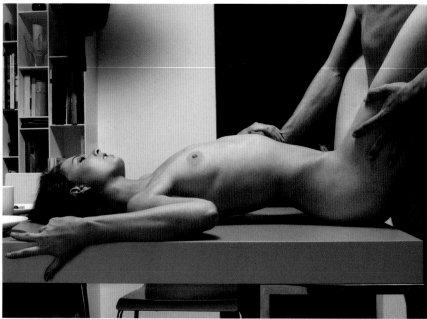

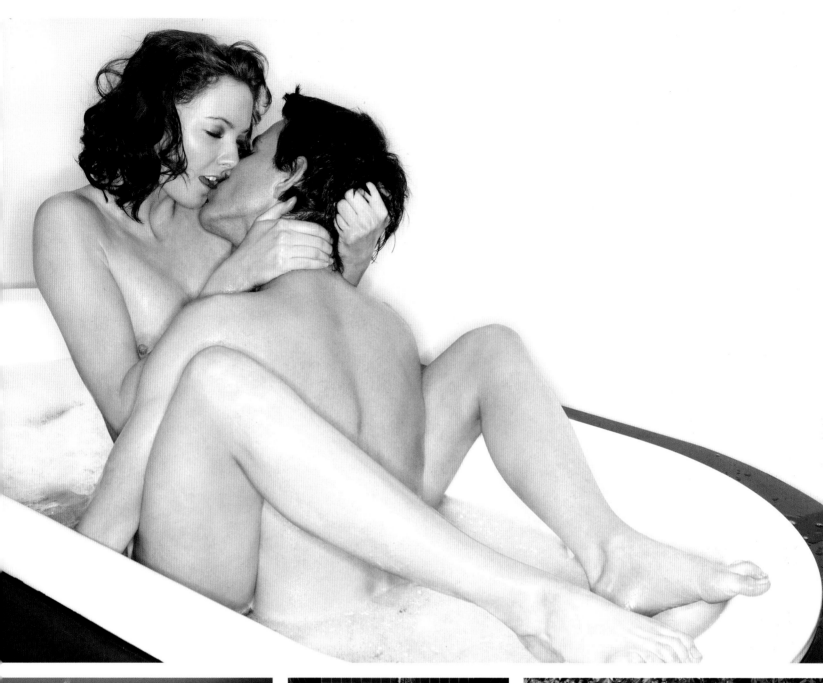

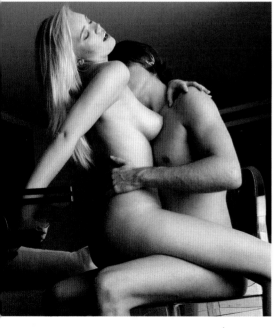

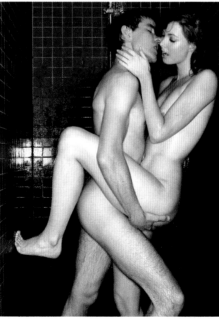

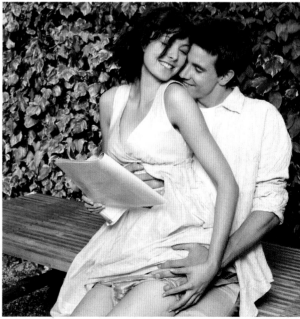

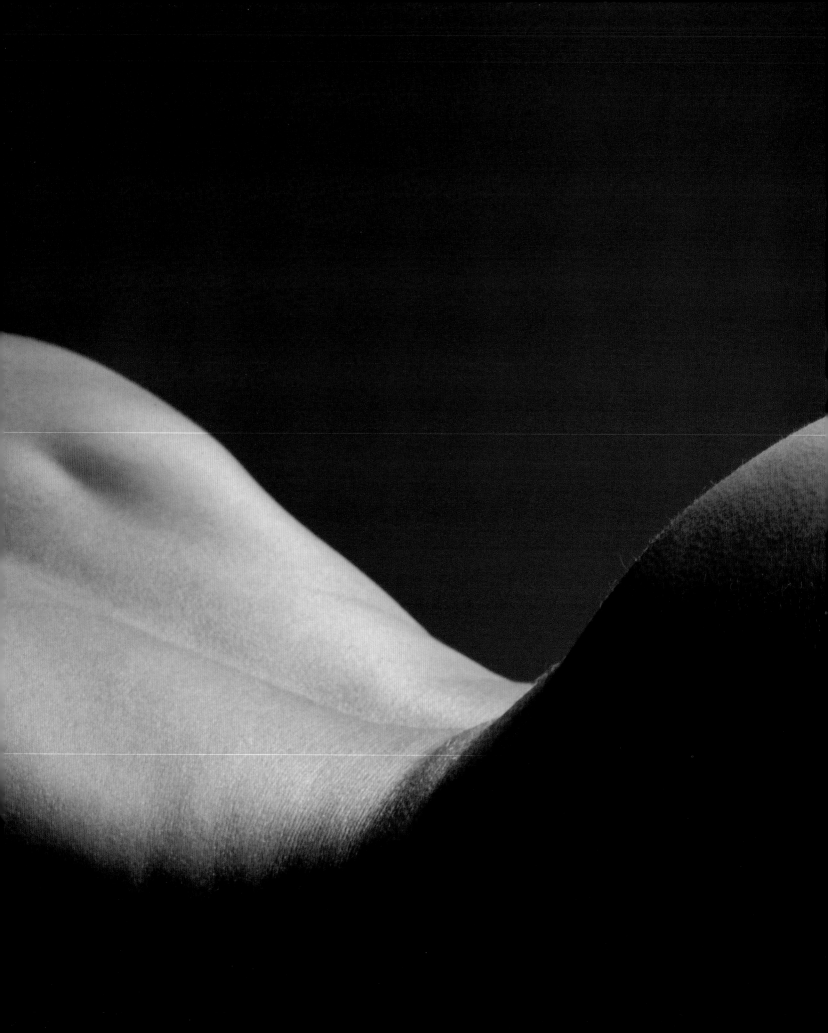

Anal Play

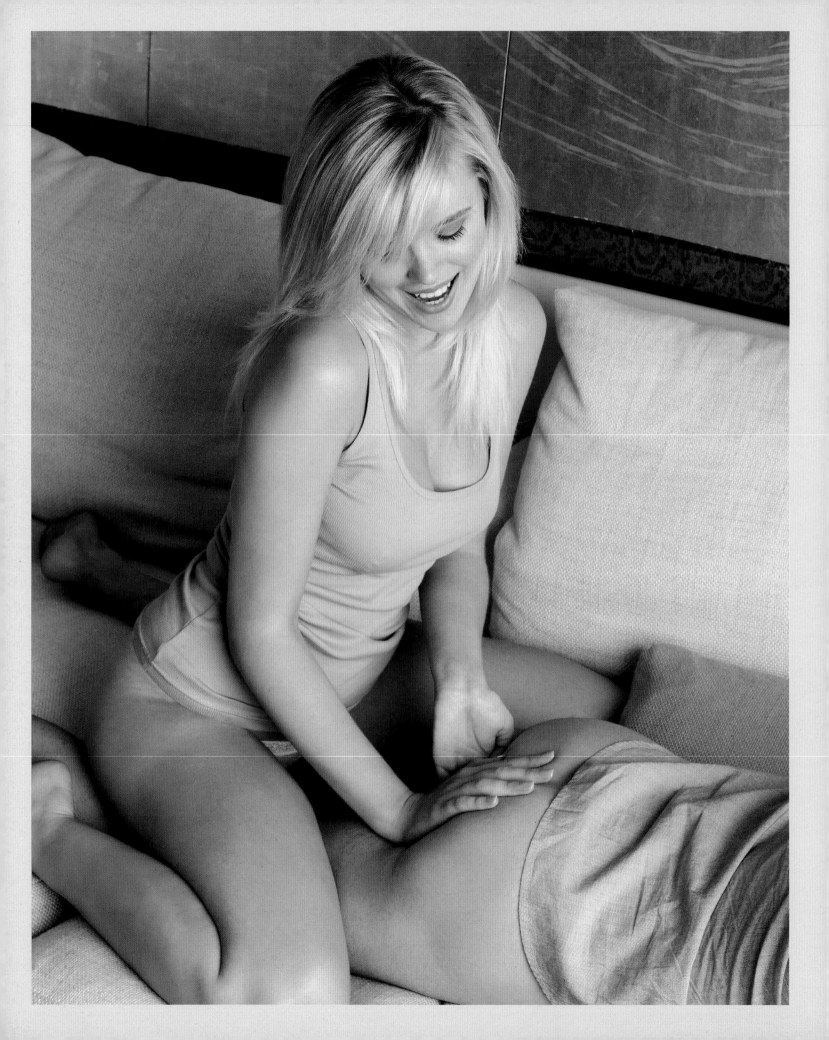

The Road Less Traveled

If ever there was a sex act desperately in need of an image makeover, it's anal play. It's the butt (literally) of jokes, it's the victim of homophobia, it's accused of being dirty in an unhygienic sense, it's approached underhandedly or with shame… in short, it gets no respect. So we're here to do some heavy-hitting PR work for backdoor play.

Exploring the orifice that dare not speak its name can bring a sort of awe back into sex. Yes, it's that intense sometimes. No matter who you vote for, who you sleep with, or where you spend your Sunday mornings, your rear is a nerve-heavy zone begging to be investigated. For the uninitiated, anal sex is not just a new position, it's an altogether new sensation.

Sure, it may not be a sensation that you want to experience every night, but making it part of your sexual toolbox means you'll have one more way to mix things up—your Saturday night special, perhaps, or something just for special days and holidays. Or, it may not be a sensation that you want to revisit at all—certainly it's not for everyone. But it's for far more people than you might think.

Still clenching your butt cheeks in dissent? Well, do yourself a sexual favor and at least reject it for the right reason—it just didn't feel good—rather than for one of a million possible wrong reasons: you don't know how, you're worried it'll make you gay, you think it's disrespectful to your partner, "that's just an exit, man," and so on. If you tried it once, years ago, and didn't like it, consider reading this chapter and trying one more time (go on… for us?). Because chances are, you or your partner missed a vital step—for example, anal sex without lube is usually unmitigated torture.

This chapter will tell you everything you need to know, from anatomy to aftermath. Afraid it's a "gay thing"? Um, only if you do it with another man—or with another woman. People are gay; sex acts aren't. Do you think it's "disrespectful"? Only if you do it disrespectfully (exhibit A: "Oops, wrong hole!"). Sure, it's not as lovey-dovey as missionary sex, but who wants lovey-dovey sex every night of the week? Even—or rather, *especially*—with your one true love. In fact, sharing an allegedly taboo act like this can actually draw you closer. And if you do it right, it's only dirty in the best possible way.

Remember, backdoor loving doesn't always have to mean hardcore butt-fucking or half an hour of rimming. Sometimes it's no more than a teasing pinkie making its way back there during oral or manual sex or even intercourse (if you're not cursed with short arms). In fact, anal play may never mean more than that for you—and that's okay, too. We just wouldn't want you to let all those good nerve endings go to waste! Ready to make some new backdoor friends?

Unlike garden-variety front-door sex, anal play isn't quite as simple as inserting tab A into slot B (though if you've read the previous chapters, you already know that vaginal intercourse should always be approached with more finesse than that, too). The anus and rectum are much less forgiving and accommodating than the vagina, so it helps to know a little bit about what you're dealing with before you go barging in there. The Anatomy & Orgasm chapter already gave you a bodily primer (if you skipped past pages 36–47 because they felt too much like homework, go back and re-read them right now!). What follows will further your anal education.

First of all, there are the two small sphincters that form the inch-long anal canal (see the illustration on the opposite page). The more nervous and uptight someone feels, the more these two muscles will clench up and say "Noooooooo!" (Resist the urge to say "Stop being so anal" if this happens to your partner.) Hence the importance of practice, patience, and site-specific foreplay when it comes to loosening things up.

Beyond the anus lies the rectum, which is not, contrary to popular belief, where the brown stuff hangs out (assuming you don't have to "go" imminently)—nope, that's what the colon is for. Apologies to those of you with delicate constitutions, but being this blunt is really the only way to convince some people that anal sex is not as dirty as they think it is. The rectum is S-shaped—and your own penis, dildo, or finger is decidedly not S-shaped. Hence the importance of experimenting with positions (p.123) until you find one that feels best—for example, any position where the receiver's legs and upper body are at a right angle will straighten out the S somewhat. But no position will smooth out the curve completely, so bear this in mind as you introduce a penis, dildo, or finger: the faster and more carelessly you go, the more likely you are to hit a curve. If you go in slowly and gently and listen to your partner, adjusting your angle as necessary, you should be able to avoid causing any discomfort.

You should also bear in mind that, unlike the vagina, the anal canal doesn't self-lubricate—hence the importance of lube (p.129). Plus, the tissue back there is much more delicate than the vaginal walls, which is what makes unprotected anal sex such a risky activity in terms of transmitting STDs (pp.178–181), not to mention causing physical damage should you rush things, use force, and/or forgo lube.

None of the above means that you'll be an unwelcome guest, however—it just means that you should be an awfully considerate one.

Anal Anatomy & Prepping

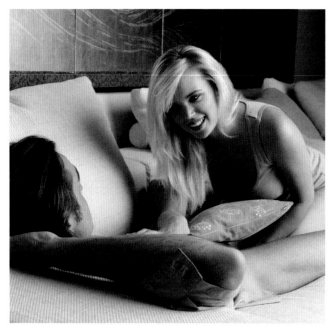

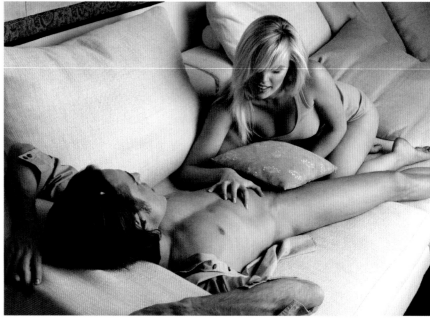

Prepping

Spontaneity and planning are not mutually exclusive in the bedroom. Rather, you plan so that you can have a rollicking good time when the spontaneous mood strikes you. Because nothing ruins the mood quite like bending over your boyfriend only to discover that there's no more lube in the top drawer of your nightstand.

Mentally—Becoming backdoor friends takes a fair amount of trust and communication—nothing feels quite so vulnerable as being penetrated back there, whether by the most diminutive of pinkies or an extra-large dildo. The power exchange can go the other way, too, of course: many men turn to complete putty at the mere idea of anal play (well, putty almost everywhere), which means that women can feel a heady rush when they get down on their hands and knees in the doggie-style position (p.94). Either way, it's not something we'd necessarily recommend on a one-night stand or at the very beginning of a new relationship. That said, this isn't rocket science we're talking about here, and it's no Wheelbarrow (p.108) either. Assuming you follow all the instructions in this chapter, there's no reason why anal play shouldn't be just another fun thing to do on a Saturday night.

Physically—In the right head space? Good. Now let's get your body there, too:
• Eat your Wheaties! A daily dose of fiber in your diet will make for more solid deposits, which keeps things cleaner and more comfy.
• Avoid brussels sprouts and other such gas inducers 24 hours prior if you happen to know you've got a hot anal date coming up.
• Drop the kids off at the pool.
• It's polite, not prudish, to shower (or at least bidet) first. No need for an enema, though—your soaped-up finger will do.
• Clip your fingernails!
• The more turned on you are, the more ready and willing your entire body will be. For women, having an orgasm first will also relax everything in the vicinity.

Accessories—Haven't you always wanted to make a to-do list that went something like "get quart of milk; pick up dry-cleaning; buy more lube"? Well, now's your chance… consider this your anal sex shopping list:
• Don't ever go near the backdoor (not even with a pinkie) without a very generous supply of manmade lube—spit's just not enough. A thick, water-based lube is ideal (though if you're going latex-free—because you're body-fluid-bonded, monogamous, and not planning on vaginal intercourse later—then oil-based will work too).
• Unprotected anal sex is the one of the riskiest forms of sex in terms of STDs, so always use a condom (unless the above exception applies to you).
• Latex gloves (or just finger cots) can help a finger slip in there nicely, especially if either one of you is a bit squeamish about what said finger might encounter.
• Oral sex dams are a nice touch for rimming—because even if you're both STD-free, other bacteria back there just might make you sick (pp.178–181).
• Unscented hand wipes are great for discreetly cleaning up toys, fingers, or other body parts, especially if the receiving partner gets easily red-faced about what their penetrator might encounter. (Chances are, they'll encounter nothing, though a little brown-tinged lube is nothing to be embarrassed about—it happens to the best of us.)

By the way, please note that neither whiskey nor any sort of "desensitizing" lotion are on the above shopping list. The key here is to avoid pain, not numb it—the latter is all too likely to land one of you in the ER (and the other one of you in the doghouse for, oh, forever).

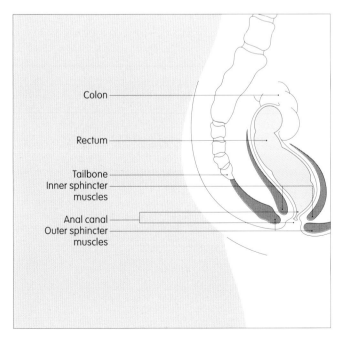

Colon
Rectum
Tailbone
Inner sphincter muscles
Anal canal
Outer sphincter muscles

Anal Anatomy (Cross Section)

No matter how open-minded you are about a little anal action, you're bound to tense up a bit the first time someone ventures back there. After all, it is an exit, most of the time—or at least, it has been up to this point in your life—so letting something in is going to feel kind of funny at first. And it's going to feel more than just "kind of funny" if your partner goes in like gangbusters, thrusting away with a penis or dildo. That's where fingers come in—yours and your partner's. It's a way to edge into the shallow end and get used to the sensation. And actually, you might decide that fingers are as far as you ever want to take things. There's no shame in that—we'll still let you into our esteemed backdoor friends club. After all, the anus has more nerve endings than any body part besides the genitals, and that puckered kiss can be fully serviced with just a digit or two.

On Yourself

Okay, so it sounds like something that only perverts or homeopathic gurus would attempt, but exploring back there on your own is not a bad way to introduce yourself to the idea of anal play. Especially if you're afraid that the first time someone goes there, you may squeak out "Oh god, no, please make it stop!" Next time you're in the shower, let a finger wander in that direction… if it helps, don't think of it as exploring, think of it as cleaning. The more often you do this, the more likely you are to enjoy yourself when the finger of a friend or neighbor is doing the wandering. Another homework assignment that may help: do your Kegels (pp.175 & 177)!

On Each Other

Given how close the anus is to a number of other much-admired body parts, it's amazing how many people ignore it completely during sex. It's like the red-headed stepchild of your below-the-waist apparatus. Perhaps it's because people don't realize what a team player the bum can be: a little stimulation back there can improve almost any sexual act. Not that you should add it into the mix every time you go to bed—but just know that you can.

One of the best times to experiment is during oral or manual sex—you're already down there, you may very well have a free hand, your partner has given themselves over to you completely, and (with any luck) they're already writhing in ecstasy and therefore open to a little suggestion. But remember, once you venture into this territory with one hand, you should keep that hand there (or else out of the way), to avoid contaminating any other sensitive areas with bacteria that could lead to infection.

Start by caressing their cheeks, just to introduce yourself in the general neighborhood. Then lube up a well-manicured finger

Fingers

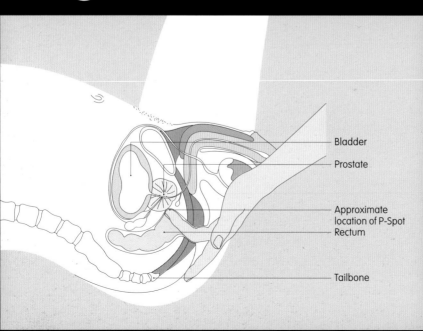

Bladder

Prostate

Approximate location of P-Spot

Rectum

Tailbone

Locating His P-spot—Push your index and/or middle fingers, palm up, two or three inches inside his rectum. Bend it/them in a "come hither" gesture. The more aroused he is, the firmer his P-spot will feel.

—your pinkie is pleasantly small and unassuming, but you'll have more control with your index finger—and let it roam in the direction of the perineum. If your partner doesn't hit the ceiling, curl into the fetal position, or leave the room in a strop, then linger there for a while—stroke, push, massage, rub in circles—before roaming a little further back, gently stroking the crack as you go. Again, watch closely for any sign that your partner may be about to lose it—the idea here is to introduce anal pleasure gradually so there are no surprises. If all seems good, start lingering on the rosebud's surface, first pressing lightly with the pad of your finger, then rubbing gently in circles—but don't actually dip in just yet. And remember: this whole time you should keep up whatever you were doing on the front porch.

This might be a good time to get your partner's permission to go further, whether explicit ("Would you like me to…?" "May I…?") or implicit (make eye contact; confirm that they are not visually pleading with you to stop). Add some more lube, then push very very very gently, so that just the tip of your finger is dipping in. This may be enough for today's lesson—you know your partner better than we do, so it's your call. When you're both ready to go further, push in slowly, feeling the two sphincters as you go. The first time you're in there, you'll probably want to hold very still—because chances are, your partner is feeling a little strange. Strange in a good way, mind you, but still…. strange. In fact, for some people, just having a finger in there is all the stimulation they ever want or need: it creates a sense of fullness that pushes them over the edge.

But for others, some movement may feel good. Some people like you to move your finger slowly in and out, while others prefer you to keep your finger in one place while gently massaging inside in different directions—up, down, around. If your partner is having a really good time, you may even want to add a second finger—but we'd ask first.

Another way to branch out without advancing to full-on phalluses is to add a vibrator (p.130) to the mix—especially if your partner seems to prefer external anal stimulation to any kind of penetration (even with a pinkie). As long as you're not going to insert the vibrator, any kind will do—try holding it against the perineum or anus during oral sex. But if you're going to push it in even slightly, just make sure it's designed for internal use, has a tapered top, and has a flared base (p.135). Or, if your partner *does* enjoy penetration and you'd like to free up both hands for more frontal work, invest in a quality butt plug (still or vibrating; see p.135) and let it do your rear work for you.

Of course, any of the above can be attempted during intercourse, too, though if you're taking a hands-on approach you'll have a more limited range of motion—there's only so far one arm can stretch, after all.

Just for Her

A finger up the bum can indirectly stimulate any number of her personal sweet spots in the vagina as well as the perineal sponge if you push in those directions (rather than just going straight in). If he's taller than she is, he'll probably find it fairly easy to reach a finger back there during intercourse—and the combination of the two may stimulate yet new places. Plus, she may well relish the feeling of being doubly filled up. But remember that any finger that has been backstage is not welcome between the labial curtains until it has been washed thoroughly (unless she likes UTIs).

Just for Him

There's a very special reason to visit his backdoor: it's the best way to stimulate his prostate gland, sometimes known as the male G-spot or P-spot (p.43). Because it's a major player in the production of ejaculate, many men find prostate stimulation makes climaxing even more intense. If he's lying on his back, you'll find it most easily by kneeling between his legs and pushing your index or middle finger, palm-up, two or three inches in, and curving it in the classic "come hither" crook (see the illustration on the opposite page). Then rub and press this area firmly—you may not feel anything initially, but the closer he gets to orgasm, the firmer his prostate will get. Assuming he's into it, he'll probably also want you to move a little faster in there as he nears his climax. If he's not "open" to penetration, you still may be able to indirectly stimulate his P-spot by pressing up firmly on his perineum. Either way, during a blowjob or handjob, try synching your back area movements with what you're doing up front.

On a final note, keep in mind that men in particular may be shy about letting their girlfriends explore, even though—go on, admit it—they're secretly dying to experience a little backdoor play. They're just not as used to the vulnerability or sensation of penetration. If you've got an apprehensive man in your life, try warming him up to the idea even earlier in the game, during a massage (pp.30–33): pay particular attention to his bum cheeks, the space between his cheeks, his perineum—and any time you sense him tensing up, return to the lower back. It's the perfect way to introduce him to all his nerve endings back there without inducing any sort of "oh-god-what-comes-next?" panic attack.

Rimming—analingus, if you want to be fancy—is when you use your tongue to kiss, caress, and probe your partner's anus. And it's all sorts of icky to a lot of people: whether they find it gross on moral grounds or for health reasons, they just don't want to go there. But rimming aficionados—those who've mustered the courage to tackle this taboo—will trap you in a corner at a party and rave for hours about the joys of salad-tossing. (Or maybe that just happens to us.) Find out what all the fuss is about…

Why to Do It

A soft, wet, probing tongue is one of the best ways to stimulate the anus's nerve endings. Plus, rimming forges an incredible level of intimacy, not only because of the taboo you're exploring together, but also because, well, you're letting someone put their *tongue* on your *asshole*.

How to Do It

On a guy, you could always test the waters during a blowjob, gradually inching along the perineum with your tongue. (Note: This will go over better toward the beginning of the bj, before he's on the home stretch and is particularly averse to any detours.) Don't try this during cunnilingus, however, as the risk of a urinary tract infection is too high. Either way, though, rimming is probably something you'll want to agree on in advance—especially because the receiving partner will no doubt want to shower very carefully if they know what's coming. (It's only polite, after all. Just be sure to rinse thoroughly afterward, as soap residue may be a little irritating—not to mention a total buzz-kill to the taboo-hunting rimmer who's all about sex being truly dirty. But if you ask us, rimming is plenty taboo even when you're squeaky clean.)

Doggie style, with the receiver on all fours or standing bent over something, is a good all-access position; the rimmer can kneel, sit, or squat behind them and spread the cheeks with their hands. Or have the receiver lie on their back with their knees bent up, even pulled up toward their chest a bit for more access. Lick and kiss the cheeks to introduce yourself, then gradually move further in. The perineum is a nice place to start, too—it's just a little less personal than the anus, after all. Lick it, suck it, nuzzle in. Then take a wide flat tongue and lick from the perineum all the way to the tailbone and back again. Getting the area wet and warm with saliva (or even an edible lube, see p.129) will make everything feel nicer. Gradually zero in on your target, trying out different moves and pressures: press your flat tongue over the starfish, take your tongue in circles around the rim, drag your tongue back and forth across the anus, dip your tongue in gently and slowly, dart it in and out really fast. When rimming a man, feel free to squeeze, lick, and rub his balls, too. When rimming a woman, a reach-around finger (or toy) to her clitoris will probably be appreciated.

Happy Ending

While some people reach orgasmic heights via analingus alone, most will probably want a little attention out front to push them over the edge. Or you could always just consider this foreplay. Wondering what goes well with rimming? Turn the page.

Tongues

What to Beware Of

Beyond prissiness (we've all got anal pubes… every single one of us… can we now move on?), there are a number of safety issues to consider. While not as risky as genital-to-genital contact, oral-anal contact can transmit almost any STD under the right circumstances (e.g., HIV and hepatitis B if there's blood around; herpes, genital warts, or syphilis, especially if there's a rash, sore, or bump in the vicinity; and hepatitis A if there's poop around, and there usually is—often on a microscopic level—when it comes to rimming). Go to pp.178–181 to read about the symptoms and treatments of the most common STDs. Beyond the traditional STDs, a rimmer also has to worry about ingesting small amounts of fecal matter that's infected with any number of bacteria (e.g. salmonella and E. coli) or parasites (e.g. tapeworm), which can result in serious gastrointestinal pain and problems. Of course, in all of the above cases, the rimmee has to have these viruses, bacteria, or parasites in the first place in order to pass them onto the rimmer. But sometimes carriers don't exhibit symptoms and therefore don't know they're at risk of transmitting some infection or disease to their beloved licker.

But let's play devil's advocate for a minute. Let's say you have none of the above infections (even though it would require an awful lot of expensive tests to determine that for sure). The question is: can germs that normally appear in the feces of healthy humans make you sick if ingested? We asked a number of doctors (you see the lengths we'll go to for you?), and, after giving us funny looks, their best answer was "probably not."

Which isn't exactly making us run right out to the doodie buffet. And that's where oral sex dams (p.182) or a even just a piece of sturdy plastic wrap come in. As a bonus, if either one of you is a little squeamish about the whole thing—whether it's giving or receiving—a barrier will probably help you to relax and enjoy yourself. And don't feel bad about insisting on one—if your partner grumbles, tell them to kiss your ass.

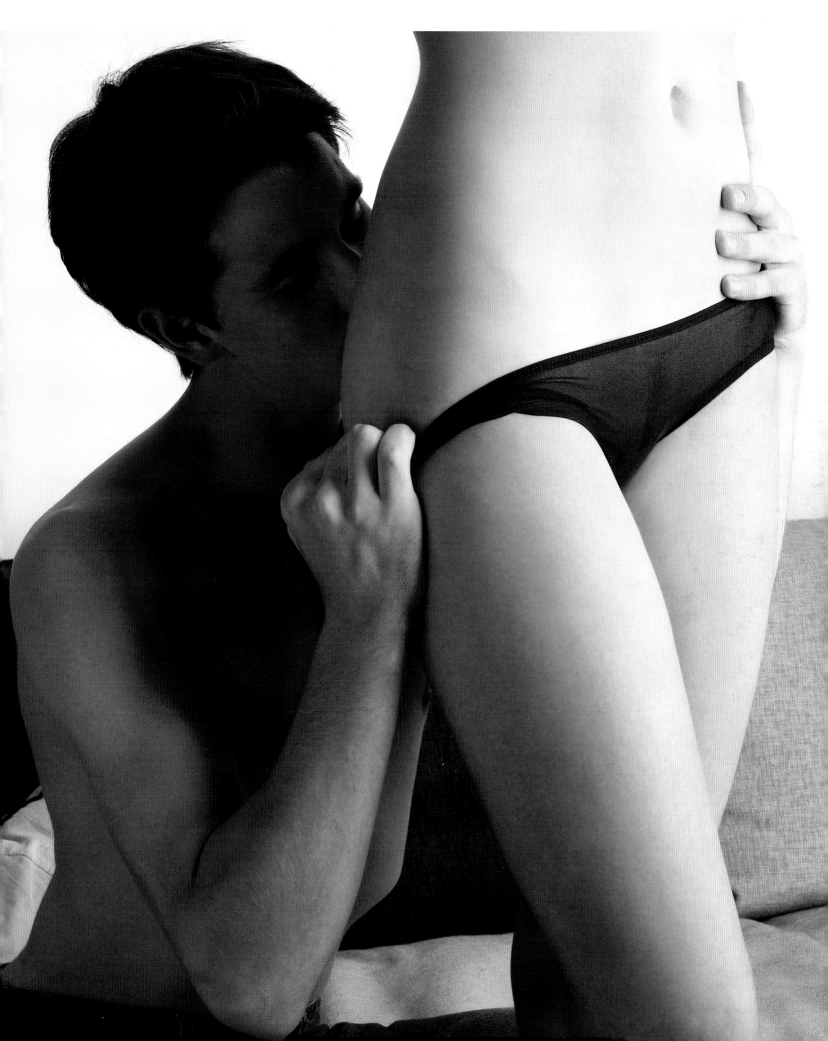

Once you're well and truly comfortable exploring each other's bums with your fingers—and, perhaps, with your tongues or with a few of the anal play-things on p.135—you may want to move onto something a little more *fulfilling*. Don't worry, there's more room in there than you'd think!

Whether you're working with a penis or dildo (let's just say "tool" so no one feels left out), bear the following in mind:
• Knock yourself out with foreplay—the more turned on your receiver is, the more likely they are to welcome your tool.
• Warm up the anus with a finger or two.
• Lube, lube, lube, lube, lube. Lube your tool, lube the anus, insert some more lube with your finger… keep reapplying, even if you think you don't need more. (Receivers, don't be shocked on your next trip to the toilet: it'll be a little lubey.)
• Go gently into that good night. Slowly, too. Inch in gradually, pausing frequently to check in with your partner.
• Remember that the rectum isn't a straight line. Don't go thrusting in and out with gusto like it's a vagina—even small, slow, contained movements feel pretty intense back there.
• The receiver is the pace-setter and gets to call all the shots. Beginners should maintain eye contact (if the position allows it) and check in with each other frequently as you figure out the best depth, speed, and rhythm. First-time receivers may even want to guide your tool in with their hands.
• If anything hurts or bleeds, stop immediately.
• Always pull out slowly and gently—the movement can feel even more intense in this direction. It might help if your receiver takes deep breaths and you pull out a little each time they exhale (they'll be more relaxed this way). Or, if it's a dildo, your partner may just prefer to remove it themselves.

Just for Penises

Never pretend that you accidentally knocked on the wrong door—unless you want your girlfriend to forever more associate anal sex with pain and suffering and never let you near her tush again. Another way to ruin the mood is to take your penis directly from her ass to her vagina, practically guaranteeing her a urinary tract infection (p.175). (That said, ladies, even the best-intentioned anal sex can sometimes cause a UTI, especially if you're particularly sensitive, so be sure to pee and maybe even shower immediately afterward.)

Gents, assuming that you want to take a kinder, gentler approach to anal sex, consider using a clitoral vibrator (pp.130–133) during foreplay so there's absolutely no doubt that she's getting the stimulation she needs to warm up. She might even find that she enjoys anal sex more after her first orgasm.

Just for Strap-ons & Dildos

As we hope we've made clear, anal penetration can be an equal-opportunity good time for all—just because she doesn't have a penis, doesn't mean he shouldn't join in the bum fun. Besides, being on the receiving end will only make him a better lover when he's on the penetrating end. And did we mention all the nerve endings—and his G-spot— that are back there? For women, getting to be the penetrator for a change is largely a heady thrill—though adding a bullet vibrator (p.132) to a harness can make it a bodily one, too.

Check out the dildo and harness suggestions on p.137—many couples consider it a kind of foreplay to go shopping together. Whether you go for a double dildo, a hand-held dildo, or a strap-on, be sure to start small. There is no such thing as an anal sex starter kit that comes with a 12-inch dong! This could go for both of you, in fact: some women like their guy to start with a diminutive dildo rather than his own tool, so she can

Phalluses

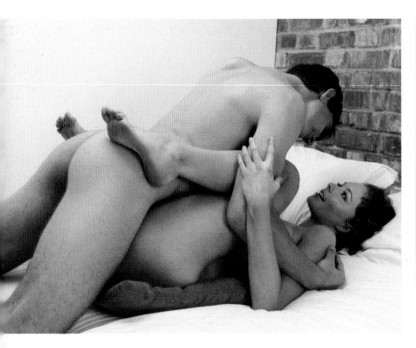
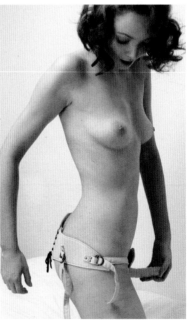
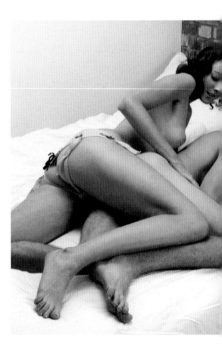

build up to his size gradually. Pick a dildo specifically made for butt play, i.e., one with tapered tip for smooth entry, a flared base, and no rough seams. Some dildos vibrate, but this isn't really necessary as the nerve endings are mostly in the anus; internally, what feels good is pressure and fullness. And don't feel you have to get a harness for your dildo—she may find that she has better control holding the dildo in her hand.

Finally, ladies, there's a very good chance he'll feel shy or self-conscious while being penetrated for the first time, so make sure you tell him how much it turns you on to fuck him!

Positions

Doing each other up the bum doesn't mean you have to get on all fours—for first-timers, there are much easier ways to do it. Here are a few to try, whether with a penis or a strap-on:

Missionary—The receiver lies on their back with their legs bent at the knee and up a little so that they're almost resting against their own chest. (A pillow under the tush may make things more comfortable for newbie receivers.) Plus it allows for unhindered eye contact and communication. If either of you is worried that anal sex is unromantic, this has all the intimacy of missionary sex, with just a naughty little twist. As a bonus, it's easy to add a handjob or clitoral vibrator to the mix.

Sideways—The receiver lays on their side and the giver approaches from behind, also lying on their side. This is another great position for beginners because the receiver can relax and the giver won't be able to gain too much scary thrusting momentum. If you find this position tricky, it may help if the inside spoon is near a wall for leverage—sometimes it just feels good to have something to push or lean against.

Doggie Style—Of course, sometimes you kind of want anal sex to feel dirty and remote—that's what makes it such

a taboo. And for this, traditional doggie style is perfect: the receiver kneels on all fours with the giver behind. Three variations on the theme: a) Downward Doggie: the giver stands instead of kneeling and places their feet outside the the receiver's legs (it looks like leapfrog). The receiver keeps their legs closer together, which can help the anus feel more relaxed and loose. Or b) Sleeping Dog: the receiver lies flat on their stomach. And c) The Ben Dover: the receiver bends over a desk, bed, back of a couch, etc., and the giver stands or kneels behind them. This is all about getting that 90-degree angle that might straighten out the S-curve a bit (p.116).

Top Dog—The giver lies on their back and the receiver kneels or sits on top. You might think this is a great beginner position because it puts the receiver in total control, but it's actually kind of tricky, because being on top will probably cause the receiver to unconsciously clench their butt—which obviously makes penetration a little awkward. If you attempt it, just be sure the receiver lowers themselves down very slowly and gently—and the giver should resist the urge to thrust upward. A variation is the Reverse Top Dog: the receiver is again on top, but they're facing the giver's feet instead and leaning as far forward as possible. You know, just in case anal sex starts to feel blah and you want to "spice it up."

Happy Ending

Gents, if you want to take her to the finish line, she may well need you to use a vibrator or your lubed fingers on her clitoris once you're inside her. Trust us, it'll be worth the arm ache! Ladies, your guy may want or need you to give him a handjob while you do him up the bum—this can feel especially good if you're coordinated enough to sync up your hand and dildo movements. You'll find the missionary position most obliging for this combo.

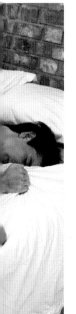
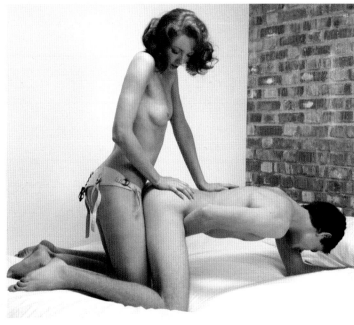
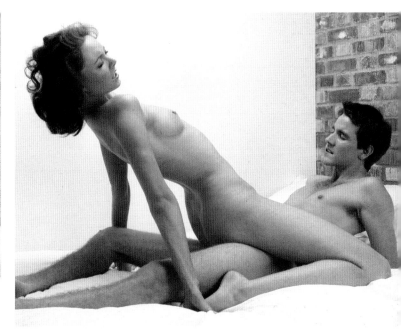

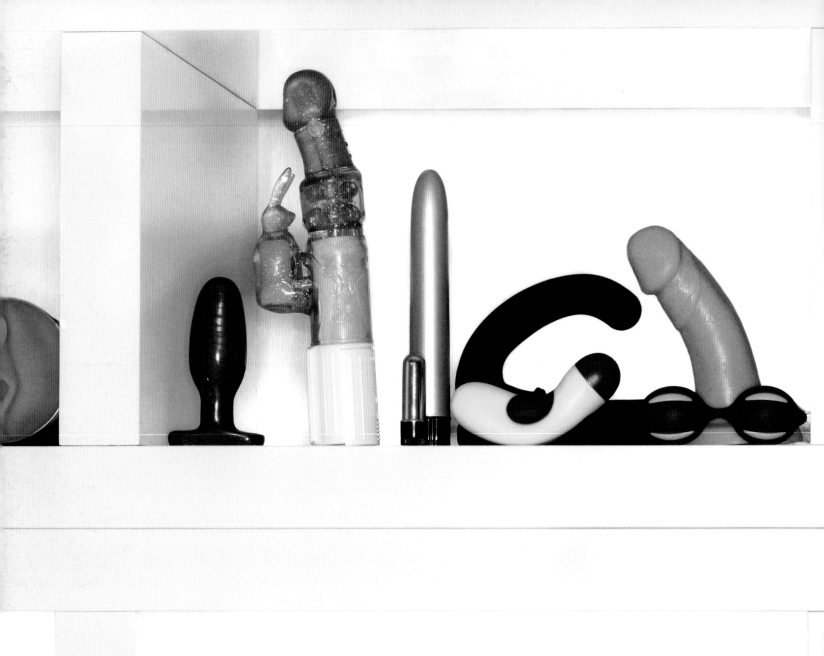
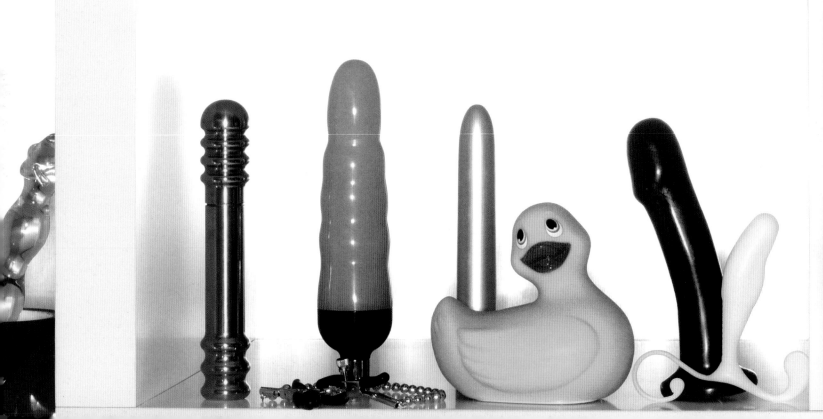

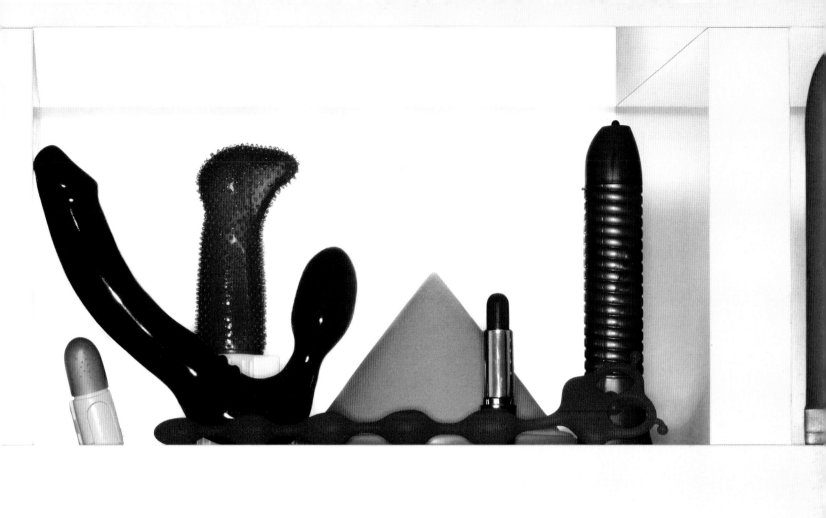

⁰⁷ Sex Toys

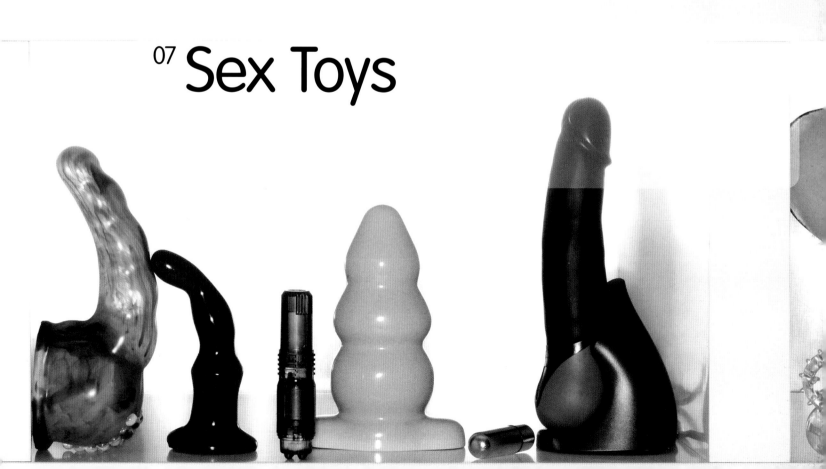

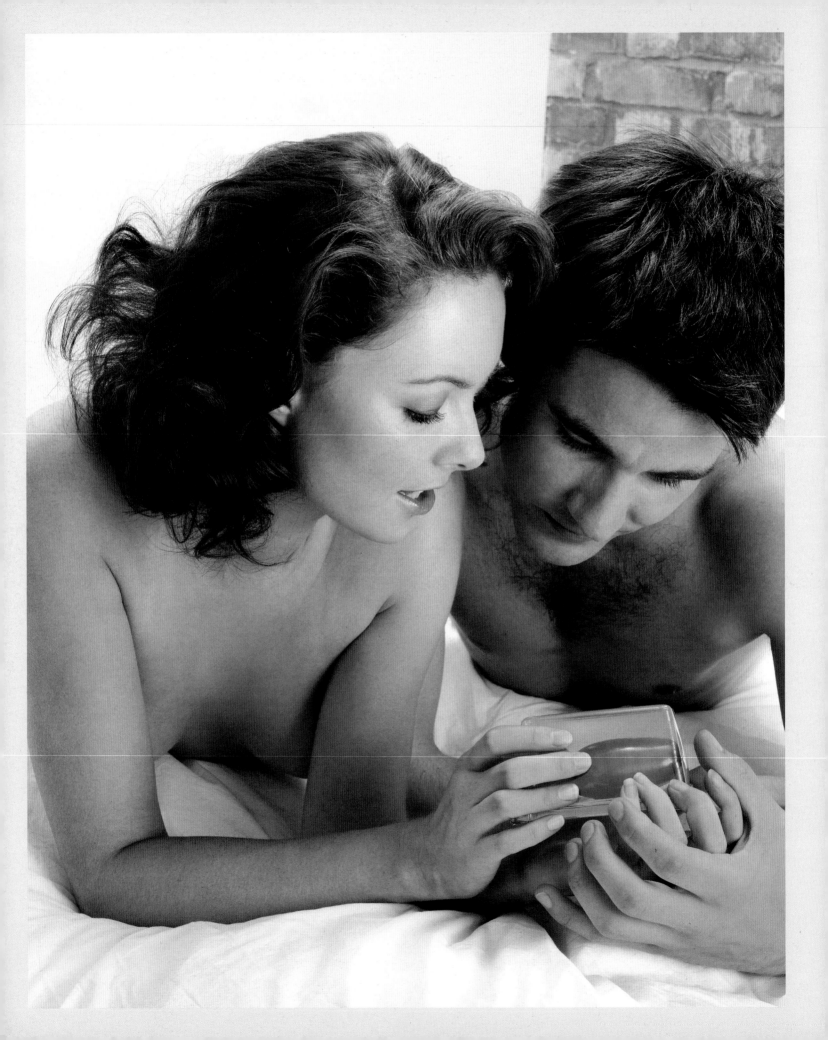

Accessorizing Your Sex Life

Just as a nice rosé complements a fresh summer salad, pearl drop earrings complete a strapless ball gown, an original piece of artwork transforms a bare-walled room, or a banner that reads "whales are nice" turns a stinky dropout into a sexy activist, so too can a new toy revolutionize your sex life. Discovering a new sensation that can be created only by battery-powered equipment may mean the difference between never having orgasms and having them at your beck and call. (And we're not necessarily talking about vibrator dependency here, though there's nothing wrong with that— after all, an orgasm's an orgasm's an orgasm. But sometimes a toy teaches you how to have an orgasm on your own, too.) Introducing a toy into partner-sex might shake up a routine that's boring and predictable. Shopping for a sex toy together makes a great date—at least for open-minded couples who are *already* sleeping together. And a beautifully designed, high-end sex toy that could pass for an *objet d'art* can be the perfect just-because gift.

If you still think that sex toys are just for creepy men in trenchcoats, "frigid" ladies, and losers who can't get a date, we'd like to invite you into the 21st century. Studies have shown that more than a third of women own vibrators or "intimate massagers," and that those who use them experience higher levels of sexual desire and more orgasms. Fortunately, procuring a sex toy no longer means venturing to the seedy side of town and slinking into a neon-lit sex shop lined with scary-looking super dongs. These days, great online retailers offer a wide selection of high-quality toys, helpful tips, and shopping discretion. And best of all, widespread sex education (namely, about how masturbation is good for you and your relationship) has created discriminating shoppers: they demand toys that are well-made, long-lasting, safe, ergonomic, nice to look at, and actually effective.

That's not to say there isn't a lot of crap out there. The sex toy industry is littered with big manufacturers and distributors who are more interested in quantity than quality. They produce cheap toys made from crappy materials—often under dubious labor conditions—and don't provide instructions or ingredient lists. Some toys are even labeled "for novelty use only," which means "don't actually use it on your genitals despite the fact that it's shaped like a penis or vagina." Which is why it's important to educate yourself about sex toy materials and safety and to shop at smaller retailers with an educated sales staff, decent customer service, and a kinder, gentler, more inclusive approach to sales (i.e. ones whose marketing materials don't exclusively feature porn stars). With some homework, you can find toys that will transform your sex life—both alone and with a partner—in all the right ways. (By the way, if you're looking to add a few kinky toys to your collection, those items are covered in the Fantasy chapter on p.140). Read on, and then plug in.

Before you start filling your, er, pleasure chest, you need to learn your sex toy ABCs to make sure you're not wasting your paycheck on toys that will crap out, toys that will irritate your parts, or toys that just won't get the job done. Oh yeah, and you want to stay out of the emergency room, too. So take a few minutes to review the basics—your genitals (not to mention the staff at your local ER) will thank you for it.

That's What Sex Toys are Made Of

Not only do sex toys come in all shapes and sizes, they're made of all sorts of materials—some better than others. At the crappier end of the spectrum are toys made of cheap jelly rubber: they often have a strong odor, feel sticky, and are impossible to clean thoroughly (because their pores can harbor bacteria). The odor is caused by an outseeping of gases from plastic softeners called phthalates, which some studies have shown to be bad for the environment and your body. That said, this squishy material is ideal for molding toys into interesting textures, and is incredibly cheap, too, so we understand its appeal. If you must go jelly rubber, then always cover the toy with a condom (it may defeat the purpose of the interesting texture, but your sexual health is more important). Better choices are non-porous, phthalate-free materials which can be sterilized, such as high-grade metals like steel and aluminum; seamless acrylic or glass; and, our favorite, 100 percent silicone—it's hypoallergenic, boilable, dishwasher-safe (if your housemates don't mind), and odorless. If you're not sure what material a toy is made of (because product

ingredients are often not listed), play it safe and always use a condom—that'll help make clean-up easier, too!

The Safety Dance

Just because toys aren't living flesh, doesn't mean you can forgo safety precautions. STDs can be transferred from one person to another via shared toys, so either a) dedicate one toy to one person only, b) make sure it's a non-porous toy that can be sterilized before it changes hands (or groins), or c) put a condom on it—one fresh condom per partner per session. And never take a toy from ass to vagina without first swapping condoms or sterilizing it (that is, if it can be sterilized). Speaking of asses, don't stick anything where the sun don't shine if it doesn't have a flared base—you could end up at the hospital in need of a very humiliating emergency extraction. Many toys are made with latex (but don't always say so on the packaging), so if you've got a latex allergy it's a good idea to use polyurethane condoms with your toys. Never use a vibrator on unexplained calf pain—you could dislodge a potentially fatal blood clot. Before fooling around with seriously kinky equipment—rope, gags, metal cock rings, etc.—do your research (which extends well beyond reading this book), because amateur dominatrixes and would-be gimps can cause or incur serious injury when they don't know what they're doing. And finally, if a toy smells toxic, starts smoking, has loose parts or rough seams, degrades over time, gives you a rash, doesn't fit with your body, or just doesn't feel right, then for goodness sake stop using it!

Care & Cleaning

Try to invest in toys that come with care and cleaning instructions—and then follow them. Unfortunately most don't, so ask or email a sales rep for suggestions. If you've got a 100

Toy Rudiments

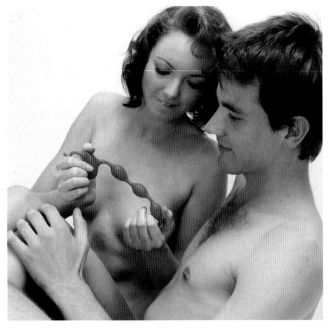

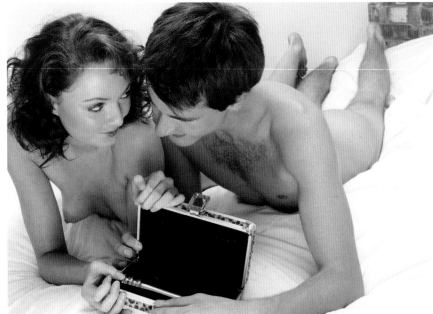

dishwasher (hold the harsh dishwashing detergent), or just wash it with soap and hot water. Acrylic, glass, and metal toys should not be boiled (unless the instructions say otherwise), though they can be sterilized with a good soap-and-hot-water scrubbing since they're non-porous. All soft toys made of materials like jelly rubber, Cyberskin, latex, etc., should also be cleaned with soap and water, but shouldn't be considered sterilized because they're porous and can therefore harbor invisible bacteria no matter how long you scrub—use a condom with them, especially if you're sharing the toy. (By the way, specially-made sex toy cleaning solutions aren't any better than old-fashioned soap and water.) Always clean a brand new toy right out of the packaging before first use, clean as soon as possible after each use, and clean before each use, too—at least if you're letting it collect dust under your bed between play dates. However, this last step may not be necessary if you're storing it correctly: remove any batteries to avoid corrosion or the toy accidentally turning on (at the wrong moment, a buzzing handbag can be incredibly embarrassing); separate any removable miniature vibrators from dildos or butt plugs; let any toy air-dry thoroughly after cleaning and before placing in its own repurposed sock or small shoebox or specially-made storage bag; and place (or hide) these bags in a cool, dry place. Don't let toys rub up against each other in storage, because some materials can nick, dent, or even melt others.

Lubes are Toys Too!

If you invest in only one bedside accessory this year, then make it a high-quality, man-made lubricant! It's affordable, easy to use, and can improve almost any sexual activity by 50 percent for anyone, male or female. Many people wrongly assume that the best and most authentic evidence of female arousal is wetness, but there are many factors which can influence a woman's natural lubrication, or lack thereof: dehydration, hormonal fluctuations, age, medications…

Supplementing that with purpose-made lube can make things more comfortable for much longer for her. Keeping things moist can help prevent condom breakage. A few drops on the inside of a condom can also enhance sensation for him. Plus, lube is what separates a good handjob from a great one, especially for the circumcised.

Lubricants come in three basic varieties. First, there are water-based lubes, which can be used with any toy, are latex-condom-compatible, and wash away easily with water (or simply just fade away). Unfortunately many water-based lubes, especially edible ones (in flavors like pina-colada or passion fruit), contain a natural sugar called glycerin (for sweetness) which may lead to yeast infections in super-sensitve vaginas, so read the ingredients list to find glycerin-free brands. Next, there are silicone-based lubes, which are thicker, longer-lasting, latex-condom-compatible, waterproof (great for shower-nozzle masturbation, but often require rinsing off with soap), and won't be absorbed by the body or react with sensitive skin (as long as they don't contain additives). There's one silicone lube caveat, however: don't use it with any silicone toys, as a weird chemical reaction might occur, destroying your toy in the process. (Though those in the biz say that if both the toy and the lube are 100 percent pure silicone, there's no problem—apparently the additives are to blame. Even if you're 100 percent sure, however, we'd still recommend a patch test first.) Finally, there are oil-based lubes, which are the hardiest and greasiest of them all, but they've got a few major drawbacks: oils—whether purpose-made or D.I.Y. like baby oil or Crisco—are *not* compatible with latex condoms or dental dams, and they're also hard to wash off, which means they can irritate vaginas and even cause infections. So the only activities we would recommend them for are male handjobs that are *not* going to end in vaginal penetration, or anal sex with a polyurethane condom (p.182). Massage oils should not be used for vaginal manual sex—stick with something water- or silicone-based. Lube—a little dab'll do you!

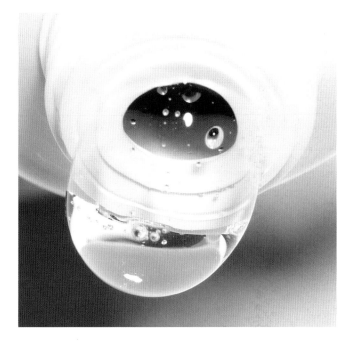

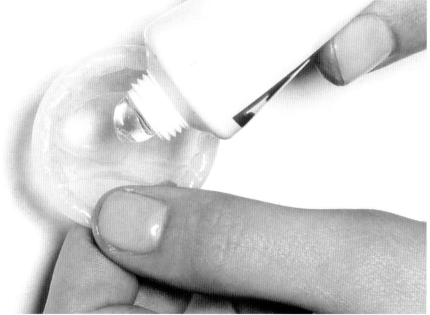

Vibrators

When you think of sex toys, you probably think of vibrators—they're the most popular masturbation aid available. Women enjoy the unique, intense, repetitive, endless, and thus guilt-free stimulation they provide (vibrators never get tired or bored)—in fact, many of them need it to reach orgasm. There's absolutely no shame in that: for some it's just a biological imperative. Which is why men should embrace vibrators, not as their replacements, but simply as extensions of their own hands. Because orgasms, no matter how they're achieved, are better than no orgasms at all.

Classic Vibes

What—These old-school, AA-battery-operated, external or insertable vibrators, often called Smoothies or Slimlines, are typically made of non-porous hard plastic, are vaguely phallic and penis-sized without being remotely realistic, and usually come in bright colors, girly pastels, or animal prints.

Why—They're affordable, fairly powerful (hard plastic transfers vibration well), and just plain cheery.

Why Not—The hard plastic may feel a little unloving, especially internally.

Which—Go for a seamless, water-proof version with multiple-speed settings. Avoid the really cheap ones with any rough seams that can harbor bacteria or those with a crappy metal-coating that might flake off.

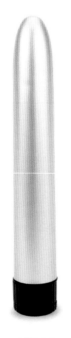

Ergonomic Vibes

What—Well-made, beautifully designed vibes that complement the contours of your body and hands in order to encourage more natural-feeling sensations and to fend off carpal tunnel syndrome.

Why—Because these toys actually have some thought put into them, they're usually made of high-quality, non-porous, safe materials that are easy to clean and, unlike most classic vibes, they won't give you numb hands.

Plus, they're easy on the eyes, and thus won't frighten your mother should she find one while snooping in your bathroom.

Why not—They're a little more expensive, but almost always worth it.

Which—The Laya Spot by Fun Factory (pictured) is palm-sized and can sit on her pubic bone, between her thighs, on her labia, or on his package. Emotional Bliss and Natural Contours are two other reputable brands worth checking out.

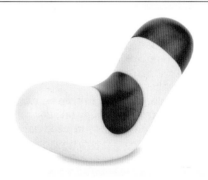

Realistic Vibes

What—Penis-shaped and sized vibrators for external or internal use. Don't be surprised if the phrase "realistically veined" appears on the toy's packaging.

Why—You love the look and filled-up feeling of a penis.

Why not—Nothing against dicks, but female pleasure doesn't always have to be male-centric.

Which—We like Fun Factory's Reality Sinnflut (pictured) because it's silicone, waterproof, *and* rechargable.

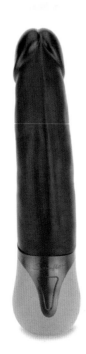

Non-Realistic Vibes

What—Internal/external vibrators that boast such un-penis-like details as smiley faces, unique textures, and un-anatomical curves.

Why—Great for those who find more realistic vibes too pornographic, or who simply prefer their stimulation to come in non-penis form.

Why not—Sometimes unrealistic designs get so cutesy and even kid-friendly (think cartoon animals with Cheshire Cat grins), they are at best unsexy, at worst completely creepy.

Which—Unfortunately the most interesting textures are often made with the worst material (jelly rubber). Try to go with a toy that's 100 percent silicone if you plan to use it internally. Fun Factory has a great selection of soft-on-the-skin silicone vibes (pictured is their Stranger 2), many of which are molded into precious animal characters.

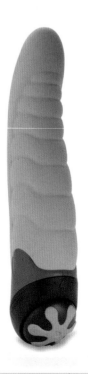

Dual-Action Vibes (a.k.a. Rabbits)

What—Popular vibes that provide simultaneous internal and clitoral stimulation. In the case of "rabbit" vibes, the bunny ears tickle the clitoral head while a shaft gets busy inside with vibration, rotation, and maybe even undulating pearls at the base of the vagina.

Why—Millions of women can't be wrong —the Rabbit is her new best friend.

Why not—This toy does so much, a man is likely to feel beside the point— so she may want to save this toy for her alone time.

Which—Thanks to numerous celebrity and pop culture endorsements, the Rabbit is the Fendi handbag of the toy world, which means the market is flooded with cheap knock-offs. But this is not the time to go bargain-hunting; opt for the phthalate-free Elastomer Rabbit (pictured) by the original Rabbit manufacturer, Vibratex.

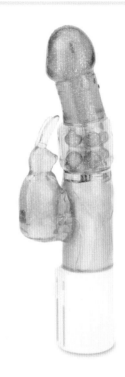

Triple-Action Vibes

What—Kitchen-sink vibrators that simultaneously stimulate the clitoral head, G-spot, and perineum/anus.

Why—You're a demanding masturbator who accepts nothing less than having all your bases covered.

Why not—Over-stimulation does not necessarily equal orgasm.

Which—Many are made of jelly rubber, which we recommend avoiding. Vibratex's Dreamboat Triple G (pictured) is Elastomer, which means it's slightly porous but not toxic.

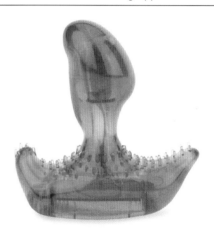

Wearable Vibes

What—Smallish vibrators, usually external, that are held in place with dainty elastic harnesses for hands-free stimulation.

Why—Great for constant clitoral stimulation during intercourse, phone sex (when you don't have a headset), or boring cocktail parties.

Why not—It might feel bulky and may not stay in place.

Which—Some wearable vibes offer external clitoral stimulation only, while others reach inside to the G-spot or around to the back, too—it all depends on how you'll be using it. Just try to steer clear of jelly rubber, especially if it's an internal toy.

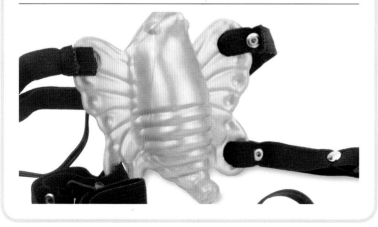

High-End Vibes

What—Sex toys that might cost up to a month's salary thanks to top-notch materials, elegant designs, extravagant trimmings, and a certain *je ne sais quoi* appeal.

Why—A high price-tag *usually* means high quality. And spending obscene amounts of money on a sex toy may make you feel less dirty using it.

Why not—If you're still waiting for grandma to die and leave you that inheritance, there are more affordable vibes that are just as high (if not higher) in quality.

Which—The Minx by Shiri Zinn (pictured is your classic high-end vibe): it's Swarovski-encrusted with a marabou tail and comes with its own display plinth. But, like yachts, why pick just one?

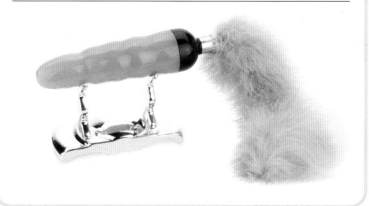

Vibrators Continued...

"Back Massager" Vibes

What—Oversized plug-in vibrators that look nothing like phalluses, are intended for external use only, and can be sold in mainstream catalogues and G-rated gadget shops because they're advertised vaguely as "tension relievers".

Why—Plug-in vibes usually last a long time, can often provide more intense vibration than battery-operated toys, and look less "sleazy" than more realistic vibrators.

Why not—They're often huge, loud, and can make the hand you're holding them in go numb.

Which—The Hitachi Magic Wand (pictured) is the category standard.

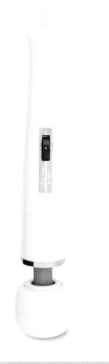

Pocket Vibes

What—Smallish, very affordable vibrators—usually made of easy-to-clean non-porous plastic and intended for external use only—that can fit into your pocket or handbag.

Why—Their demure size is non-threatening to newbies and men, they typically require only one battery, and they're good for orgasms on-the-go.

Why not—The gentle buzz may not be enough to push you over the edge.

Which—Doc Johnson's "Pocket Rocket" is the original pocket-sized vibe and comes with different textured tops to vary clitoral sensation, but we prefer Vibratex's well-made waterproof "Water Dancer" (pictured).

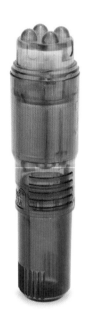

Bullet Vibes

What—Teeny-tiny vibrators: the smallest kind look like suppositories; the largest like oblong eggs, though they're not usually intended for insertion, just external stimulation. They're used alone or in conjunction with a vibrating love ring (p.136). They're either self-contained with watch batteries, or attached to a remote control/battery console via a cord.

Why—They're inexpensive, travel-sized, discreet, and non-threatening.

Why not—In the self-contained versions, the tiny watch batteries usually don't last very long (and are a pain to replace). Those with cords can get pulled on (and thus broken) more easily; plus, they're harder to clean well.

Which—Go for a cordless version that's waterproof and/or offers variable speeds.

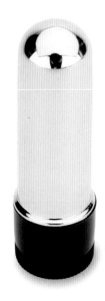

Pebble Vibes

What—Small external vibrators (i.e., smaller than pocket vibes, slightly bigger than most bullets) that sit in the palm of your hand as pleasantly as a sand-buffed pebble you found on the beach.

Why—Their elfin size makes them discreet, non-threatening, travel-friendly, and great for use between two bodies during intercourse.

Why not—They feel this nice because they're incredibly well-made, and you pay for what you get.

Which—The Swedish design company Lelo makes a series of *gorgeous* pebbles (pictured is the Lelo Lily): they're rechargeable, silky smooth, and come in impeccably tasteful packaging.

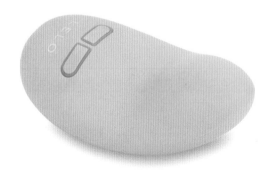

Multi-Vibes-in-One

What—Full-size, plug-in vibrators, occasionally advertised as "muscle massagers", that come with various attachments to create different sensations for external stimulation and sometimes (if specified) internal penetration.

Why—It's like getting several toys in one, allowing you to more easily and cost-effectively determine what kind of sensation your genitals like best.

Why not—Those sold as back massagers, like the popular Wahl, claim not to be intended for genital use (yeah right!), so use at your own risk.

Which—The light-weight, oscillating Eroscillator (pictured) claims to be the only sex toy endorsed by the famous German-born sexologist Dr. Ruth.

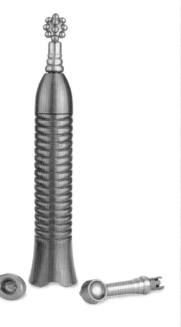

Metal Vibes

What—Vibrators made of chrome, brass, titanium, aluminum, stainless or surgical steel, silver, or gold.

Why—They're non-porous, phthalate-free, firm on the G- and P-spots, incredibly smooth (especially with lube), and great at transmitting vibration and temperature (though don't freeze them 'cause they'll stick to your bits!).

Why not—The best metal vibes tend to be some of the priciest.

Which—Avoid toys with cheap metal coatings (which can flake off), and invest in solid, high-grade metal numbers. For instance, Elemental Pleasures creates high-end vibrators (pictured) made of either stainless steel, titanium, or anodized aluminum; they're all quiet, multi-speed, waterproof, and, amazingly, boilable.

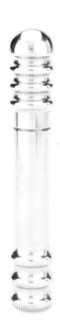

Finger Vibes

What—Small vibrators that attach to one or more fingers in order to turn your hand into a love machine.

Why—Finger vibes can make you feel more connected to the vibratory pleasure you're providing yourself or your partner—the toy is just enhancing your own first-class manual sex skills, rather than taking you out of the stimulation equation altogether.

Why not—Numb fingers. And they might remind you too much of a waterproof finger bandage.

Which—The Fukuoku 9000 (pictured) is the original finger favorite.

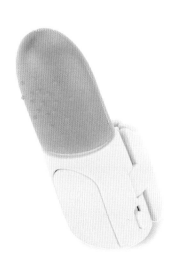

Bendable Vibes

What—Insertable vibrators with flexible spines that can be bent to create angles customized to your own sexual preferences.

Why—Rather than one shape fitting all, you can shape it so it fits your *individual* anatomy—because not all G- and P-spots are created equally. Play around with different angles for different sensations.

Why not—Many bendable vibrators and dildos are made of soft porous rubber, which makes them bacteria-friendly and harder to get really clean. So use those with condoms.

Which—Look for (and be prepared to invest in) the rarer silicone versions. Some are even waterproof, like the Bendi (pictured).

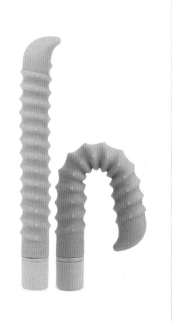

G-Spotters

As we learned in the Manual Sex chapter (p.48), the G-spot can be stimulated through the top wall of the vagina—you can feel the spongy area with the pad of your finger by pressing toward the navel an inch or three inside. But G-spots often like fairly firm, repetitive stimulation that can be hard to keep up with fingers alone—and traditional straight-as-an-arrow vibrators can miss the G-spot completely. That's where these toys come in: they all feature a nifty curve, they all vibrate, and—as long as you've got enough batteries on hand—they won't ever get a "cramp."

Vibrating G-Spot Toys

What—Internal vibrators with a pronounced curve at the tip to target the G-spot.

Why—You want to find out if you like having your G-spot stimulated.

Why not—You already know you don't.

Which—The pure silicone, multi-speed G-Swirl (pictured), designed by the legendary sex toy shop Good Vibrations and manufactured by Fun Factory, features sculpted bumps along the shaft as well as a ridged base so the clitoris, labia, and perineum don't feel too left out.

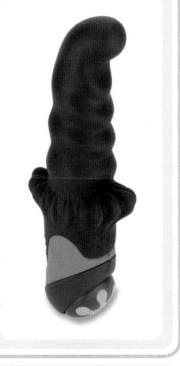

G-Spot Attachments

What—G-friendly attachments for "back massagers" or multi-vibes-in-one.

Why—Sometimes you feel like external clitoral stimulation and sometimes your G-spot wants a turn, but you don't necessarily want to buy a brand-new vibrator for each mood.

Why not—The intense vibrations of these toys might be a bit much on the inside.

Which—Just make sure it's pure silicone, like Vixen's Gee-Whiz (pictured), which attaches to the Hitachi Magic Wand (p.132). Some versions include ridges at the base for labial and clitoral attention, too.

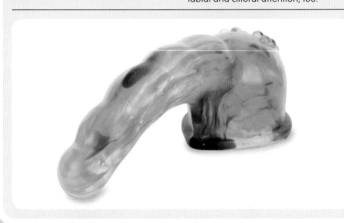

Come Hither G-Spot Toys

What—While shaped just like standard vibrating G-spot toys, these toys have a shaft which actually moves up and down, replicating the "come hither" gesture often employed during manual stimulation of the G-spot.

Why—With a regular G-spot vibe, you'd have to move the toy in and out yourself to create this motion.

Why not—They can feel very mechanical, are often loud, may be incapacitated by squeezing from strong pelvic floor muscles, and *cannot be inserted anally* (so keep away from his P-spot!).

Which—The Pixie vibe by Vibratex (pictured) is made of phthlate-free (albeit porous) Elastomer, features hundreds of tiny nubbins for all-over internal stimulation, and may come with a vibrating clitoral attachment (depending on the model).

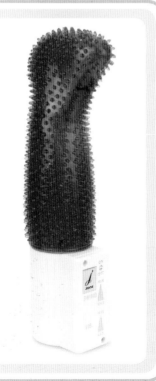

Rocking G-Spot Toys

What—U-shaped vibrators that simultaneously target the G-spot (the long, curved end) and the clitoral head (the wider, ridged end), while maintaining constant genital contact along the area between these two spots.

Why—Unique ergonomic design means you can forgo traditional in-out thrusting for female-friendly rocking and rubbing. Plus, for once the clitoris isn't just an afterthought—this is an equal opportunity vibrator.

Why not—It's kind of scary looking, like a clamp.

Which—The Rock Chick (pictured) is made of soft, safe silicone; comes with a removable bullet vibrator you can make pulse with just the touch of a finger; and can be used in the shower, even *with* the vibe.

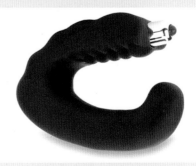

Anal Play-Things

The anus contains more nerve endings than any other part of the male body, and any part of the female body save for the clitoris. Plus, your pelvic floor muscles wrap around the anus, and anal toys give them something to clench onto during voluntary and involuntary contractions of pleasure. Opt for easy-to-clean silicone bum toys; start small and work your way up; never go from ass to vagina or ass to someone else's ass without sterilizing first (or swapping condoms); and be sure to use purpose-made lubricant with all of the below. Ready, set, bend over!

Basic Butt Plugs

What—Anal insertables, often with a tapered entry-end for easy insertion and always with a flared base (so as not to get lost up there). They are smaller than dildos and designed to be left in place during other stimulation.

Why—Sometimes it's logistically difficult to deliver two kinds of stimulation (one in the front and one in the back) at the same time with your own body parts—a butt plug does half the work for you!

Why not—Go too small and it might wriggle out at the wrong moment; go too big and it might turn you off butt plugs forever.

Which—Go for any butt plug made by the industry leader, Tantus—because all their products are hand-made from the highest quality silicone.

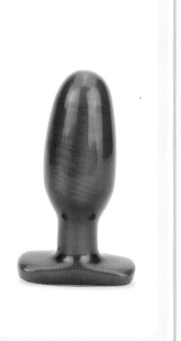

Vibrating Butt Plugs

What—Same as basic plugs, except with miniature vibrators, either built-in or removable.

Why—Many people like to up the ante on their anal stimulation. The sensation can reverberate throughout the entire genital region.

Why not—You might find that vibrations back there feel funny in a bad way.

Which—Tantus's Pro-Touch vibrating plug (pictured) replicates the shape of a large, curved finger to target his P-spot. Sterilize it (remove the vibrator first) and it can serve double-duty as a G-spotter for her.

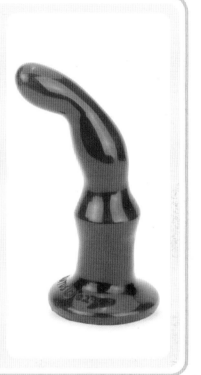

Textured Butt Plugs

What—A cross between anal beads (see next) and a miniature dildo.

Why—You get the gradually-bigger-bump sensation ot anal beads with easier insertion.

Why not—They may not have the flexibility of anal beads or the curves of other anal insertables to conform to the contours of your rectum.

Which—Try Tantus's biggest seller, the harness-compatible Ripple butt plug (pictured).

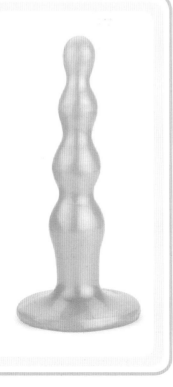

Anal Beads

What—A string or stalk of beads or balls, which usually graduate in size (small olive-sized to large grape), that are inserted into the anus one at a time.

Why—They bunch up to make you feel full and can enhance pleasure when gently—we said *gently*!—pulled out by the un-insertable ring-like handle right before or at the moment of orgasm.

Why not—The cheap kinds come on nylon chords (which get nasty fast) and are made of plastic (which have rough seams, ouch!).

Which—One of the best sex toy manufacturers, Fun Factory, makes a great, soft, 100 percent silicone version on a bendy, seamless stalk that's super easy to sterilize (pictured).

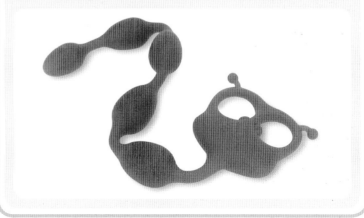

Toys for Boys

"Sex toys for boys" have come a long way since the days of blow-up dolls with thousand-yard stares. Just as manufacturers are finally considering the real sexual and anatomical needs of women in their toy designs, they're also finding new and innovative ways to keep guys from having to steal their girlfriends' vibrators. We've still got a way to go, but the following are all great places to start. Gentlemen,

Non-Vibrating P-Spot Toys

What—Anal insertables—butt plugs or dildos—specially curved to target and stimulate the male prostate gland (a.k.a. the P-spot, a.k.a. the male G-spot): the toys are inserted about three inches and curve toward the belly button, stimulating the prostate through the rectal wall. He or she can move the toy by hand, or the contractions of his pelvic floor muscles and anal sphincters can provide safe, hands-free stimulation.

Why—Prostate massagers can help keep the gland flushed (and thus healthy); can be worn during masturbation, manual sex, oral sex, or intercourse for added sensation; and can increase the intensity of orgasms.

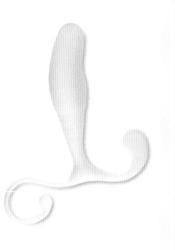

Why not—Many heterosexual men feel like anal penetration is just a gay- or girl-thing. But they'd be wrong—it's one of the most successful toys for boys available.

Which—The hard, plastic Aneros (pictured) was designed by scientists to promote prostate health by massaging the gland via the rectum and perineum. But then users fortuitously discovered how *good* it actually felt to use.

Vibrating P-Spot Toys

What—Same as the still version, except—you guessed it—vibrating!

Why—Many men enjoy the extra sensation of reverberation throughout the whole anal and genital region that can be achieved only from a battery-powered, insertable vibrator.

Why not—Sometimes you *can* get too much of a good thing.

Which—The Rude Boy (pictured), brother of the Rock Chick (p.134), is made of 100 percent silicone that's non-porous, easy to sterilize, firm but silky to the touch, and hypoallergenic. Plus, it's waterproof, even with the removable bullet vibrator. See also Vibrating Butt Plugs on p.135.

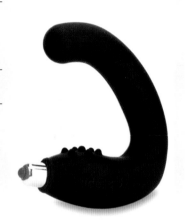

Masturbation Aids

What—Any of the following: masturbation sleeves which mimic the feel of a vagina, anus, or mouth; molds of vaginas, anuses, or breasts, usually of particular porn stars; cheap blow-up dolls best suited for bachelor parties; high-priced, custom-made, life-size Real Dolls; and vibrating penis cups and huggers.

Why—Sometimes it's nice to give your hand a break.

Why not—The selection of high-quality male masturbation aids with an eye toward design (and away from creepiness) is very limited.

Which—The gimmicky Fleshlight (pictured)—which looks like a giant flashlight but feels (or, at least, is *supposed* to feel) like a textured vagina, anus, or mouth—is a bestseller among boy toys.

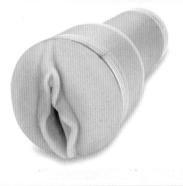

Vibrating Love Rings

What—Soft, stretchy cock rings worn around the base of the shaft or around both the shaft and the testicles, with a miniature vibrator either built in or added to a top loop on the ring. The buzzing ring stimulates her labia and clitoris during intercourse and gives him nice genital vibration too.

Why—Hello, hands-free clitoral stimulation during intercourse? Why use a regular cock ring when you have this! Plus, any kind of ring may give him firmer, longer-lasting erections, due to the snug fit around his package.

Why not—Despite their very friendly designs, new penis rings still have to overcome their old kinky gimp image. Plus, many versions come in cheap jelly rubber—not the greatest material, but at least you're not inserting it anywhere, so not too bad.

Which—Disposable versions offer a cheap introduction. If you find you like love rings, buy a soft silicone version

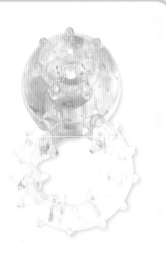

(pictured) or even a medical grade-steel or silver one, like the PVibe—it lasts longer and is easier to clean. Avoid rings made from unbroken metal, as they can't be removed in a hurry! Don't wear a ring for more than 20 minutes (and take it off if it's not comfortable).

Dildos & Harnesses

A dildo is a phallic, usually non-vibrating object, often with a flared base, used for poking a vagina, a bum, or even a mouth. Throw in a harness and *voila!*—you've got a strap-on, meaning you can wear the dildo where a penis would normally pop up and use it to be the penetrator for a change (or just to penetrate with something different). Wearing a strap-on doesn't automatically mean you always wear the pants in the relationship, and being on the receiving end does not make you gay, deviant, or henpecked—though if it feels dirtier to pretend so, don't let us stop you.

Realistic Dildos

What—Dildos that look and feel like flesh-and-blood penises (some with balls!). They can be wielded by hand, used for strap-on sex (if they have a flared base), or just worn under your trousers (if they're floppy enough).

Why—For some, the whole point of sex-toy penetration and play is to mimic the look and feel of a real, naturally sexy penis.

Why not—For others, sex-toy penetration is more palatable when the "tool" in question *couldn't* pass for a penis in a dark alley. Small, purple, and glittery may be a lot less intimidating.

Which—If you're going to insert your dong anywhere (rather than just using it as a fun paperweight), make it a silicone one. Newer versions of this material can be quite flesh-like: try the Tex by Vixen (pictured) or any of Tantus's realistic dildos. And if it's going in a harness or in a bum, make sure it's got a flared base.

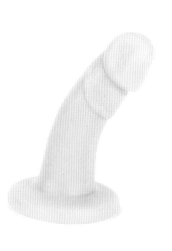

Vibrating Dildos

What—Phalluses—with a removable, often multi-speed, miniature vibrator in the base—that can be used anywhere a penis would be welcome, either strapped into a harness or hand-held.

Why—The addition of a mini-vibe makes your dildo more than just a second-rate penis. Plus, both partners can benefit genitally from the vibrations when it's worn in a harness.

Why not—Strap-on sex is kind of a big deal as it is—adding vibration might be just a bit too much for beginners.

Which—As with any dildo, opt for a silicone version (and one with a flared base, if it's going in a harness or a bum). You can't go wrong with anything from Tantus, like the Buzz (pictured).

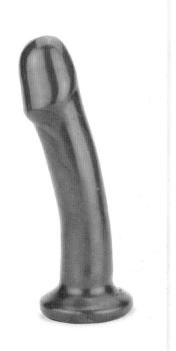

Harnesses

What—Contraptions for making a dildo an extension of your own pelvis. The one-strap versions fit like a G-string, while the two-strap versions fit like a jock strap.

Why—A harness allows for hands-free dildo-penetration by a partner, which may be the closest she gets to experiencing what it feels like for a man (save for using a double dildo). Most harnesses fit different sizes and shapes of dildo—experiment with what works best for you. Some even come with a tiny pocket that holds a bullet vibrator for clitoral stimulation. Plus, you might like the skimpy, kinky look of a harness—it gives a whole new meaning to the term "crotchless panties."

Why not—If the base of the dildo doesn't fit securely into the harness or the harness itself isn't easily adjustable or the right size for you, you'll have trouble controlling aim and movement.

Which—A nylon harness (pictured) is machine-washable and easily adjustable on the fly, but a leather, vinyl, or rubber one that buckles can up the kink factor.

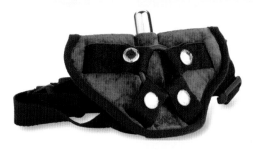

Double Dildos

What—It's all dildo, all the time: one end for each partner for simultaneous, mutual penetration.

Why—You two might feel more organically connected since you'll both feel internal stimulation as you move (her in her vagina, him in his tush), without having to use a bulky or kinky-looking harness.

Why not—Old-school versions— long, straight shafts with tapered or penis-shaped ends—require you to get into impossible positions and move awkwardly just to keep them simultaneously inserted. New-and-improved versions are more ergonomically designed with angles that take advantage of the way bodies actually move together, though the "penetrator" will still need strong pelvic muscles to maneuver and may find she needs help steadying the dildo with a harness or a pair of undies.

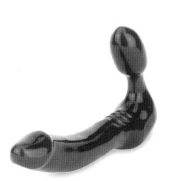

Which—The Feeldoe (pictured) is a bestseller in this category with an optional vibrator and a bulb-like end for her G-spot; the ridges at the centre may also stimulate her clitoris.

Quirky Toys

We're living in a golden age of sex toys: each year we travel a little further away from the cheap plastic trinkets that are good for a laugh at a bachelorette party but pretty much useless in the orgasm department. Toy manufacturers are now using better materials and their designs are increasingly creative, ergonomic, and attentive to mutual pleasure. Here are a few of the more inspired recent developments in the assisted orgasm industry.

Glass Dildos

What—Dildos or butt plugs made of sturdy glass. They may not be vibrating workhorses like, say, the Hitachi Magic Wand, but they're sure to be the prettiest toys in your collection.

Why—Their heft and rigidity make them great for Kegel exercises or G-spot/P-spot stimulation (the latter only if there's *no* way the toy will get lost up the bum). Plus, glass holds temperature really well, so try running it under warm or cool water before use for a new sensation (*do not freeze*).

Why not—You have to be prepared to do all the work, because these toys don't come with on/off switches.

Which—It should be made of Pyrex or labeled "medical grade" glass. The ridged kind are easier to get a grip on once you've lubed up.

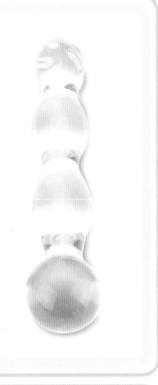

Remote-Control Toys

What—Vibrators that are worn by one partner and operated by the other partner from either a small distance or a remote location.

Why—You can play at home or, if you like surprises and have an excellent poker face, you can take your play out on the town (the rest of the bar doesn't need to know that the earth is moving for you). Remote-control toys leave one partner at the mercy of the other—great for teasing or power plays (p.154).

Why not—They're not for people with control issues.

Which—The Vibra-Exciter (pictured) has two parts: a silver bullet vibe that can fit between your underwear and any favorite erogenous zone, and a battery pack receiver that looks like a mobile phone. When you send or receive a text message, the bullet automatically vibrates for 20 to 30 seconds; when you make or receive an actual phone call, it vibrates for the duration of the call—great for phone or text sex with a partner who's away on business. If your phone isn't exactly ringing off the hook, you can always switch to manual mode.

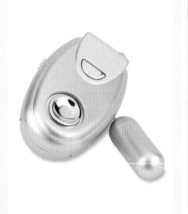

Insertable Balls

What—Two (or occasionally three) balls the size of large marbles, either free-floating or attached to a cord, that are inserted into the vagina. Some are solid, some contain loose weights, and some even vibrate.

Why—Great for a) exercising her pelvic muscles, b) providing a very subtle kind of internal stimulation that could work as foreplay (before or during a date, say), and c) giving her vagina something to squeeze onto during an orgasm (e.g. when used in conjunction with manual sex or an external vibrator).

Why not—They don't really move around so you might not feel a lot.

Which—"Ben wa balls" have been around for centuries. Avoid ancient carved ivory or cheap seamed plastic with absorbent cords in favor of Fun Factory's Smart Balls (pictured): the casing and string are non-porous and phthalate-free, and the balls contain loose weights for added sensation.

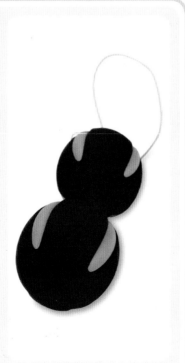

Cone Vibes

What—A cone-shaped, hands-free, over-sized external vibrator for her or him: sit on it, lie over it, or rub against it during masturbation or partner sex.

Why—It's the most novel sex toy in decades—it'll stimulate your curiosity, if nothing else.

Why not—It may be a little bulky, especially for partner play; you might prefer something with more targeted vibration or greater insertion capability; plus, it's pink.

Which—There's really only one version right now ("The Cone", pictured), but we're sure knock-offs are coming soon. The Cone is made of soft, medical-grade silicone, comes with a handy instruction manual, and has 16 power levels (from barely-there to bed-shaking) with a nifty "orgasm button" that takes you straight to 16.

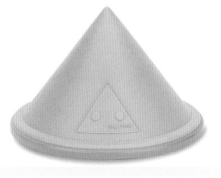

PG-Rated Toys

There's no rule that says every sex toy in your treasure chest should make you blush. And if you've never brought an accessory into the bedroom before, we're guessing you don't want to start with a 9-inch strap-on. Get used to the idea of props with some of the following low-profile items. (You might even find a birthday present idea for your Aunt Edna!)

Edible Body Dust

What—Light, fragrant, edible powder that's dusted over your bodies before you go exploring with your tongues (for external use only).

Why—It provides a yummy excuse to slow things down; offers a nice alternative to the full-body massage for lazy bums; stimulates your senses of smell and taste as all great sensation play should (p.164); and can be worn simply as regular body powder.

Why not—The smell may be overpowering to sensitive noses and the sweetness may be irritating to sensitive vaginas.

Which—Kama Sutra's Honey Dust (pictured) is shimmery gold, hypoallergenic, made from real honey (though it's far from sticky), and comes with a sensual feather applicator.

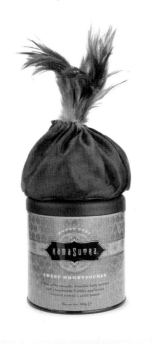

Undercover Vibes

What—Vibrators that can pass for far more innocent objects: nail polish, lipstick, pen, mascara, hairbrush, cell phone, etc.

Why—They are easily camouflaged in a handbag; are non-threatening to guys who worry about being replaced by realistic penis-shaped toys; make great gifts for your prudish female friends in dire need of an orgasm; will fool nosy houseguests snooping in your cabinets and drawers; and may even make it past airport security (though we wouldn't try it).

Why not—These toys tend to be high on gimmick and low on vibratory capacity and life-span.

Which—Whichever product is most likely to blend in with your surroundings.

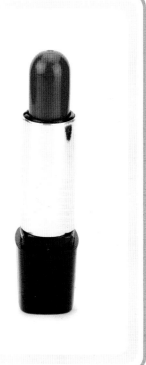

Bath Toys

What—Undercover toys that are waterproof, such as vibrating shower scrunchies and sponges; sensuality enhancers such as bubble bath, fizzy balls, and edible chocolate soap; even waterproof erotica collections and underwater sex manuals that you can take in the tub with you.

Why—The bath is the perfect place to relax your mind and prepare your body for sex (see p.19 for more on this topic).

Why not—Baths make for great foreplay but aren't always conducive to female orgasms, especially since water will wash away her natural lubricant. So make sure you bring along some waterproof silicone lube.

Which—Sure, there are innumerable waterproof vibrators on the market, but if you don't want to have to hide your toy between baths, try the ever-popular vibrating rubber duckie (pictured). Though if you get the one that's dressed in leather with a studded collar (no joke), your cover will be blown.

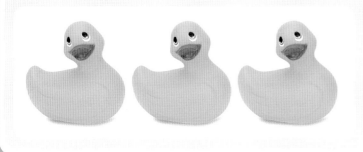

Massage Creams

What—Massage products that start in a solid form (some are like a bar of soap, others like a tub of butter) and turn into a smooth, non-sticky moisturizing lotion as you rub them in.

Why—They're less messy than traditional liquid massage oils.

Why not—These creams are actually oil-based, so don't use them on her genitals or with latex.

Which—Good Vibrations' Body Butter (pictured) is not only edible, it's actually tasty—a rarity among so-called edible bedside accessories (and it's vegan to boot).

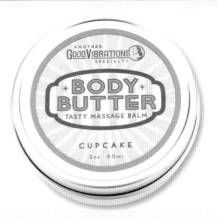

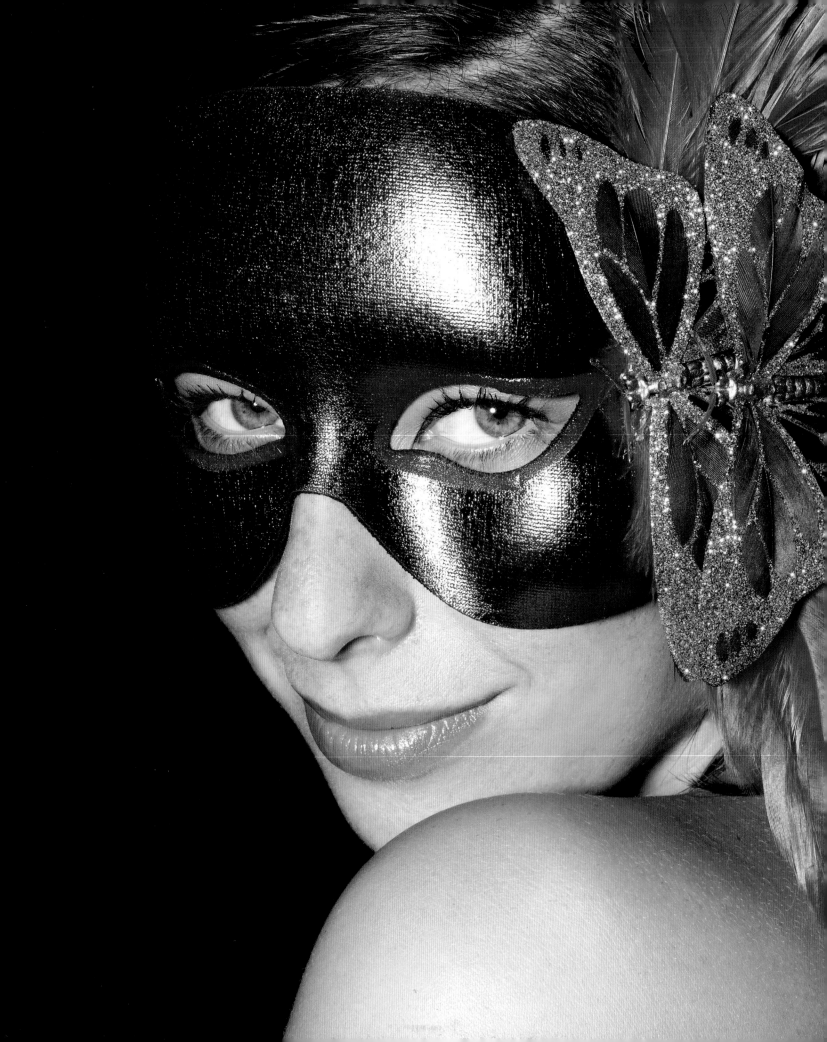

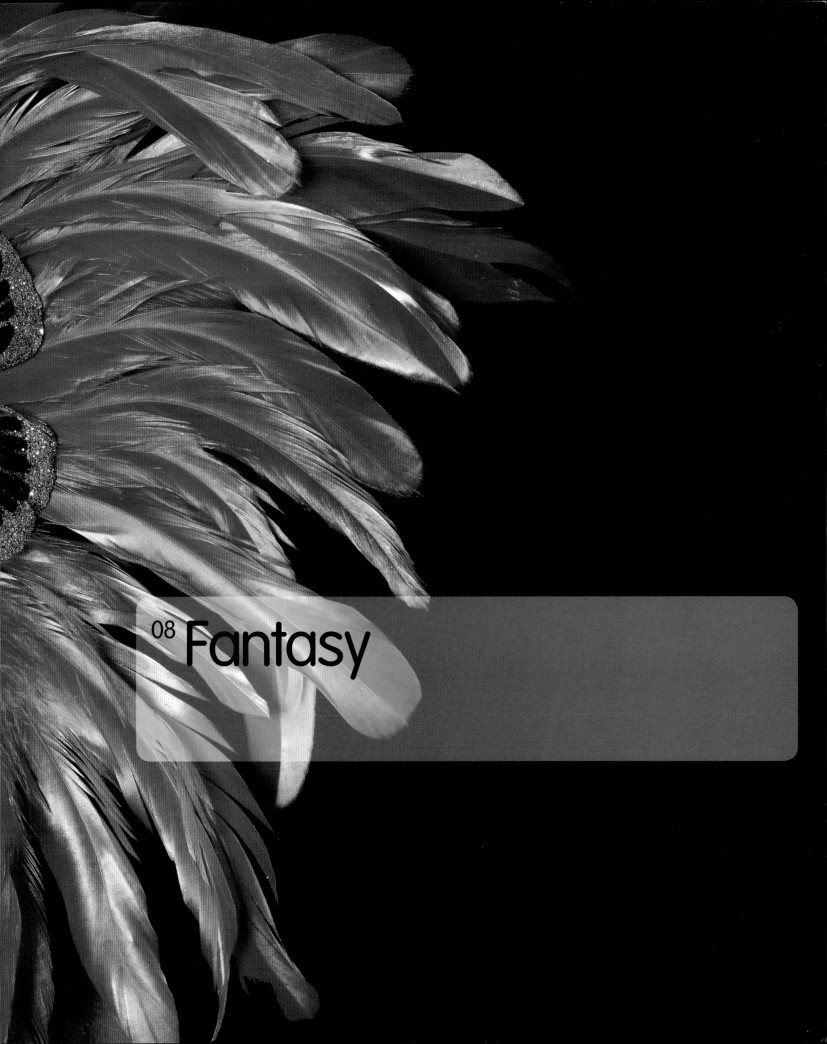

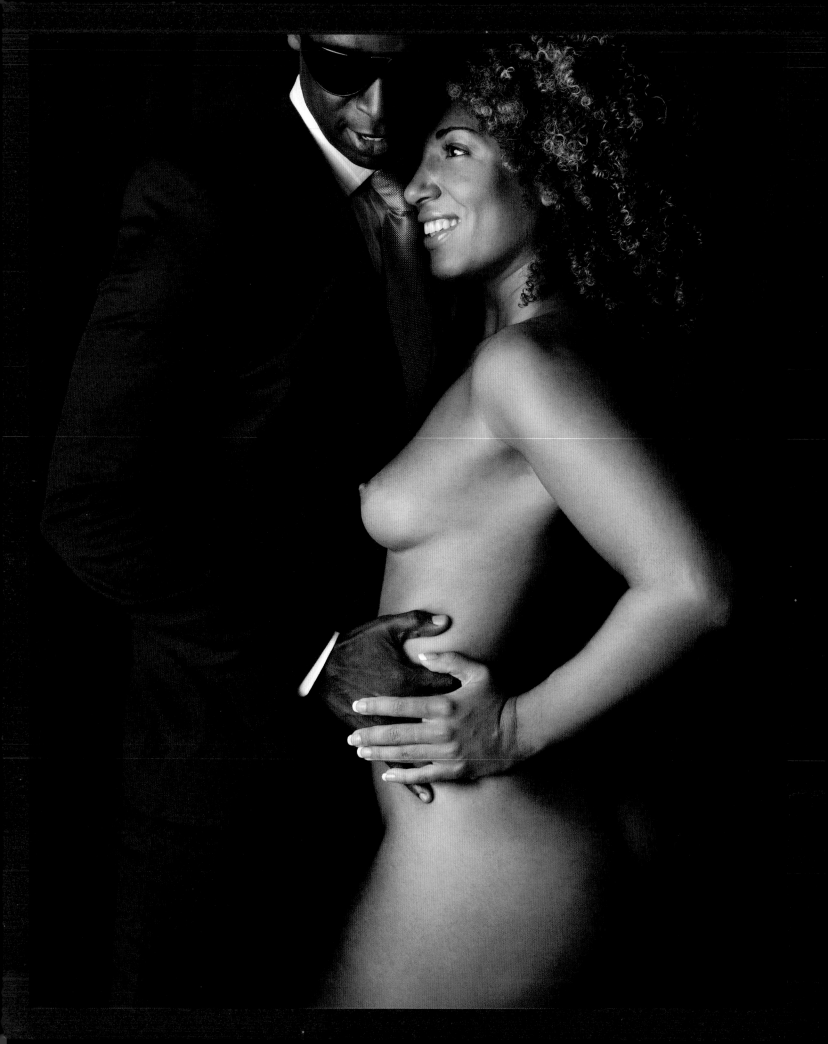

The Spice of Your Sex Life

The phrase "spice up your sex life" is enough to cool even the most ardent desire to get kinky. You're probably imagining your old school teacher in a gag, your parents' friends spanking geriatric flesh back to life, Kathy Bates wrapped in plastic wrap in *Fried Green Tomatoes*, essentially platonic couples grasping at erotic straws. The assumption is, "spicy sex" is the sole domain of the desperate, the boring, the unskilled.

But we highly recommend you not put limits on your sexual repertoire out of a fear of being clichéd. There's too much fun to be had! Variety is the life force of the bedroom, so the license to become someone else in this space is paramount. Roleplaying need not involve complicated scripts or costumes (though if you are so inspired…); it only requires a commitment to suspend your disbelief, to trust in your partner, and to allow yourself to be transported to another time and place. And the right dirty thoughts and props can help you get there.

A leather paddle gives you the courage to coax your partner into sexy submission, an old-fashioned Polaroid camera nurtures your inner pornographer, rope cuffs teach a diehard giver how to be more selfish in bed, a masked partner lessens your self-consciousness when trying something new, a shared fantasy lets you explore a taboo together. This kind of sex is dramatic, deliberate, and dirty—an entirely new brand of pleasure.

So why would you want to save all that for when you're "in a rut"? That'd be like holding off on sex until the seventh year of marriage, for when you really needed a morale boost. In fact, we've always thought that the sooner you experiment together, even just a little, the more naturally it'll come *throughout* your relationship. Because nothing spells "awkward" quite like breaking out the gimp suit after 25 years of the missionary position.

Exploring your dirtier, darker fantasies with a partner requires a boatload of trust and communication and can actually bring a couple closer together—closer than even the most teary-eyed, face-holding, make-up sex. Think of kink as the X-rated version of that trust-falling game you used to play as a kid. Sure, you could get kinky with a near stranger: sometimes anonymity is what gives you the courage to try spanking or dirty talk for the first time. But we think that most of the activities in this chapter are safest and hottest with a long-term partner. After all, it's way more fun to break a taboo with someone who knows you just crossed a line.

It comes down to this: leaving your comfort zone every now and then and crossing your own personal boundaries—wherever they may lie—is one of the best ways to keep things… we won't say "spicy", but how about "steamy"? Or at least entertaining. We believe that every person's sex life should contain at least one act they'd never share over brunch or beers—if nothing you currently do makes you blush that much, then keep reading. John Waters once said, "I thank God I was raised Catholic, so sex will always be dirty." In the absence of a vengeful higher power, consider this chapter a friendly reminder of how dirty sex can be.

Taboos provide structure and boundaries. But they also encourage inhibition—the arch-nemesis of passion. By cultivating, sharing, and even acting out your fantasies with a partner, you'll learn to let go of your more useless inhibitions and generate some psychic heat. You could try roleplaying—or just playing games. You could dress up—or dress down… to music. And, if you're brave, turn a camera on each other for some exhibitionism/voyeurism. Just remember, what you do with your hands, mouth, and other essential organs is only half the story: stimulating each other's gray matter is the rest. In fact, kinky sex starts with your mind in the gutter—and your mind might just be as far as the kink ever goes.

Let's Pretend—You can have a threeway with a friend or an orgy with the neighbors without any awkward morning-after small talk. You can break the law (or the laws of physics) without repercussions. And you can experiment with taboos that you're on the fence about, or those you'd never venture near in real life. Even missionary sex can feel dirty if you're sharing a fantasy while you do it. The heady experience might convince you that you're ready to act out the fantasy—or it may confirm that you can't go there. Either way, you've tested a taboo and should therefore feel very pleased with yourself.

99 Percent Inspiration—If you don't have a favorite fantasy, then you haven't spent enough time dirty–day dreaming. Inspiration surrounds you—you just have to seek it out. Browse a sex toy shop, in person or online, for some new gadgets, accessories, videos, or books. Kinky erotica like Anne Rice's *The Claiming of Sleeping Beauty* or anthologies like *Best Bondage Erotica*, *Best Fetish Erotica*, and *Sweet Life: Erotic Fantasies for Couples* can be read alone or together before bedtime (many come as audio collections so you can truly defile your MP3 player). For a more how-to approach, try Violet Blue's *Ultimate Guide to Sexual Fantasy*. Or buy a card or board game that's designed to inject a little creativity into your play: it's as easy as rolling the dice, pulling a card from the deck, and following the instructions. (If you're too shy to visit a sex toy shop, you'll often find these games in party supply shops that specialize in bachelor and bachelorette parties.) Even a simple game of strip poker with your own deck of cards can give you permission to be naughty ("I have to, it's the rules!"). Adult videos might help stir things up, too, whether as a source of fantasies and tricky new moves, or as a naughty activity in and of itself. There's a vast sea of porn out there, much of it clichéd, tacky, or downright disgusting (which may turn out to be just your thing). But if you're looking for something a little more female- or couple-friendly with higher production costs, fewer fake boobs, maybe even a little plot, try browsing the video sections of female-owned and operated sex shop retailers for suggestions. Or seek out female producers and directors (such as Maria Beatty, Candida Royalle, Tina Tyler, Tristan Taormino, Audacia Ray, Stella Films, and Veronica Hart)—the by-women-for-women porn field is expanding by the year. You might also find porn classics like *The Opening of Misty Beethoven* easier to stomach—it's not cheesy, it's retro chic! (Plus, back then, balloon boobs and the scorched earth approach to pubic hair had yet to sweep the porn world.) For popcorn-friendly activities that are a little less hardcore, rent kinky mainstream films like *Secretary*, *Kama Sutra: A Tale of Love*, *Crimes of Passion*, *Wild Orchid*, *Sex, Lies & Videotape*, *9½ Weeks*, *The*

Playing & Posing

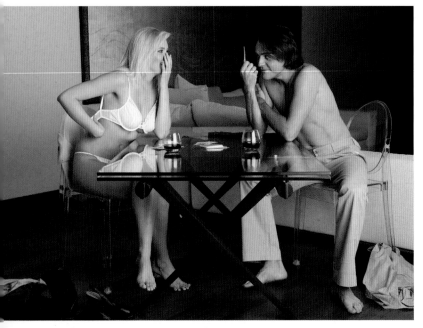
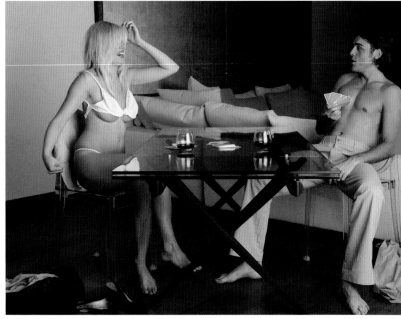

Pillow Book, Y Tu Mama Tambien, Basic Instinct, Bound, Eyes Wide Shut, Body Heat, Henry and June, The Unbearable Lightness of Being, 9 Songs, Betty Blue, The Lover, Shortbus, Crash (1996), *The Dreamers*… Whatever you rent, keep one hand on the remote to speed through anything that threatens to ruin your mood. And finally, if real people getting fucked (or pretending to get fucked) on film just isn't your thing, you might prefer adult graphic novels—no live humans are harmed or humiliated in the making of their truly naughty illustrations!

Making Peace with Your Perversion—Don't be embarrassed about what turns you on. It's your fantasy, so own it! (That said, the hottest fantasies will usually make you blush a bit.) Remember, fantasizing about something *doesn't automatically mean you actually want it to happen.* For example, imagining what sex might be like with your favorite A-list celebrity doesn't mean you want to cheat on your partner or that you would cheat if given the chance (especially as celebrities are notoriously narcissistic—a recipe for dreary sex!). Another example is the rape fantasy, which is one of the most common fantasies out there, especially for women. Let's be clear here: fantasizing about rape does not mean you actually want to *be* raped; it simply means you get off on the notion of erotic power plays (p.154) within the confines of your own mind, where you control everything that happens (even if you're imagining you have *no* control). In the same vein, mentally experimenting with a same-sex partner doesn't automatically make you gay, dreaming about receiving a spanking doesn't mean you've got self-esteem issues, and picturing yourself with Fabio under a waterfall doesn't make you weak in the head (if it did, then a billion romance-novel readers would have the world's therapists booked solid). Don't worry about making your fantasies fit your day-to-day values, your real-life hopes and ambitions, or your notions of political correctness. As long as you don't find your fantasies distressing or intrusive or obsessive-compulsive, then give yourself permission to lie back and enjoy them.

Know When to Hold Them—There's no rule that says you have to share every single dirty thought that crosses your mind. Maybe that gangbang fantasy you enjoy during your self-love sessions is hot precisely because nobody knows about it. Or if your partner's the jealous type, then they don't need to know that you occasionally rub one out while imagining their best friend, or worse, their parent (actually, even if they're not the jealous type, we might keep this one under wraps). And you know what? Though some therapists might tell you otherwise, we think it's alright if you secretly fantasize about someone else during sex with your partner every now and then, too. Lifelong monogamy can be a slog sometimes, and if we'd all cut ourselves a little slack in the fantasy department, we reckon the world would be a happier, sexier, less adulterous place.

Sharing Is Caring—Of course, sharing a fantasy with a partner can be a cheap and easy way to foster trust and intimacy, and kink things up. But it takes courage. What if you think yours is too mundane to put into words (remember Meg Ryan's faceless stranger fantasy in *When Harry Met Sally*?). Or what if you're afraid your partner will be jealous or even disturbed? Or what if they laugh? Set the stage for safe sharing by asking your partner to tell you one of their biggest/darkest/strangest masturbation fantasies, explaining that it'd be such a turn-on. Promise them you won't judge or giggle (and keep that promise). If they're reluctant, set a brave example by offering up one of your own (insist that they honor the no-giggling rule, too). Or the next time you're having regular old comfort sex, talk about something you'd like to try now, something you'd like to try eventually, or something you'd never want to try but are simply turned on by. Then suggest that your partner do the same (no pressure though!). Or just recount a dirty story you read. The fact that you're having sex at the time will mean awkward pauses can be filled with moans. And when you're both distracted by physical pleasure, there's less pressure for your fantasy to make narrative sense. Just a sentence or two here and there will get the point across.

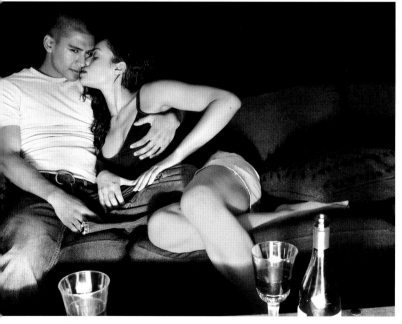

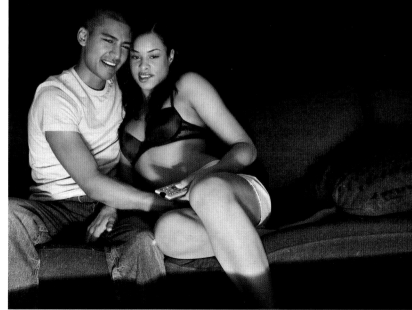

Roleplaying

Why do we like to watch Hollywood blockbusters and reality TV, read trashy novels, hear all the gory details about our co-worker's one-night stand, or download Internet porn? Because we like to live vicariously! Well, roleplaying is like that, except the thrills are experienced first-hand. Pretending to be someone you're not, in a safe, predetermined, sexual scenario, gives you a break from being your own bad self. In other words, if you're kind, giving, shy, and timid in your daily life, then roleplaying grants you permission to be cruel, selfish, confident, and bold (at least for as long as the sex lasts). If you're a career-minded, tough-talking go-getter, then roleplaying gives you an excuse to be a weak, vulnerable, sexual doormat. You get all the benefits of being "bad," with none of the soul-fattening guilt! So how do you turn this fantasizing into hot, kinky, real-life roleplaying? Read on.

After Party—If you hate karaoke, and if public speaking is one of your greatest fears, then the whole idea of acting out your fantasies probably sounds about as appealing as, well, karaoke and public speaking. If that's you, then use Halloween or your next fancy dress party to test the sexual benefits of roleplaying: wear something a little out of character that makes you feel sexy and use it as an excuse to act a little differently. When you get home with your partner, keep the costume on and stay in character while you start making out. The stupendous sex will practically happen by itself. And then you'll be a convert.

Making a Scene—No costume parties in your datebook? You'll just have to jump right in. But that doesn't mean you can show up in a ski mask at your new girlfriend's place one night—something that heavy must be figured out in advance. Lighter forms of roleplaying—with a blindfold or a pair of fuzzy handcuffs, say—can be negotiated on the fly, especially in a long-term relationship. But you'll usually have to do *some* planning.

Before you start complaining about sex being so much work, think of it this way: the planning is just part of the foreplay. Once your imagination has been sparked, start exchanging dirty emails, text messages, and late-night phone calls about how the scene is going to go down. Leave out books for each other and mark the pages that caught your eye. Make a saucy to-do list and slyly show it to your partner under the table during drinks with friends. Surprise your partner with those props you've been ogling. The point of doing all this ahead of time is so that you can lose yourself in the moment (instead of worrying, "Am I pressing too hard? Am I saying the right thing? Do these assless chaps make my butt look big?") .

If the planning still feels duller than Excel spreadsheets, take consolation in this: the more you get into the kinky swing of things, the less communication it all takes, and the more natural it feels. If you successfully negotiate a strict teacher/naughty student scenario, and it turns out that you both love it, then the next time you want to get into character it'll come a whole lot more naturally. Eventually you'll get to know each other's kinky mood swings so well that you'll be able to tell whether it's a good day for roleplaying.

Getting into Character—Roleplaying can give some helpful context to the kind of kinky sex you're engaging in: if it feels weird to spank a grown man, then pretending he's a naughty boy might make things feel more believable. If you're using costumes, get dressed in separate rooms to cut down on the giggle factor. But you don't necessarily need a new look—just a new attitude. A shot or two (*max*) of tequila might help (and allay some "oh my god what are we doing" fears). And then, well, just see where the mood (or the costumes) take you. If you're cringing just reading this, don't attempt extended dialogues (complete with accents) or narratives. Sometimes just having sex in costume may be all the roleplaying you need. But don't be surprised if you find yourself overcome with the urge to crawl, beg, smolder, boss, or spank, you devil you. For more on dressing up, turn the page.

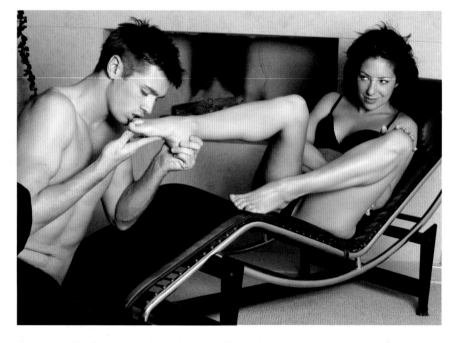

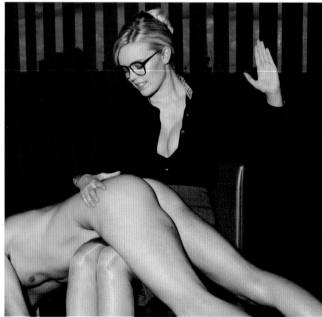

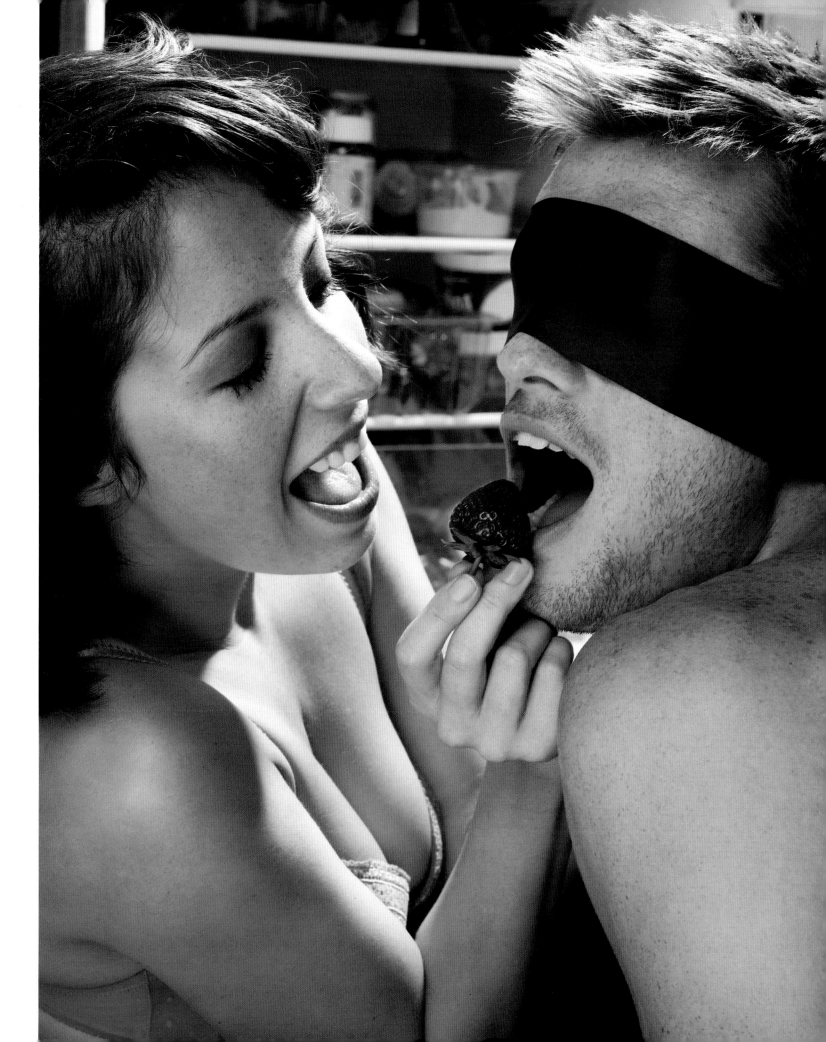

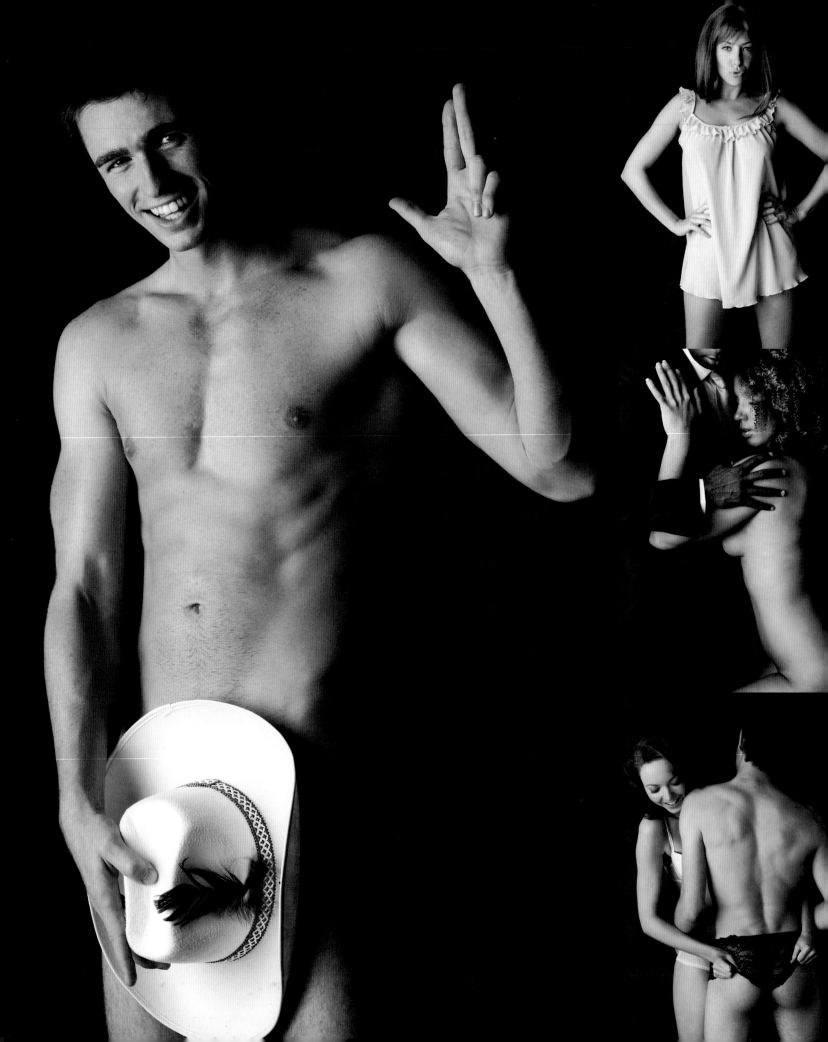

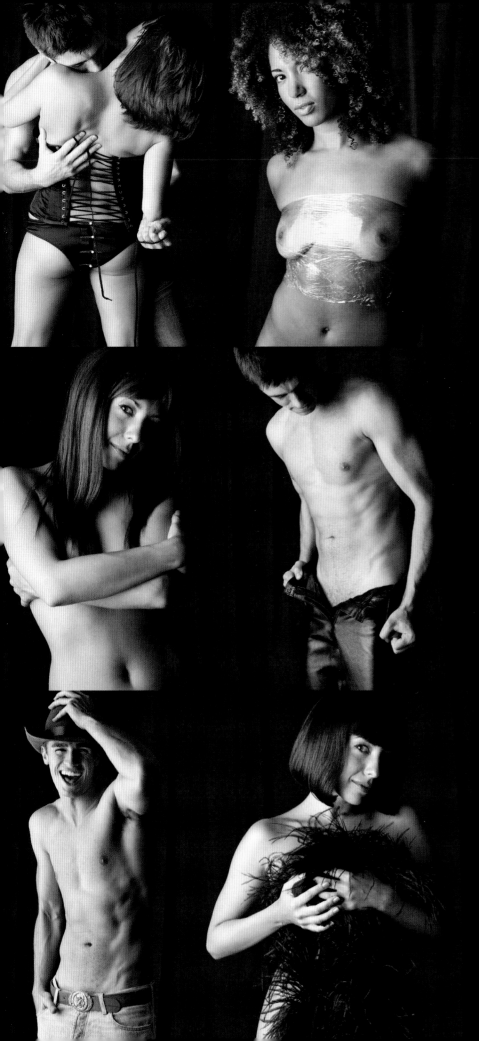

Dressing Up

You know the old joke: "Are you into casual sex or should I dress up?" Well, why *not* dress for sex? And we don't mean the kind of "dressing to get laid" outfit we discussed in the Seduction chapter—we're talking full-on, for-your-partner's-eyes-only kinky gear. Here's why: certain items of clothing are almost guaranteed to make you feel naughty. And when you feel naughty, who knows *what* you'll get up to…

Fancy Dress—Most "uniforms" at sex toy outlets tend to be tight, revealing, and made of latex. If realistic is more your style, go DIY or rent a costume from a fancy-dress party outfitter. For 100 percent authenticity, try industry supply shops or eBay. Popular costumes (whether latex or real) include: doctor/nurse, patient, priest, nun, military personnel, interrogator, police officer, law breaker, vampire, Victorian, school marm, school girl/boy, cheerleader, governess… in other words, anything that helps create or emphasize a certain sexual power dynamic. By the way, if you do decide to go latex, you may need a little powder or lube to help you slip into the outfit (hey, it's nothing to be ashamed of—scuba divers need lube, too).

Wig Out—If you're not the costume type (are you always "busy" when your friends throw fancy-dress parties?), you can simply accessorize your way to kinkier sex. Leave your hat on. Wear your sunglasses at night. She can throw her hair in pigtails and he can go crazy with the gel to create an old-fashioned pompadour just for fun. A wig is also a quick and easy way to transform sex for both of you: most gals like to play around with different looks (without making a cut or color commitment), while most guys like the illusion of partner variety that a new hairdo provides. Also, the treacherously high stiletto is totally impractical for walking (at least for most women), which means you can't really do anything in them but fuck… or at least look pretty. And a free make-up application by one of the tacky ladies at your local department store might be all it takes for you to live out your crack-whore fantasy when you get home. Or rather than wearing your "nice underwear" as we recommended in the Seduction chapter, pick up some truly "naughty" underwear— the kind made to be taken off. Basically, just wearing even one item that's slightly out of character will make you feel like a new one.

Clothes Make the Man-Slave—The right outfit can help you suspend your disbelief and facilitate some of that roleplaying we discussed on the previous page. When you're wearing your six-inch, buckled-up boots, you *will* feel powerful like a proper dominatrix should; when your girlfriend convinces you to try on her panties or your boyfriend wraps you in plastic wrap*, you *will* feel owned like a Ken or Barbie doll; when you secretly wear a corset under your power suit, you *will* feel deviant; an authentic-looking police uniform *will* make frisking come more naturally; when you're wearing your little French maid costume, you *will* feel like bending over to do some light dusting, "accidentally" exposing your frilly-bottomed panties on the way; and in your naughty nurse's outfit, you *will* finally muster the confidence to poke your boyfriend with a well-lubed, latex-gloved finger (p.119). You don't necessarily need a script and a scenario to act out: an outfit can be enough to affect the way you touch, kiss, and talk.

Because we care: plastic wrap is a form of bondage, thus you should follow the standard bondage safety guidelines on p.156. In a nutshell: don't cut off circulation, don't cover breathing passages, and watch for overheating.

Exhibitionism & Voyeurism

Dressing Down: The Striptease—The traditional striptease is not for everyone: some consider it the ultimate display of female sexual power, while others find it embarrassing or even demeaning. One thing's for sure: many a man truly enjoys the visual, so an erotic dance can be a generous gift. This is not to suggest that the ladies don't like to look too. Or that a striptease can't be a joint effort or a male endeavor (we think it should be, and often). But for the sake of simplicity, the following do's and don'ts are written assuming the lady in the relationship *wants* to be the first to perform. You go-go girl!

Do

—rent *9½ Weeks* to learn from Kim Basinger's striptease: the outfit/moves/music/shy-cheeky-sexy attitude.
—slow down. Fancy moves are less important than simply taking your time with each layer.
—dance to a song that you'll both enjoy—you should feel sexy moving to it, but he shouldn't be thinking, "I can't believe she's still into boy bands."
—maintain eye contact. If your back is turned, glance over your shoulder. If you need a break, look down coyly then back up at him, like, "Who me? Strip?"
—wear a shirt with buttons: it automatically creates 10 extra moves! Play peek-a-boob with each side. Once it's undone, turn your back on him and shimmy it off your shoulders before dropping it to the floor.
—put your hair in a loose updo that you can pull out.
—use the wall: lean your back against it and writhe, or slide down into a squat and up again (so long as you're sure your thighs are strong enough to get you back up effortlessly).
—use the door jamb: span the gap with your arms and legs and move your hips.
—use a chair: straddle it backward or sit in it sideways to remove each thigh-high stocking with pointed foot in the air.
—practice removing your stockings ahead of time. For extra balance (and teasing), place your toes between his legs or on the arm of his chair while you push the stockings down.
—throw clothes in his direction as you remove them.
—feel free to tell your fella, "You first" or "Now your turn!"

Don't

—think you need the body of a model or stripper to dance suggestively for your partner. He'll be focused on the show, not on your so-called imperfections.
—forget that a strip is in the hips: keep them moving.
—let your arms hang limply. If you're not undressing, put your arms up in the air and cross your wrists while you move your hips side to side, or trace a body part—thighs, stomach, opposite arm, hips, breasts—with your fingers.
—wear tight trousers. Because if you can look sexy while taking those off, then you can quit your day job. Instead, wear a pencil skirt that you can push down (while bending forward with your back or side to him) and then step out of.
—take off your heels (except to remove stockings—and you could put the heels back on once the stockings are off).
—forget the *tease* part of "striptease": pull your skirt up or your underwear down a few inches before removing, push your bra straps off your shoulders before turning away to unclasp, and don't get completely naked until the very end—and even then, tease him with a back view until he can't take it anymore.
—forget your audience. Walk toward him (one foot all the way in front of the other, like you're on a catwalk) and loop his tie or a piece of your clothing around his neck to pull him closer to your face or cleavage.
—install a pole in your bedroom.

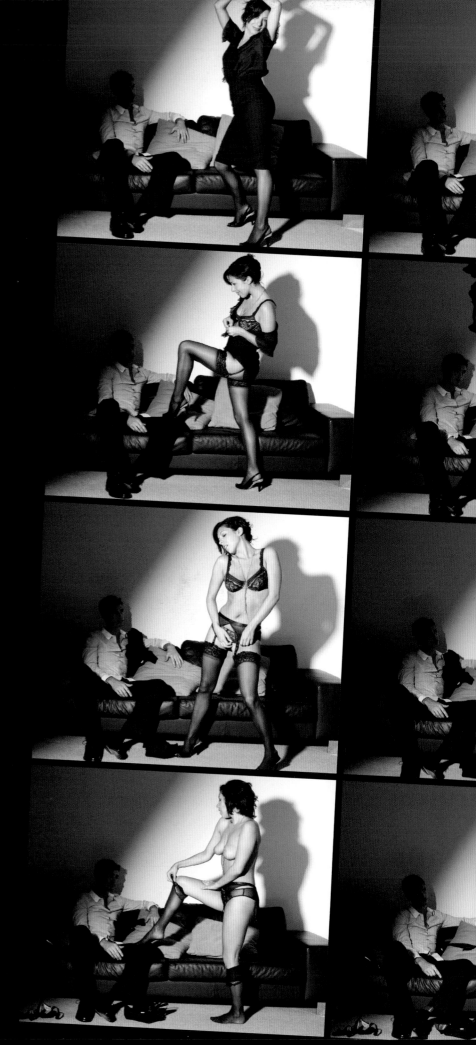

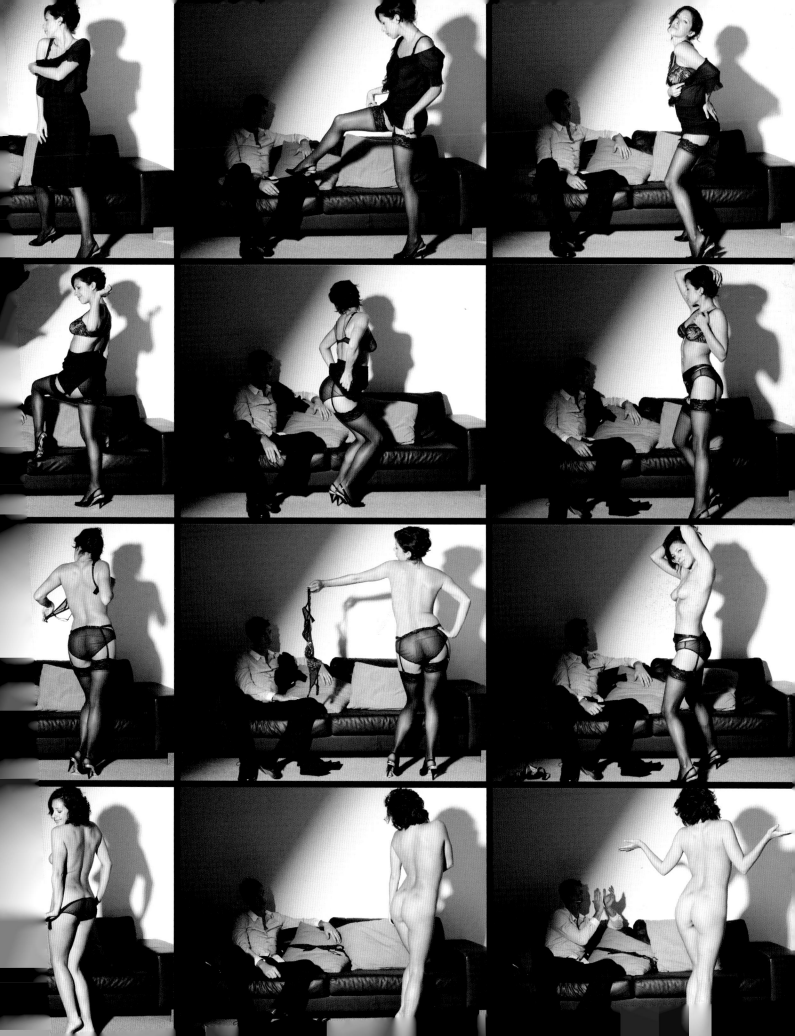

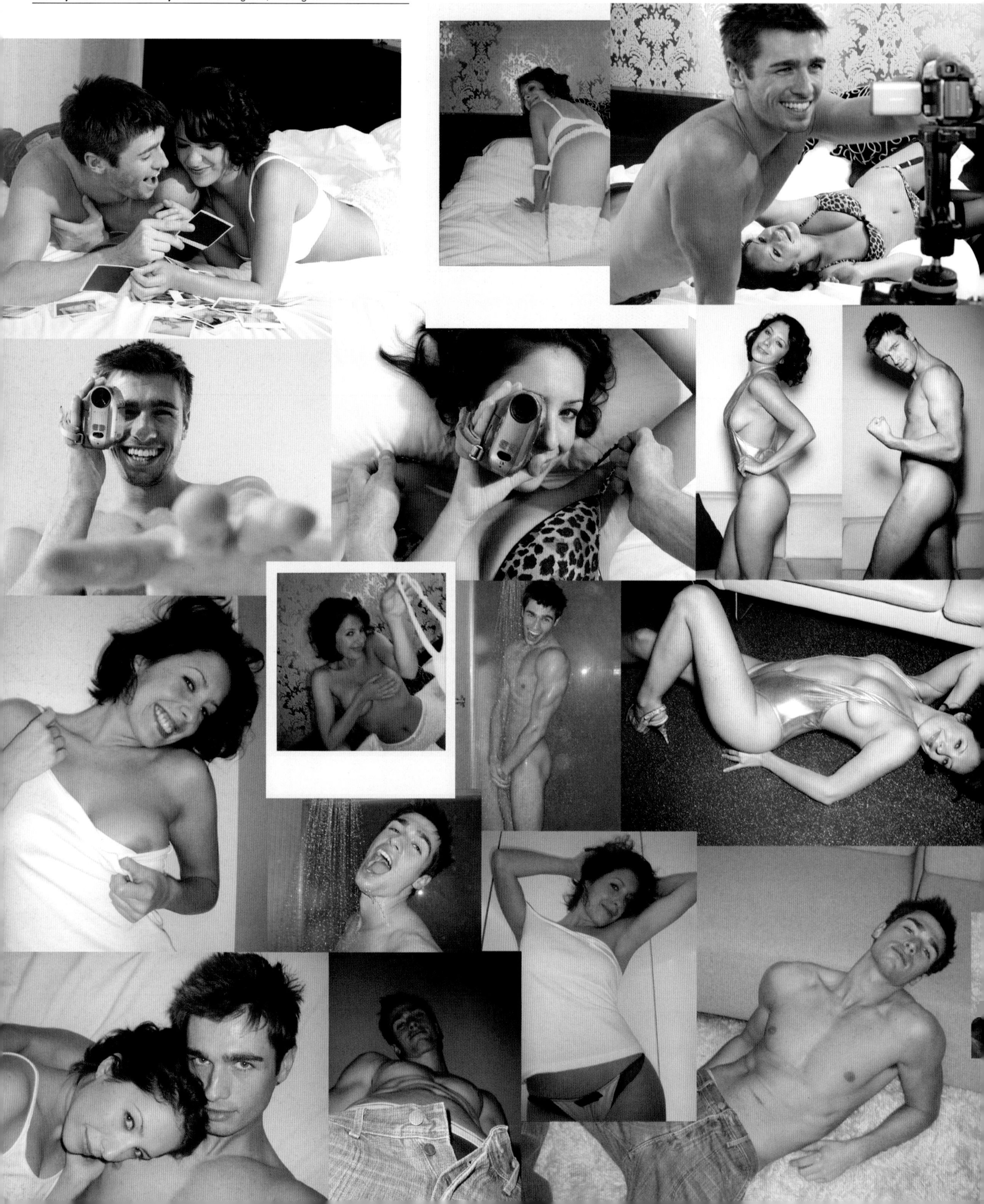

Taking Pics, Making Vids

You don't have to look, sound, or act like a porn star or producer to whip out a camera during your next romp in the bedroom. In fact, you don't even have to like pornography to enjoy making your own. After all, creating naughty pictures and videos together is more about the process than the end result: engaging in your own sexual shoot, whether as the star or the director or both, automatically makes things more dramatic and theatrical, even if you end up keeping most of your clothes on or refuse to make any cliched "orgasm faces." You could erase all incriminating evidence immediately afterward and still have the pleasant memory of an amazing show-and-tell session. Plus, that way, there's no chance that a family member will ever stumble upon your "art," that an insensitive partner will show it to friends, or that a bitter ex will post it on the Internet as payback for a broken heart.

Very Candid Camera Tips—

• Whether you're shooting photographs or video, start off slowly, leave some clothes on, tease—there's no need to get totally naked and go for the full-on spread-eagle or "money" shots. Sometimes showing less is more.

• In fact, if you have any body parts you're self-conscious about, then by all means use an item of clothing, a blanket, a pillow, dramatic chiaroscuro lighting, or your partner to hide them.

• A tripod is your friend. Use it to photograph or film yourself when you're alone so you can practice poses and moves. When you create something you like, make it a surprise present for your partner (assuming you trust them implicitly): hide it in their suitcase before a business trip or (e)mail it to them as a promise of things to come. When you're together, use a tripod so you can both be in the shot.

• That said, it's also fun to pass the camera back and forth, so you can experience both sides of the exhibitionism/voyeurism coin. Plus, you'll probably capture a better sense of action and movement than you might with a static, tripod-mounted camera.

• If you're behind the camera, don't shoot your subject from below, or from any unflattering angles for that matter. Consider your subject and try to make them look as good as possible—and not just what you think looks good, but what you think they'll think looks good.

• If you're in front of the camera, don't slouch (it creates rolls), do flex your muscles (it masks flab), and do work your good side (you know you have one).

• Ladies: arching your back, pointing your toes, and lifting your arms over your head are all feminine slimming tricks.

• Avoid harsh, overhead, or florescent lighting—it tends to highlight imperfections. Experiment with daylight from a window, low-wattage lightbulbs in lamps, and candlelight.

• Review the pictures or the film together. Delete anything that makes you feel uncomfortable, whether it's for reasons of vanity or caution. But don't be too hard on yourself or too overprotective—in 20 years you'll wish you had that body back again and might appreciate it captured for posterity.

pHOTography—

• For still photography, don't use film that needs to be developed by a professional. Go with instant-gratification gadgets like digital cameras and Polaroids.

• In fact, we highly recommend Polaroids for their retro factor, their built-in suspense mechanism, and the fact that they're not great with detail, which is good news for imperfections and modesty.

• Avoid using a harsh flash that lights up the whole room. Go with ambient light: that'll mean you'll have to hold the camera very still to keep the picture from turning out blurry, but the improved aesthetics of the picture will be well worth it.

• Speaking of blurriness, sometimes that's not a bad thing. For example, you could both hold still save for her pumping hand around his unit and then take the pic—chances are that focal area will come out blurry and end up looking a little more arty (i.e. less porny). Blurriness can also nicely capture the motion and drama of, say, intercourse.

• If you're standing for the camera, pose at an angle (rather than straight on), have good posture (it makes you look thinner), and do something with your arms (other than keeping them at your sides).

• Respect the laws of gravity: taking a picture of your partner when you're on top and they're on the bottom usually looks better than when you're in the reverse positions.

• Don't feel like you have to strike a pose for every shot. Just like when you're on vacation, the best pictures are the action shots (when you're in the middle of doing something, moving, or laughing) rather than those boring, stiff, head-on shots in front of landmarks.

Id Vid—

• When filming video, you don't have to include your full bodies in the shot. You don't even have to show anything that dirty. Try a cool angle, like from the head of the bed (but remember, never from below lest you look like beached whales) or a close head-&-shoulders crop: the focus can be on your expressions, your sounds, and the intimacy of the moment. Or shoot everything but your faces.

• Turn on the night-vision feature—it obscures any imperfections and creates a funky, sci-fi look. Plus, you can shoot entirely in the dark, which is a tequila-free method of loosening inhibitions.

• If your squeaky mattress gives the video a slapstick feel, then cut the sound and replace it with your favorite in-the-mood song. (A million Hollywood directors can't be wrong.)

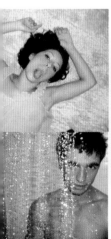
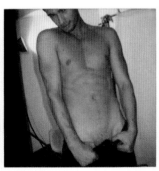
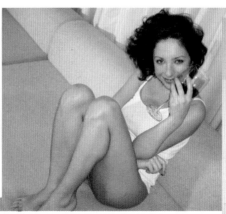
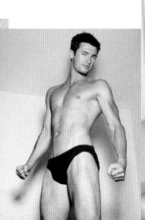
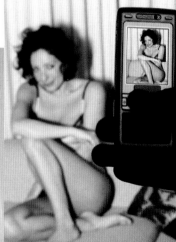

Once upon a time, "kink" meant deviant sex, which implied that those who did things a little differently in bed were touched in the head. But that meaning has gone out of favor with open-minded people who like sex. The new rule is, as long as something is safe and consensual, then it's fair play. These days kink is more often thought of as any sex or erotic play that's off the beaten path. This has less to do with fucking in the woods near a hiking trail (though that could count too) and more to do with BDSM—in fact, the word "kink" has come to serve as a friendly synonym for any non-mainstream sexual interaction. BDSM stands for bondage & discipline, domination & submission, and sadism & masochism.

Sexual power plays are the glue that holds BDSM together—the creamy center of all kink. If good sex is about a mutual give and take, then good kinky sex is about deliberately manipulating that give and take together (i.e. consensually) in order to create psychological and/or physical drama in the bedroom. Typically, one partner—"officially" referred to as the top, or the dom—agrees to take control (and thus most of the responsibility for the couple's physical and emotional safety) while the other partner—referred to as the bottom, or the sub—trustfully agrees to relinquish it.

These terms derive from the gay male community, wherein "bottom" means "receptive one" (the partner being penetrated), and "top" means the partner doing the penetrating. Traditionally, these roles were assumed to be set in stone, and when they were first adopted by the official kink community, they were taken very seriously. But kink's not just for specialists anymore: anyone can do it (no matter what their sexual orientation), being a top or bottom doesn't have to be a permanent state (you can trade places from one session to the next, or even mid-session), and you don't even have to use the official lingo. If you should relinquish control to your partner for an hour or two, you don't have to be penetrated, or get *literally* on the bottom *à la* missionary sex, or even be in a particularly submissive mood either (though the two frequently go hand in hand, kind of like Paris Hilton and sex tapes). And if your partner agrees to give you control, you don't have do any penetrating, or get *literally* on top, or even be in a particularly dominant mood either (though, again, the two frequently go hand in hand, kind of like piety and side-partings). No, the bottom is simply the one receiving stimulation while the top is the giver. Stimulation can be a spanking, an icy-hot rubdown, 30 feet of rope, a pinkie finger, a butt plug (p.136), or a good ol' tongue licking while tied up.

So why would a loving couple in a relationship that's based on mutual respect want to put each other in such compromising positions, ones that might result in vulnerability, embarrassment, or even a bit of pain? Because those things make sex exciting, especially for long-term couples who've lost the suspense of the unknown that automatically comes with brand new partners. And taking turns being the boss can serve as a reminder not to take each other's naked willingness for granted. Even though playing with power in the bedroom creates the illusion of an unequal or unfair erotic relationship, the goal is that both parties get off on their respective roles. Because each role actually—and in the top's case, ironically—puts the pleasure of the other first and foremost.

BDSM

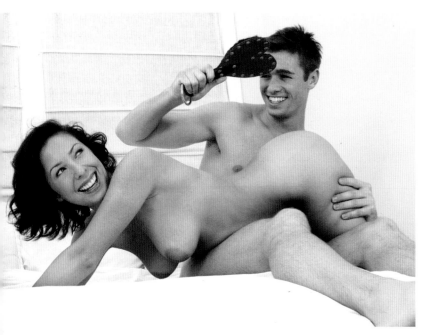

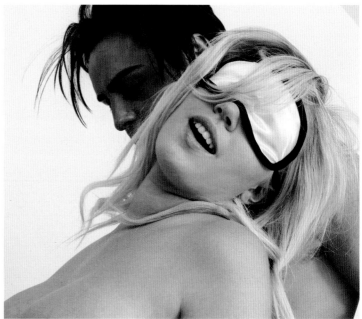

You'll still hear plenty of people today declare that kink is pathological or immoral or anti-feminist or "largely a gay thing" (and we'd bet that at least one of them keeps a gimp in the cellar). And you'll hear plenty more people declare that BDSM is just plain weird (and we bet a good chunk of them can't have sex with the lights on). But without the poo-poo-ers, this stuff wouldn't be half as fun. Still, we pity them: when you compare kink to the alternative—sex in the same position 2.4 times a month, lying back and thinking of England—who wouldn't want to get their kink on? What follows are some easy ways to do just that.

Bondage—The "B" of BDSM, bondage involves restraining someone during an erotic exchange in order to limit their movement, and thus their control. Because bondage requires the least amount of creativity and theatrics (hey, if you've got a wide silk necktie and a willing partner, you're good to go), it's the most common form of kink. Your parents have probably even dabbled (we know: *eeeeew*). Still, it demands you follow some serious safety rules. Turn to pp.156–163 for techniques and guidelines.

Discipline—Discipline is bondage's loyal sidekick, at least as far as the BDSM acronym is concerned. That said, you might enjoy bondage for years without ever bringing any discipline into it. As an umbrella term, discipline covers pretty much everything kink-related that you might do to a partner besides restraining them, from the physical (e.g. spanking) to the psychological (e.g. sexual orders such as "Bathe me… go down on me for 10 minutes… now kiss me, you fool!"). Whatever form the discipline takes, and whatever the "reason" (pure physical pleasure, pure physical torture, sexual mind games, etc.), the general idea is the same: the dominant partner is creatively exerting the power that the submissive one has handed over to him or her.

Domination & Submission—The "DS" of BDSM. While bondage and discipline occasionally have nights out without each other, domination and submission are entirely codependent: "D/S", as it is symbolically known in the kink community, is essentially the psychological element of BDSM— the power exchange that takes place in just about all kinky play. A dominant type gets off on power—but first you have to get your partner to give you that power (it's all about consent, remember?). Submissive types get off on yielding control— but first your partner has to be willing to take it (it's not just bottoms who have to give consent).

Sadism—The "S" of SM and BDSM: deriving sexual pleasure from inflicting physical—and, way less commonly (especially where this chapter is concerned), emotional—pain and abuse on a willing recipient. While a masochist can happily exist without a sadist in their life (that's what masturbation is for…masturbating with nipple clamps, that is), a sadist needs a willing masochist. After all, any self-respecting sadist's pleasure is dependent on the knowledge that the recipient of their erotic "torture" is truly enjoying it. (Getting off on an accidental 5-car pile up is not what we're talking about here.)

Masochism—The "M" of SM and BDSM: getting your rocks off on physical—and, way less commonly (again, especially where this chapter is concerned), emotional—pain and abuse. Contrary to popular belief, you don't have to hate yourself to befriend erotic pain. While masochism was once associated with mental illness, it's considered fair play these days, so long as it's "safe, sane, and consensual" (p.156). Some people theorize that masochists are genetically predisposed to enjoy pain, while others think masochists are made (and not necessarily born), whether through early childhood "imprinting" or a series of life experiences. Just as you can be a submissive who's not interested in pain, you can be a masochist who's not interested in submission. And accidentally slamming your finger in a door isn't likely to evoke multiple orgasms: the pain must be delivered and received in an erotic context. See pp.164–167 for more on how light erotic pain *might* work for you.

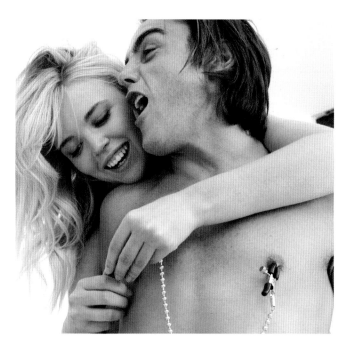

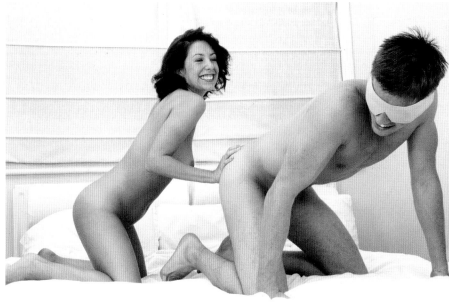

Playing It Safe

Communication is essential to any kinky scenario, but especially so when it comes to BDSM. Because this kind of play can involve heavy emotions and some physical risks (if you don't follow the rules), you need to establish your expectations and limitations ahead of time, and reaffirm them as you go, in order to make sure that everything continues to feel sexy throughout your kinky play, even if you're tied up and being spanked! To do that, make sure you've got all of the following...

Understanding—Before roleplaying, exchanging power, or inflicting painful-pleasure, make sure you each comprehend what the other would like to happen, what they would hate to happen, and what they would break up with you over. Do this explicitly by talking things through beforehand, exchanging do's & don'ts lists, and asking questions. For more on kinky communication, turn back to "Making a Scene" on p.146.

Empathy—When it comes to kinky play, you should be able to take what you dish, to see things from the other side, to say you've walked a mile in your partner's 6-inch stilettos. Even if you determine you are a dominant for life, you should know what it feels like to be spanked or paddled or tied up or anally poked or whatever it is you want to do to your partner. Being the recipient of a sensation will only make you a better provider (kind of like how shrinks are required to get therapy themselves). Besides, if you try it, you just might realize you like it!

A "Safe, Sane, & Consensual" Philosophy—"Safe, sane, & consensual" is a BDSM motto that emerged in the '80s (along with shoulder pads, a-ha, and political correctness) to distinguish kinky play from the kind of sadomasochism found in the classic shrink handbook *Diagnostic and Statistical Manual of Mental Disorders*. "Safe" means taking care to avoid injury, playing within the limits of your expertise and experience, and using common sense (e.g., never letting a complete stranger or a vengeful ex tie you up). "Sane" refers to your frame of mind, i.e., don't play when you're drunk, high, sad, mad, or otherwise incapable of operating heavy machinery. And "consensual" means that all involved parties agreed to the activity (and no one was stumbling drunk when they gave said consent).

We'll Say It Again: Consent—For those of you who like the obvious to be made super obvious, consent is what makes kinky activities legal. Therefore, it should come before anything else in this chapter. A bottom is only a bottom if they consent to be a bottom—and they're not really a bottom unless their partner consents to be a top. (Because what are two bottoms going to do for fun—sit around blowing sunshine up each other's asses? "You are my all-knowing Master, I'm yours." "No, you're too wonderful to be anything but my god-like Mistress, how can I please you?" "No, how can *I* please *you*?"...) But even if given, consent may be withdrawn at any moment with the deployment of the safeword.

Safewords—These are the BDSM equivalent of crying uncle. A safeword is a pre-agreed-upon term that means "game over" (or at least, "time out") during a kinky session, so that "no" doesn't have to mean no. After all, in the world of kink, the word "no" is one of the sexiest tools at your disposal— why spoil the fun by making it actually do its job? A safeword means you can beg and moan all you want, you can cry for your mommy, you can yell "Stop it, you bitch", you can whisper, "Oooh that hurts, Pookie", but your partner's going to keep on going—and you'll like it, damn it. A safeword should be something you would never actually yell during sex—like, say, "Grey Poupon" or "snakes on a plane". Some people use the traffic light system, where "yellow" means "Could you ease off there a little buddy?" and "red" means "Stop everything right now". And we should mention that safewords aren't just for bottoms—the top might invoke it to mean, "Woah, heavy shit, I need to break for a Mountain Dew". Of course, not all kinky scenes require a safeword. For example, if you've been married for 10 years and have got that whole communication thing down, then it's pretty safe to say that you could experiment with ankle and wrist cuffs or a little spanking without a full-on scene negotiation or safeword. We'd like to think that in long-term committed relationships, people know each other well enough to be able to tell the difference between an ecstatic "no" and a panic-stricken or pissed off "seriously, no". That said, the more intense the play gets or the less you know each other, the harder it is to tell the difference—so, if in doubt, pick a safeword.

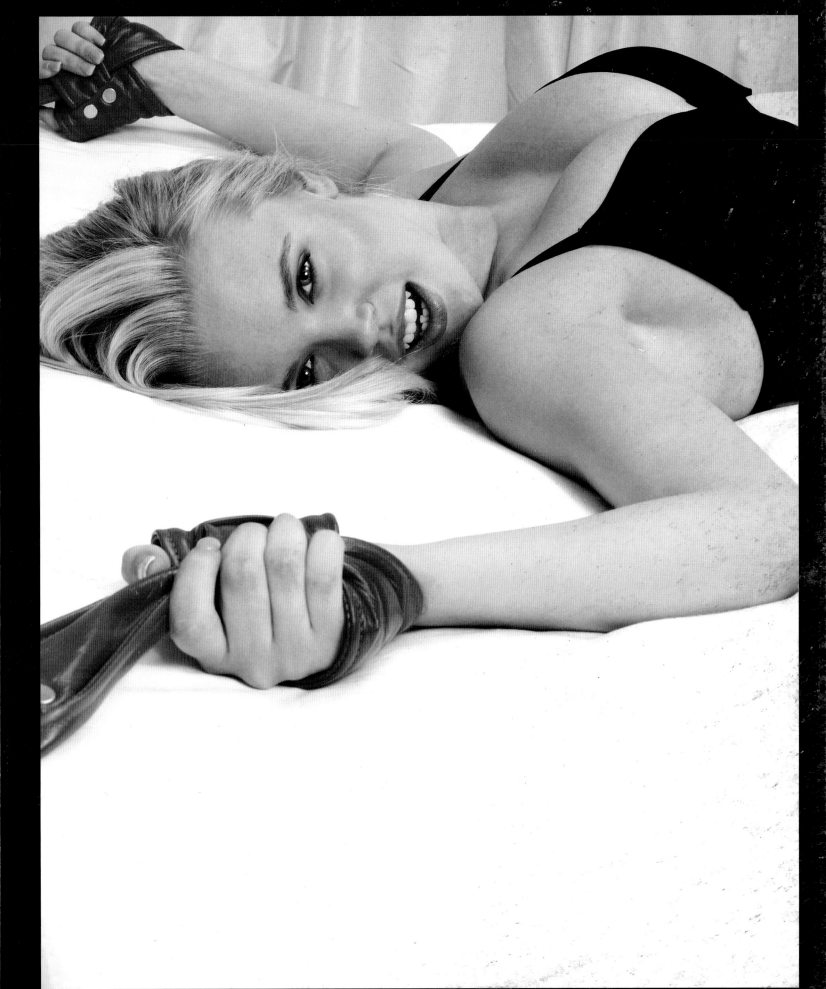

Bondage

Restraining or being restrained in an erotic context is one of the cornerstones of kink. Bondage is a great on-ramp to kinky play because you don't have to get into character or find your motivation in order to do it. In fact, quite the opposite—the ties that bind can actually bring on a kinky mood: a pair of made-for-play cuffs (p.160) can really help you indulge that bad cop fantasy ("No donuts for you!"). And when you tie up your partner with the Ted Baker silk tie that he wore all day while slaving for the Man? Let's just say that someone's in a *lot* of trouble for screwing up the PowerPoint presentation. And as for bondage's frequent traveling companion, discipline? There's nothing like some bondage tape to make sure your bad boy or girl stays put while you give them the spanking (verbal or otherwise) that they deserve.

Not that bondage has to be accompanied by a fantasy that "explains" the situation at hand, of course. Sometimes the appeal is purely aesthetic: a series of well-tied knots can end up looking like sculpture; thick leather wristbands call to mind a rockstar's bad-boy/girl aesthetic; masks, blindfolds, and nipple clamps are accessories just like sunglasses and necklaces. Besides looking good, bondage can feel good, too—like a cozy, heavy, X-ray blanket.

Other times, the simple fact of being rendered helpless—or being responsible for this state of affairs—is enough to send you over the edge. If you tend to be too much of a giver in bed (especially true of women who worry about how long their partner spends chasing down their elusive orgasm), then a dose of bondage will force you to lie back and enjoy that partner's administrations. It's hard to stress about returning the favor when you've got about 20 feet of intricately wound rope between you and your "turn." Alternatively, if you're a bit of a sheep in the sack and always let your partner set the pace, then tying up your shepherd will force you to make some damn decisions for a change. It's the best way to find

out what you really like (speed, position, depth, angle, mayo vs. salad dressing, etc.). You may think you're not confident enough to fly solo like this, but there's nothing like being the only one who can move to make you feel like you've got all the moves. The most common and user-friendly form of bondage is the kind that you'll be familiar with from cop movies, old westerns, and the lesbian-lite film, *Bound*: tying various parts of the body to each other or to foreign objects (a chair, a bed, a large house guest, etc) to restrict movement, using rope, cuffs, neckties, or bondage tape (p.160). Technically, the term bondage also encompasses several other activities—variations on the theme, if you will—such as suspension and mummification. But such play is typically reserved for more advanced players, and we can't in good conscience recommend it for beginners or anyone who hasn't done a hell of lot more homework on the topic than this book can offer.

Bondage Safety—Even if you're just dabbling with made-for-play cuffs, bondage tape, or the simple rope techniques described on p.162, keep all your extremities intact by following these bondage do's and don'ts:

01 There's no rule that says bondage should be uncomfortable: it's not like you're illegally detaining someone at Guantanamo. In fact, if something hurts (and not in a good-pain kind of way), stop immediately. You should be playing with drama, not death—think Criss Angel rather than Houdini.

02 If something turns blue, purple, numb, or cold to the touch, it's the body's cry for help (and oxygen): release the bondage, stat! The top should check for these symptoms frequently, and the bottom should report numbness or tingling immediately.

03 Distribute the tension evenly over a wide area of flesh with the appropriate materials. Good = thick padded cuffs or several coils of thick rope tied properly. Bad = a single coil of rope, silk scarves and stockings, twine, or electrical cord —they can all cut off circulation and are a bitch to untie.

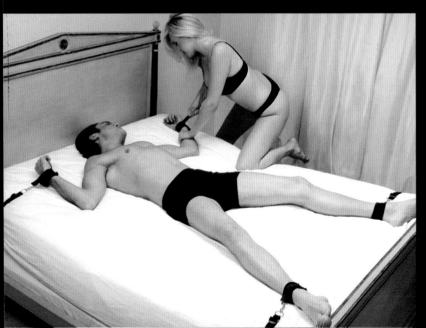
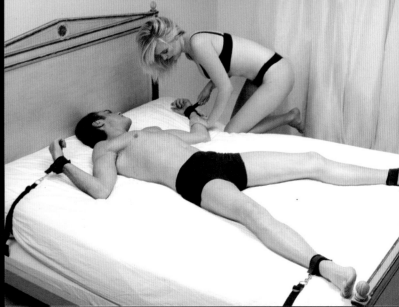

04 The more of a newbie you are, the briefer the bondage should be. Start out at 10–15 minutes—less if you spot any symptoms listed in point 2, obviously. Once you've worked on your craft and form, you can keep a healthy, willing partner in a comfortable position for half an hour or so.

05 Don't start something that you can't finish: you need to be able to release someone quickly and safely in case of an emergency (see point 2). So make sure you have medical scissors handy for cutting bondage, use the kind of rope knots that are secure but can be untied quickly (p.160), and keep keys for locks nearby. Actually, you don't want to end up nervously fumbling with your keys during an emergency —the way victims in horror movies always do when the serial killer is right around the corner—so why not stick with heavy-duty Velcro?

06 To avoid nerve or circulation damage, always leave a finger's width between skin and the ties that bind. And when binding two body parts together (e.g. wrist-to-wrist), leave a little space between those parts.

07 Bondage doesn't have to be actually inescapable (for example, your captive could probably undo two Velcro cuffs that are hooked together). But while you don't want the bondage too tight, you definitely want it to be secure and stable. If it's too loose, it can cause chafing. Plus, if your captive is struggling against their bonds and they suddenly come undone, they might hurt themselves or you —an accidental punch in the face is neither kinky nor cool.

08 Never restrain someone by the neck, suspend someone off the ground, or tie them up while in a standing position (could be a problem should they faint).

09 Don't ever abandon someone who's all tied up (you can *pretend* to abandon them to mess with their head a little, but never actually let them out of your sight or earshot).

10 Don't ever agree to be tied up by a stranger you met on the internet (or a stranger you met anywhere, for that matter), anyone who fails the finger-to-nose sobriety test, or a vengeful ex.

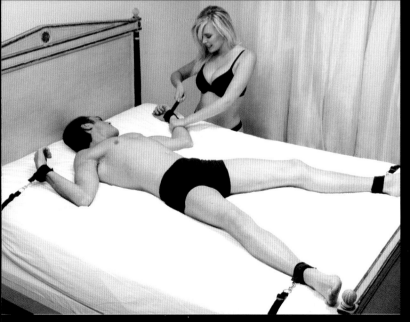
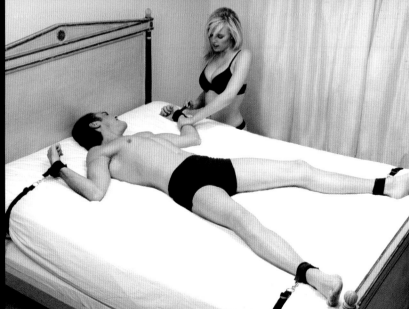

Ties That Bind

There are plenty of things you can tie your partner up with, but that doesn't mean you should. Steer clear of silk scarves, household twine, thin rope, and electrical cord—the knots will tighten with stress ("stress" being a euphemism for "your partner writhing around in torturous ecstasy") and will be hard to undo in a pinch. Plus, the thinner bindings will cut into the skin and can cut off circulation or cause nerve damage. And as for duct tape, it can take off hair and skin, so keep it in your junk drawer. The following materials are safe for simple use, so long as you follow their instructions and safety guidelines to the letter:

Bondage Tape—Did you ever wonder what office life might be like if nobody had ever gotten around to inventing Post-Its®? Not nearly so pleasingly yellow or easily adhesive, that's for sure. And that's how we feel about bondage tape: soft, stretchy, reusable, and often brightly colored PVC tape that sticks only to itself (i.e., not to skin, clothes, back hair, etc.). Sure, people have been tying themselves up since the *Kama Sutra* without it, but was it ever this much fun? And because bondage tape binds only to itself, it doesn't get tighter once it's in place—plus, no need for tricky knots! Oh yeah, and it's waterproof, too. It's possible to accidentally cut off circulation, so don't overdo it. You should also keep blunt-ended medical scissors handy in case emergency release is required. Its only real drawback? PVC ain't great for the environment, as it can't be readily recycled.

Made-For-Play Cuffs—If restraining someone by their wrists and ankles is the meat-and-potatoes of bondage, then made-for-play cuffs (sold at any sex toy store) are bondage's frozen dinners: quick, easy, and surprisingly satisfying. Bondage cuffs are way safer than handcuffs and provide instant gratification—unlike rope, with its admittedly high learning curve. Most cuffs are made of either leather (for meat-eaters) or nylon (for kinky vegans) and are often lined with faux fur or padding (for comfort even during marathon sessions). And before you complain that faux fur is "not me" or "so last season," just try writhing around in a pair of police-issue handcuffs first (on second thought, don't). Bondage cuffs feature either buckles or Velcro (the former gives a stronger hold, the latter a quicker release) and are fairly wide (at least two to three inches) to ward off the nerve damage that is a risk of traditional metal handcuffs (see, we *told* you not to try them). Avoid anything that locks with a key—those little suckers always go missing. As with any form of bondage, the bottom should speak up as soon as he or she notices any numbness or tingling, and the top should allow for at least one finger's width between cuff and skin. And bondage cuffs should never be used for any kind of suspension. For self-contained bondage, just attach wrist to wrist and ankle to ankle. You can even attach bound wrists to bound ankles (either in front or back) for an instant hogtie! For attaching cuffs to something, see "Being Tied Down" on p.163.

Rope—It's cheap, versatile, and readily available. You can certainly hop on over to the hardware store for some basic rope, but it's worth the time (and, in some cases, the money) to get higher-quality materials: poly-blend bondage rope from a sex-toy retailer, nylon boating line from boating stores, the nylon tubular webbing and accessory cord sold at climbing stores, magician's ropes made of 100 percent cotton (including the core) from magic stores, Twisted-Monk.com's hemp rope that's colored using a vegan conditioning process, and twisted rope made of soft flax or rugged promilla fibers available at KinkyRopes.com—all are washable and easy to work with. Ropes made from synthetic fibers are very smooth on the skin, long lasting, and easy to loosen, though you might have trouble getting knots to stick; keep their ends from unraveling by melting them with a candle flame. Natural fibers look and feel more rugged, are pliant, and knot tightly (though sometimes too tightly, making them difficult to undo); keep the ends from fraying by dipping in glue or nail polish or wrapping with duct tape. Many bottoms like the comfort of nylon rope, even though it can stretch out and loosen during wear; some like the tell-tale pattern twisted rope can leave on the skin; and others (especially advanced Japanese rope bondage enthusiasts) prefer the rough texture and grassy smell of hemp. Whichever material you go with, get about 50–100 feet so you can cut it into several shorter pieces. The thicker the rope, the less likely it is to cause circulation problems: beginners, stick with something between half an inch and one and a half inches in diameter. In addition to following all the rules of bondage safety, remember to distribute the tension over a wide area to avoid too much concentrated strain on muscles or joints at a single point: use several coils, a.k.a. "wraps", of rope spread evenly over an area, keeping room between rope and skin. One wrap is never enough; three to six wraps should be fine; too many and you won't be able to keep them from bunching up or overlapping (a no-no). You should always leave a finger's width of space between skin and rope. A single turn of rope around all the wraps (running perpendicular to them) can comfortably and safely provide a snugger fit while maintaining this finger's width of space. Finally, when untying (or even tying), make sure you don't whip the ends of rope around and accidentally hit your honey in the face. For more in-depth safety and technique info, check out Jay Wiseman's *The Erotic Bondage Handbook* or, for more advanced players, *The Seductive Art of Japanese Bondage* by Midori.

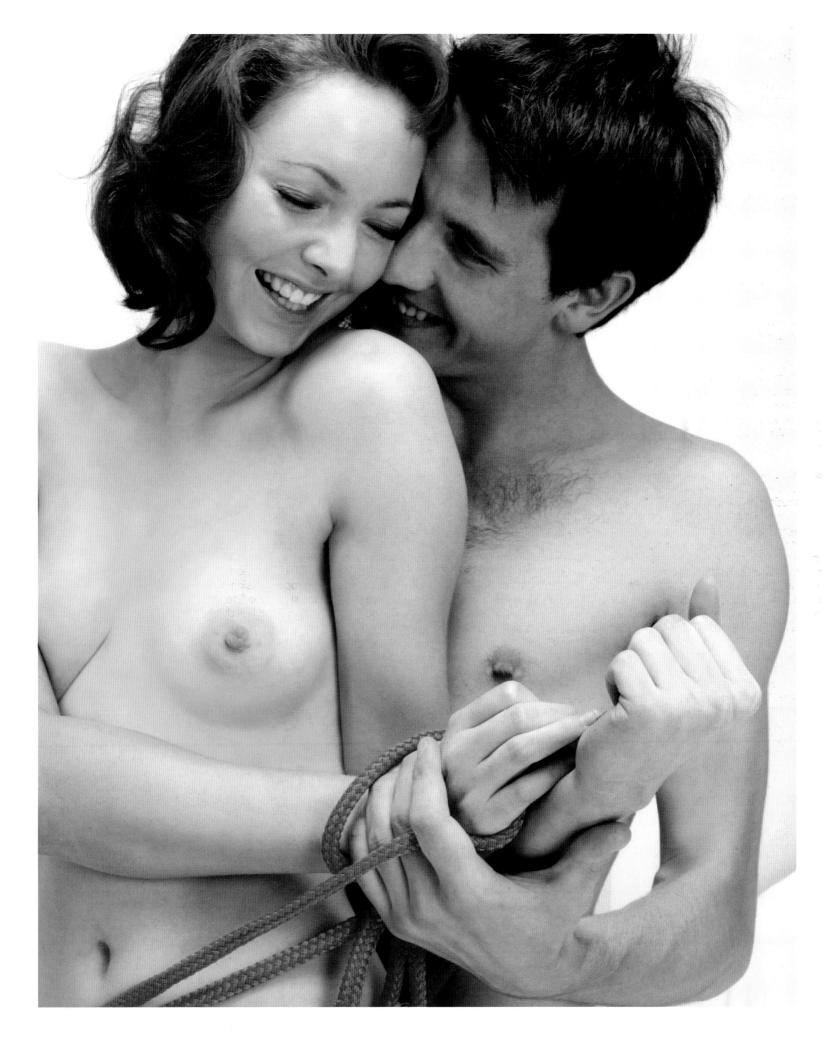

Knots

Rock climbers don't use the same knots as sailors, fisherman don't use the same knots as cowboys, and grown perverts shouldn't use the same knots as 11-year-old Boy Scouts. So drop the camping manual and get yourself Jay Wiseman's *Erotic Bondage Handbook*. In the meantime, here are the two basic knots you'll need to know in order to accomplish the techniques described in the "Rope Cuffs" section below. Use them exactly as instructed: don't go applying them willy nilly or they won't work properly or—more importantly—safely.

01. Square Knot—To make this knot, also called a reef knot, you twist the right end over and around the left; the end that started on the right should now be in your left hand and vice versa. Take the end that's now in your left hand and twist it over and around the right; you should end up with a symmetrical loop inside a loop. Good for rope cuffs and securing them to a post that's within reach of the bottom's hands (since simply tugging on one tail won't release it).

02. Bow Knot—When tying one end of rope to an object that's out of the bottom's reach, it's handy to use a knot that will come undone with a quick pull of one tail, in case of an emergency (or just an urgent desire to fuck without constraint). Simply wrap each of the tails of the rope around the post at least one time each. (Unlike with wrapping limbs, it's okay—actually it's preferred—if these wraps overlap each other, as pressure put upon them will secure them.) Then simply tie with a bow knot, the kind you use to bow your shoelaces (i.e. the first half of a square knot, and then the bow bit).

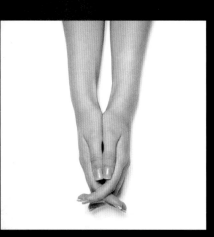

Rope Cuffs

Step 1—When binding wrist-to-wrist, put the palms face-to-face and lace the fingers together—this will help create a natural gap between the wrists for circulation room.

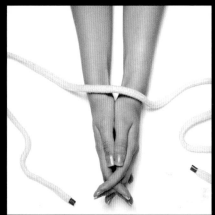

Step 2—Get about six feet of rope (a few feet longer if you plan on securing the cuff to a sturdy object later—see "Being Tied Down" opposite). Then center it over the two limbs that you're tying together.

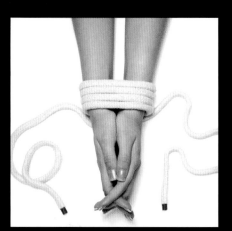

Step 3—Wrap each end around both limbs several times (at least three or four). Line the coils side-by-side and distribute the tension evenly over the skin, leaving a bit of room between the limbs—one and a half to two inches—so circulation does not get cut off and so you can cinch later.

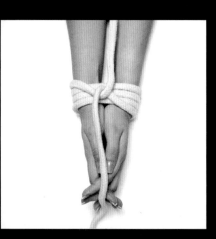

Step 4—Twist the two ends around each other at a central point between the limbs (as opposed to the side of one limb) to position the rope at a right angle to the initial binding.

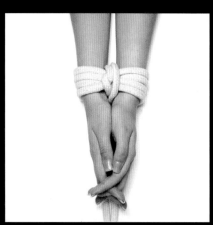

Step 5—Like a ribbon around a gift, wrap those ends in opposite directions once or twice around your initial coils of rope, between the two limbs. (If there's enough space between the wrists and you're not planning to secure the cuff to anything, you can continue to wrap at right angles to the first set of coils until you run out of rope.)

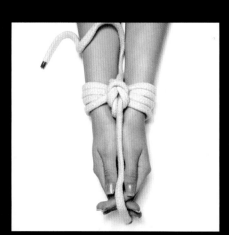

Step 6—Gently cinch the two ends to make everything evenly snug and tie them together with a square knot. When you're finished, there should be enough room between skin and rope to easily slide a finger through. You can certainly stop there, but if don't want your bottom nibbling their restraints, or if you'd like to secure the cuff to something, then see "Being Tied Down."

Being Tied Down

"Object bondage" involves restraining someone to something, like a chair or a bed. The challenge with this is to make sure that tugging won't result in a) tightening the bondage around the limb, and b) the object falling over on top of them. For this reason, your safest beginner bet is to stick with restraining someone who's lying on a bed to that bed: they'll be in a comfortable position, they won't fall should they faint, trip, or get tired, and, assuming there's no earthquake, the bed isn't going anywhere.

Made-for-play cuffs (p.161) often come with straps that can be tied or Velcroed around sturdy bed-posts, -frames or -legs. If not, they should at least have D-rings: loop some rope through these rings, wrap the two tails around the post a few times, and finish with a bow knot.

"Under the Bed" restraints, available at sex toy shops, include two pairs of Velcro cuffs, each attached via snap hooks to a long, adjustable strap that fits under any mattress (a prop almost everyone has), so you can quickly and easily secure all four limbs in a spread-eagle position without needing the right length of rope, knot knowledge, or a secure post. The downside of these is that Velcro cuffs can be weaseled out of fairly easily, and the hooks are often fairly cheap, making them less than ideal for heavy tugging. So shop around for brands with wide, padded, adjustable cuffs whose hooks and straps are strong and sturdy.

If you have the time and the inclination, rope is much more secure—plus, it's got that whole damsel (or dude) in distress aesthetic. There are innumerable options with rope (if you have the right bondage handbook), but here is one quick and easy method to master. Take about 10 to 15 feet of rope and tie two limbs together with a "rope cuff" (see previous page); then wrap the two ends of the rope, or the "tails," around a bed-post, -frame, or -leg a few times, and tie off with a bow knot if out of reach of your captive or a square knot if within their reach (see "knots" on previous page).

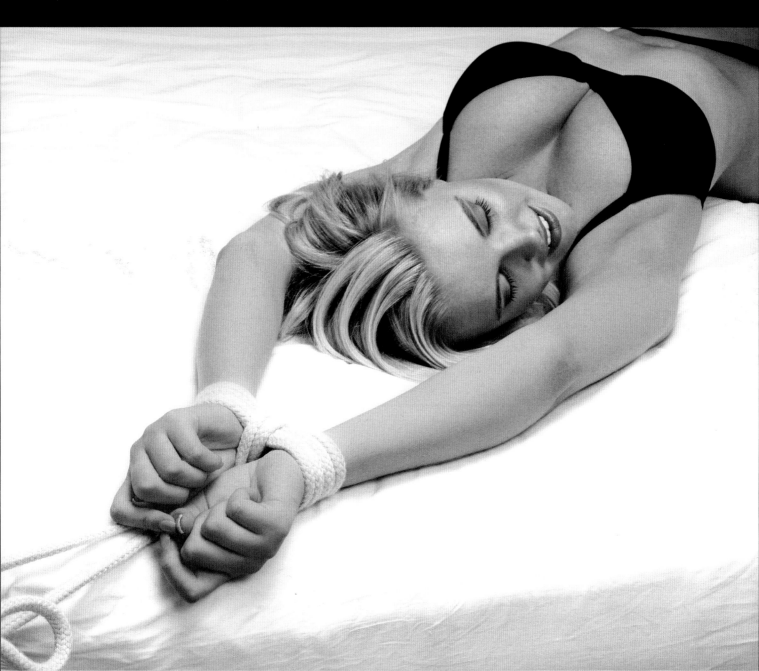

Sensation Play

Remember that game you played in elementary school where you closed your eyes or stuck your hand in a box and had to identify various objects just by using your sense of touch? Well, in the case of sensation play, you're using your whole naked body for the tactile experience, you're probably blindfolded, and it might hurt, just a little. Bare hands on your body feel good, no doubt; but sometimes you want to mix things up, arouse your nerve endings in new and unexpected ways, pretend you're having sex with Thumper, C-3PO or the Abominable Snowman. This can include being touched, tickled, teased, or tormented—with an ice cube, hot wax or tea, a fur glove, a hairbrush or comb, menthols like Ben Gay or peppermint toothpaste, a feather, an emery board, and other textured objects—pretty much anywhere on the body except internally (or on delicate external bits, either, in the case of harsher props). Alternating contrasting sensations can be quite a mindfuck. A pleasant sensation might even cross wires with a painful one, helping to lessen the latter's sting or having a Pavlovian effect on it, whereby the pain becomes associated with the pleasure. But please understand, sensation play is not meant to scar, break skin, or be excruciating—this is the softer side of BDSM. We cannot endorse the intense (read: "really fucking dangerous") forms of sensation play: blade or knife play, fire play, branding, and play piercing. While we think sex is pretty damn important, it's not worth bleeding to death or singeing off your eyebrows for.

Sensory Deprivation—By restricting your partner's ability to see, hear, and/or move, you can create a unique sensual and even psychological experience. Limiting one or more senses automatically heightens the unrestricted ones, especially touch. The simplest way to achieve this is with a blindfold: pocket the sleeping mask you get on transatlantic flights, or invest in a silk or satin version. If you go with a homemade blindfold, tie it to one side of your partner's head so they don't have to lie on the knot. The suspense created from not knowing what you're doing—or are about to do—to them can add erotic tension to otherwise routine sex. Up the ante by giving them some iPod earbuds, and they'll swear you took a Tantric workshop on erotic handwork! Or torture them by temporarily withholding touch. For some, this can be a deeply profound, moving, and even spiritual meditation; for others, it's one of Dante's levels of Hell. You'll never know until you try. Just be sure to work out a safeword (p.156) ahead of time: "turkey" means "Take me out, I'm done!" And we wouldn't recommend gagging your partner: there are too many risk factors—blocked breathing passages, gagging reflexes, miscommunication—to make it safe for beginner BDSM play.

Temperature Play (T.P.)—Turning the heat up or down on the skin can turn the heat up in the bedroom. The most common form of T.P. involves hot wax, but don't grab just any old candle. Scented and colored candles may contain plasticizers, which make them burn very hot—i.e., way too hot to be safe. Black candles and beeswax candles burn the hottest of all. We know black is the new, well, black for BDSM activities, but you're better off with the plain white paraffin candles sold at grocery and hardware stores. Better still are soy candles, which burn cleaner and at an even lower temperature than paraffin. To use: blow the candle out before dripping the wax (not a candle that's been burning for hours or else it'll be too hot); test the wax on the back of your hand first; hold above your target area (the higher you hold the candle, the cooler the wax when it touches down); when the wax hits the skin, rub it in to disperse the heat; don't drip wax on your partner's face, orifices, or hairy bits (unless they want hair removal the hard way). A great way to get your feet wet in hot wax, if you will, is to try a massage candle, available in most sex toy shops—its wax melts into a body oil when rubbed, without any messy buildup. (Turn to pp.30–33 for more massage ideas.) On the other end of the temperature-play continuum is ice: cheap, readily accessible, non-staining, and just baby-step kinky. One cold cube—traced down someone's back on a hot summer's day, or strategically placed on a lazy nipple—

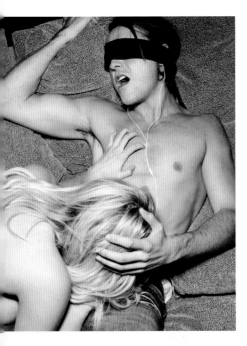
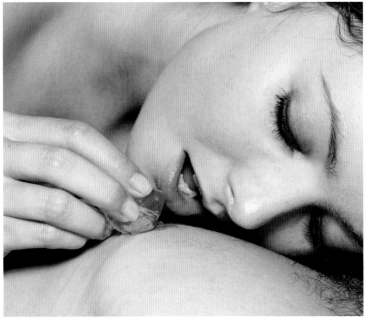
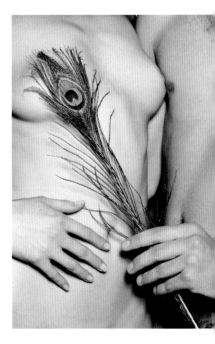

can make an otherwise ordinary session extra hot (er, cool). You can even buy aromatic ice cubes (e.g., from Kenzoki.com) or go D.I.Y. with an ice tray and some water enriched with essential oils. Just be sure to keep the actual ice on the outside of the body and away from delicate internal linings.

Other tools for temperature play include menthols, hair dryers, wet towels warmed up in the microwave… You can even take a sip of hot herbal tea or ice cold water (or suck on an ice cube) right before an oral administration to make them feel warm and cozy or send chills up their spine. Extreme forms of T.P. include fire play and branding, otherwise known as "really bad ideas."

Erotic Pain—You know "Hurts So Good" by John Cougar (Mellencamp)? Yeah, we hate that song too, but you gotta admit the lyrics make a good point: "Sometimes love don't feel like it should." When you're really turned on, pain can feel a lot like pleasure. Have you ever enjoyed rough sex or a little hair pulling during intercourse? See? Same thing. You don't have to get a Marquis de Sade–style ass-kicking to get a kick out of pain—just a nipple pinch or one well-timed spank can be enough to heighten the sexual tension.

But don't be surprised if you want a little more. Pain triggers the autonomic nervous system, which produces endorphins (opiate-like chemicals in your body) and increases your heart rate, breathing, and blood pressure—all of which is a lot like sex. This endorphin rush, also known as runner's high, can make the pain feel like intense, even euphoric sensation. If it wasn't clear before: *this* is why people like to get tied up and flogged for an hour. Add to this the eroticism of the power dynamic involved in a pain exchange, the intimacy engendered by the trust necessary for such an exchange, and the sexy vulnerability (or even humiliation) of being spanked while naked, and it's no wonder some people (admittedly, a minority) can actually orgasm from erotic pain alone. Remember, the key word here is "erotic": getting kicked in the

nuts or punched in the face is neither sexy nor safe. There's good pain and then there's bad pain—you're only interested in the former. And you get it by going slowly and always erring on the side of love pats. If good pain starts to feel like bad pain, stop immediately. Breathing steadily, making some noise, and relaxing your muscles will also help you better appreciate how pleasure and pain, like love and hate, are two sides of the same coin. Beginners shouldn't get greedy, though: one kind of erotic pain at a time. It's either nipple clamps or a spanking, but not both.

Speaking of nipple clamps, made-for-play pinchers can be a great introduction to this side of BDSM (for spanking, turn the page). Besides accessorizing the breasts (or labia, or scrotum, or even earlobes), clamps can supply varying degrees of erotic pain to the area in question, first when they're applied, but then especially so when they're finally released and all the blood goes rushing back in! Once removed, the areas may experience a period of increased sensitivity and may stand to attention more than usual. Go for varieties which allow you to vary the amount of skin you pinch (the more skin, the less painful it is) as well as the amount of pressure you apply. Tweezer-type clamps, with padded tips and a connecting chain, are a very popular choice. Just don't wear them for more than 10 to 15 minutes at a time (less if you notice anything getting blue or cold).

Of course, pain in any form, even a lightly pinched nipple, may not interest you at all: you can be into submission and only ever want soft and fuzzy touches; you can be into spanking and never want to try anything with more of an edge. Either way, make sure you've got a responsible, well-informed partner who'll treat you wrong in all the right ways. Talk about what you do and don't want to happen, and insist on lots of post-session care: namely, fixing you a cup of tea and giving you a good cuddle when it's all over.

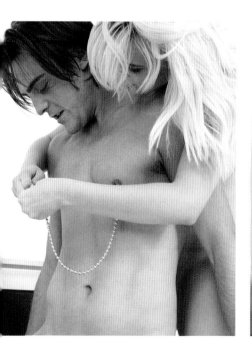
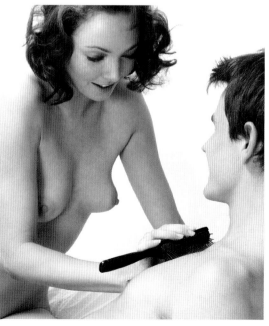
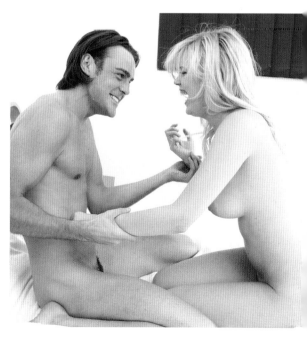

Spanking

We can't in good conscience recommend any kind of flagellation beyond what you might administer playfully with a pillowcase. Whips and floggers are serious business, and should be wielded only by serious kinksters with lots of experience. But hand-to-bum contact? Now that's something we can get *behind*. Not only is spanking more intimate and way less scary than any other type of flagellation, it's definitely safer for newbies, since you have much more control over (and better aim with) your own hand or a small paddle. Try a few spanks during a particularly passionate bout of intercourse to add some kinky flavor, or make spanking the main goal. If you're keen on the latter, then follow these important guidelines:

01 Have the spankee lie across your lap, kneel on a bed, stretch out stomach-down, or bend over something they can put their full weight on for comfort.

02 Remove all bracelets and rings.

03 Start with a tush massage to warm things up.

04 When it comes to actually spanking, start slowly and build up intensity gradually with your partner's permission, varying your pressure and strokes. You may even want to begin over jeans or underwear first.

05 Contain your spanking to the lower, fleshier halves of each cheek and the backs of the upper thighs (even if you're just having a spanking snack during sex, this area should be your target)—the lower back, tailbone, and back of the knees are your enemies in this endeavor.

06 Follow each blow with a short massage, too, to spread out the pain and keep things nice and warm.

07 A woman might like particular attention paid at the intersection of butt crack and crease, with the vibrations reverberating throughout the vulva, but definitely steer clear of his family jewels.

08 Remember that, because of your close proximity to your partner, spanking is especially great for pleasantly diddling their front side while whacking their backside.

09 If you don't want your hand to get numb, let a paddle do the work. It's easy to control the aim and the force (way easier than whips, which are too dangerous for dabblers).

10 Made-for-play paddles are available at any sex toy shop: get two paddles in one with a version that's got fluffy faux-fur on one side for a delicate touch and hard rubber on the other for a stinging slap (pictured). Or try paddles that feature shapes (like stars) or words (like "slut") cut out to help you leave your mark on your partner's bum, as if you were some kinky Zorro. However, there's really no need to invest in a pricey paddle when you've got a variety of household items that'll do the job: a wide plastic spatula, a rubber-soled slipper, and, of course, a ping pong paddle.

For more info, visit SpankingCream.com, a cute site on "honey buns" with vintage photos, advice, and yes, even "spanking cream." Also, GoodVibes.com's "Whipsmart" video has a good visual how-to chapter on love patting. SpankingBlog.com will keep you posted on all the latest breaking spanking news. And for inspiration, read *Naughty Spanking Stories from A to Z* by Rachel Kramer Bussel.

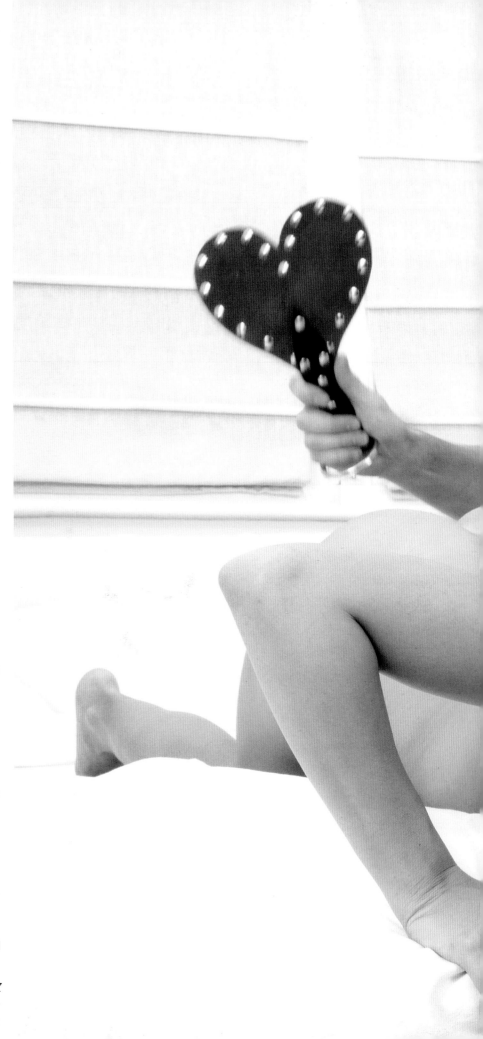

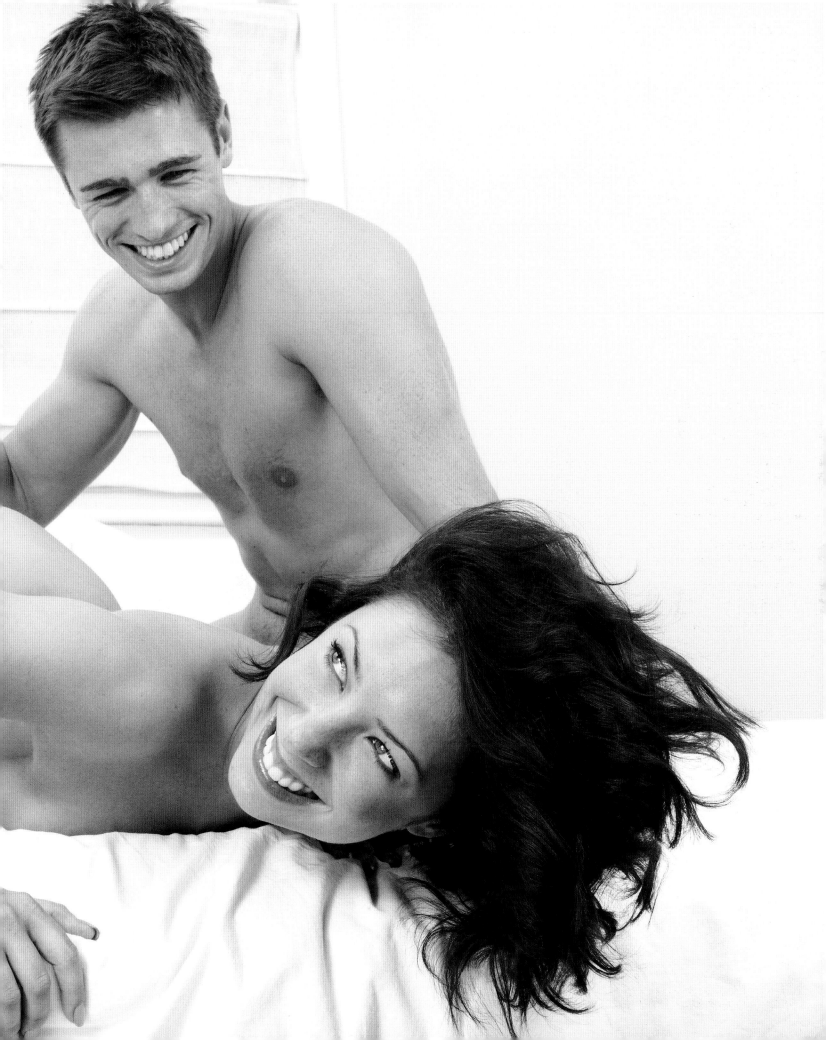

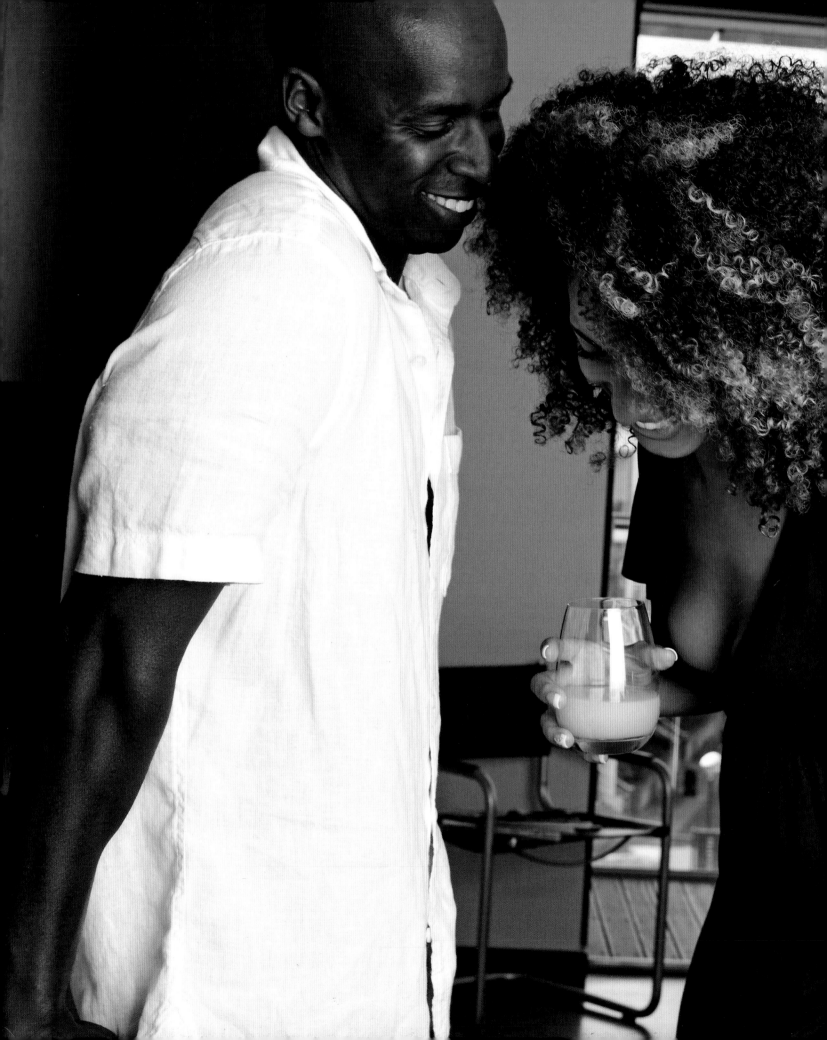

⁰⁹ Sexual Health

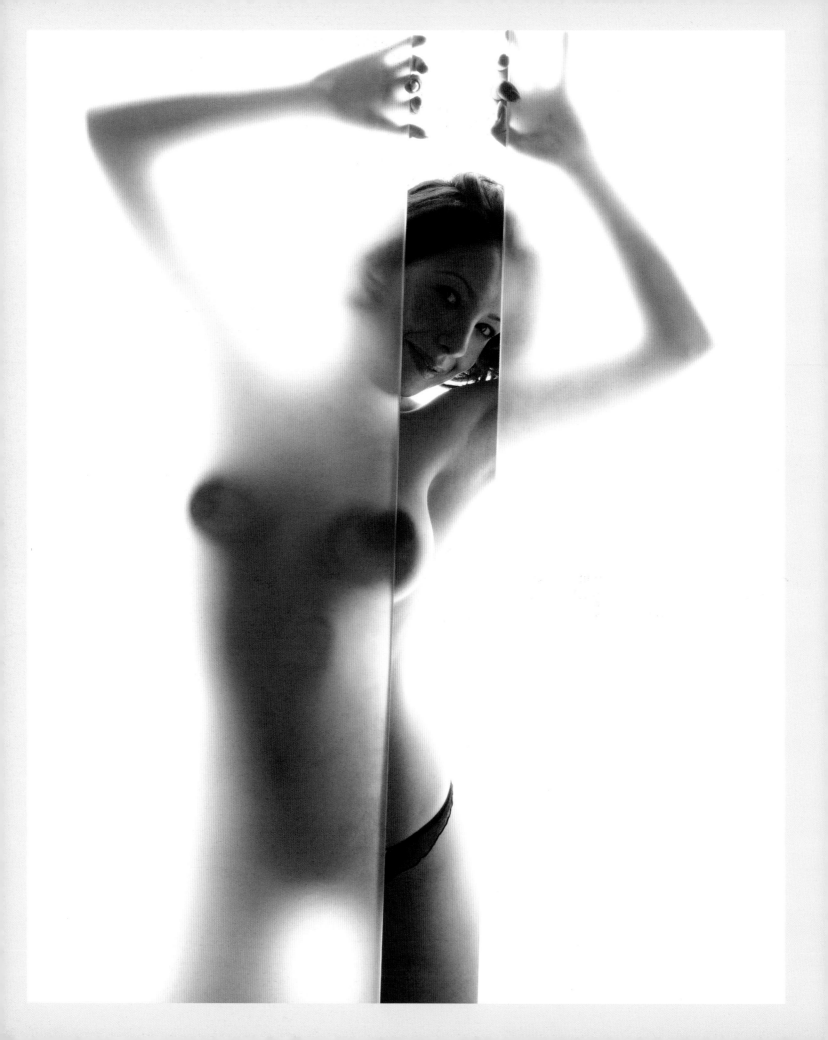

Taking Good Care

Let us guess: your first thought upon seeing the title of this chapter was "Bummer," right? Apologies for killing the mood, but we happen to think that there's nothing quite as sexy as honest, safer* sex. Think of it this way: there's nothing quite as *un*sexy as dishonest, unsafe sex that leads to bad vibes or viruses. So, logically, the opposite of all this has got to be sexy. Of course, translating this sexy logic into actual foreplay is not always such a simple equation.

Sex is messy, on many levels. And it's easy to forget just how messy when your hormones are raging, your nerve endings are all a-tingle, and your loins are on fire. So it's imperative that you educate yourself about the best ways to care for yourself, both emotionally and physically, before you get in a sexual tizzy. That way, self-preservation is second nature when desire turns you dumber than a doorknob.

And remember that a "healthy" sex life doesn't just mean you're getting it all the time. It's about quality, not quantity. Anyone can learn how to drive a car, but that doesn't mean they'll do it well or safely. You can certainly follow all the techniques outlined in this book, but if you're not starting from a place of respect, humility, open-mindedness, and plain old street smarts, the orgasms just aren't going be that good. Okay, not as good as they could be. If you're stressed out or distracted—about your body, about catching an STD, about the risk of unintended pregnancy—you won't be able to fully enjoy the sexual experience. And if you're not careful, those orgasms could actually end up hurting you —either emotionally or physically.

So learn to love your body; eat right, sleep plenty, and exercise (pp.172–173); have a straightforward conversation about your sexual history before having sex and get tested for STDs (pp.178–181); always use protection (pp.182–183) and birth control (pp.184–185) when you're with someone new… Basically, respect yourself and others. Or, at the very least, respect each other's genitals.

(*We're sticklers for grammatical accuracy, hence our use of the term "safer sex" rather than simply "safe sex". Because outside of masturbation, there's really no such thing as 100 percent safe sex. But that's no excuse not to make the sex you are having as safe as possible. Hey, it's either that or an exclusive, long-term relationship with your dominant hand.)

Healthy Living—

Good sex isn't just about putting your right hand in and taking your left foot out—a more holistic approach may be just what it takes to make the earth move for you. There are numerous aspects of your daily life that can affect your sex life, from stress levels to sleep habits, and most especially, diet and exercise. A healthy lifestyle increases your energy level and self-esteem—and both are great for your sex life. In fact, anything that does a body good will do your sex life good. As the hippies like to say, everything's connected.

Attitude

You've heard the old chestnut that your biggest sexual organ is your brain? Well, that saying has stuck around because it's true. And if you don't have your head screwed on right, you certainly can't screw well. Depression or other mental imbalances can squelch a sex drive (though, it's important to know, certain medicines can further dampen those drives). Festering resentment and miscommunication can foster bad vibes—often the enemy of intimacy. Abusing sex as a tool of power or manipulation demotes pleasure from its rightful top spot (unless all parties are on board with the power play, in which case it's just kinky, p.154). Insecurities about perceived physical flaws or inabilities, often just the result of unrealistic expectations, can sabotage a libido. The list of internal factors that can make sex more frustrating than fun goes on and on—especially, it must be said, for women. For all these reasons, it's important to check in with yourself (hey, don't laugh, crystal-wearing new-agers have great sex): analyze your motivations, communicate honestly (not critically) with your partner, and seek therapy or treatment when needed. It's all about clearing your head of anything that might get in the way of a good time for you or your partner. See the Relaxation (p.19) and Communication (p.20) sections for a good place to start.

Sleep

Make sure you're getting enough quality rest. Because the more tired you get, the more your body will start to crave sleep over sex. A nap becomes the erotic, and anything that prevents you from napping becomes, well, the opposite of erotic.

Diet

A sexy diet begins with the proper care and feeding of your libido. If you're on one of those starvation diets, you won't have the energy or stamina for sex, or even for getting in the mood. Again, this is especially true for women, whose bodies have a self-defense mechanism to prevent pregnancy when they're not physically up to it. As their weight plummets, their womb shrinks, menstruation stops, and their libido dwindles along with their dress size. This is not a free pass to eat at Mickey D's, however. Improving your cardiovascular health and lowering your cholesterol with a diet that's high in fiber, fruits, and veggies and low in fat improves blood flow to your genitals—which is exactly what happens when you get turned on. So, more blood flow means getting in the mood faster, heightened sensitivity, and possibly even stronger erections for him. Broccoli, who knew? Plus, all that fiber can do wonders for your digestive process, keeping things, shall we say, tidier, so you'll feel more confident having *all* your nooks and crannies intimately explored. You heard it here first: bran flakes and prunes may just revolutionize your sex life!

Exercise

Of course, diet is nothing without exercise. Regular workouts are just as important—if not more so—when it comes to improving your cardiovascular health, cholesterol, and thus blood flow to your genitals, and all the good stuff that entails. And that's not the only reason to hit the gym. For one thing, more stamina means more energy for hot and heavy marathon sessions—wheezing after a minute on top isn't exactly sexy. For another, many people find that when they're in better shape, their orgasms are stronger and easier to attain. And over the long-term, exercise boosts your sex hormone levels. Plus, working out just makes you feel more confident about your body, which tends to translate to hotter sex—as opposed to employing the same old position every time because it doesn't make you jiggle.

Then there's the more immediate impact of exercise: if you jump each other's bones right after a bike ride or a run, you'll have a jump-start on the foreplay, since the increased blood flow, increased heart rate, and change in breathing from a workout mimic the increased blood flow and heart rate and change in breathing due to sex. Plus, you probably associate each other's sweaty bodies with really intense sex anyway—so let those associations flow! A revved-up body just gets aroused more easily—and often lubricates more, too. Also, testosterone levels rise in the half hour after a workout, which boosts your sex drive. (All of which might explain the tales we've heard of partners who like to do naked push-ups or jumping jacks in front of each other to get in the mood, or of women who get turned on dancing around their bedrooms.) So either get fit together, or—if you don't want to be one of those cutesy couples "spotting" each other in the weight room—just warn your other half to be ready and willing on your return from the gym.

If you've worked out together, you can segue into sex play with some contact stretching: press the soles of your feet against each other's, then hold each other's hands and slowly rock back and forth. Next, one of you lies back while the other uses their body to slowly press against the back of their partner's legs, gently pressing each leg closer to their torso. Finally, help each other do side stretches, like a naughty personal trainer. In addition to acting as foreplay, all this stretching will make you more limber, so you don't pull anything in bed—important if you're attempting a "fancy" position like The Wheelbarrow (p.108).

On a final note, while there are many, many reasons to hit the gym (or the bike, or the yoga mat…) on a regular basis, we would be remiss in our duties as sex advisors if we didn't tell you about how to occasionally short-cut your way to revved-up good loving. Anything that triggers your fight-or-flight mechanism will cause your body to mimic a sexual response and turn up the heat in the bedroom: a pillow fight, riding a rollercoaster, even watching an intense action flick. So don't ever complain that good sex is all work and no play.

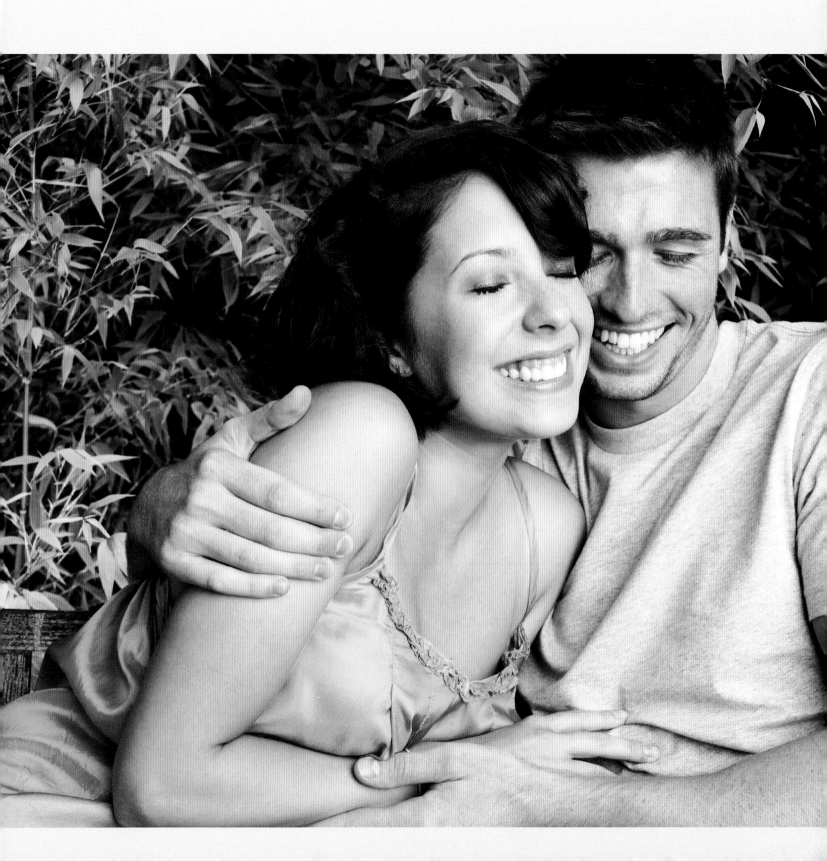

Lady Parts—

The features of female genitalia that make them so sexy and mysterious—darkness, warmth, moisture, introversion—also make them more susceptible to bacterial imbalance and infection. Lady parts are also particularly susceptible to fascist beauty standards. Read on to figure out how to keep things in check, in balance, and in perspective.

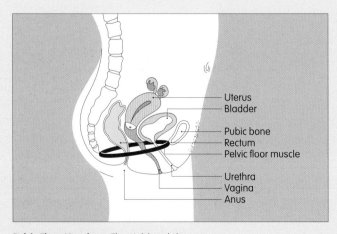

Labels:
- Uterus
- Bladder
- Pubic bone
- Rectum
- Pelvic floor muscle
- Urethra
- Vagina
- Anus

Pelvic Floor Muscles—The pink band shows your pelvic floor muscles wrapping around your internal genitalia.

The Great Size Debate

It has been brought to our attention that genital size-induced stress is now a co-ed affliction. Yay, equality! Let's start with the labia: apparently the mainstreaming of porn has led some women to conclude that their lips are not "sexy" enough. What's next, prettifying our vital organs? Yes, labia come in as many shapes, sizes, and shades as penises. Sometimes the left is larger than the right, sometimes the inner lips protrude further than the outer, and most of the time they don't look a thing like the trim, pink lips you see in those airbrushed magazine "spreads." Which is where labiaplasty comes in: surgery to "fix" the labia. It started in L.A. (where else?) but has since spread (ahem) worldwide. Can we all please agree that this is toad-licking crazy? First of all, your labia are packed with nerve endings—do you really want to slice those away, just to get a neater look? Second, one of the possible side effects is complete loss of sensation. (So much for "sexy".) And third, it's surgery. On your labia. Here's our non-surgical solution for labia that get in the way during sex: add lube and use fingers (yours or his) to spread the lips before penetration. And here's our non-surgical solution if your partner suggests there's room for improvement down there: date someone else. It shouldn't be difficult: our informal research found that 99.9 percent of men who find you attractive enough to take to bed couldn't give a shit what your labia look like. And the other 0.1 percent watch way too much porn.

The other size issue is one of elasticity in the vaginal canal. Childbirth can sometimes weaken or even severely injure the pelvic floor muscles, causing nerve damage, incontinence, even prolapse (when your uterus literally falls out of your vagina—no joke). More often than not, a strict regimen of Kegel exercises (see below) can really improve the situation and make surgery—what's known as vaginoplasty or vaginal rejuvenation—unnecessary. There *may* be legitimate instances when the procedure can help. But too many insecure women seek it out because they're too lazy to do Kegels or they think this will make them more "attractive" or they're suffering from some kind of sexual dissatisfaction and think this is a miracle cure. Critics, including the American College of Obstetrics & Gynecology, warn that there are no scientific studies which prove the safety or efficacy of such treatments—a pretty damn good reason not to jump off that cosmetic surgery bridge. Now get Kegeling!

Pubic Hair Care

First of all, let's get one thing straight: pubic topiary is not a requisite for sex or sexual health. It's a simple aesthetic preference. If pubic hair doesn't bother you, why waste your time and money living up to someone else's definition of "sexy"? Why deny yourself, and your luvva, the fluffy fun of sudsing up a super soft bush in the shower, playfully tugging on it during sex, or absentmindedly running your fingers through it after an orgasm? Who needs razor burn and ingrown hairs down there? And does he want to risk post-oral sex beard burn? Embrace your treasure trail and unruly bikini line as a symbol of your maturity and sexuality: confidence trumps a hairless crotch pretty much everywhere except Brazil. That all said, it's okay to want trimmed, shaved, or waxed nether regions. After all, shaving everything down there is labor intensive, which makes for some quality time with your genitals: you really have to look your vulva in the face and like what you see to go for such a brazen display of labes. Perhaps you want an unimpeded view, easy access for cunnilingus, a new sensation, a "cleaner" feeling (if you're not into normal bodily secretions and the sexy musk they create), a dirtier feeling, or simply a new look. Or maybe you think of prepping for sex via genital pampering as DIY foreplay. Do whatever makes you feel sexiest, whether that's total topiary, or nothing at all.

Grooming the Locks—There are countless products dedicated to waxing, shaving, clipping, and trimming—all things designed to destroy the pubic rainforest—but good luck finding a single one that pays homage to the pleasures of playing in the garden of mother nature's delights. So our advice is: just treat it as you would dry, frizzy head hair. Try shampoos specifically made for extra softness, deep conditioners (especially after washing with soap, which can be drying), V05 Hot Oil treatments (just not too hot!), warm olive oil applications—hell, we'd even recommend running a comb through it to work out any kinks and/or fluff it up. Or clean your pleasure junction with mineral oil—it's less drying (not to mention less irritating) than soap. We'd avoid leave-in hair products, since we don't know of any de-frizzers that are edible or flavored like vanilla. And make sure that oils and fragrant shampoos don't actually get inside anywhere (vagina, uretha, anus), as this could lead to irritation or infection.

Just a Trim—Like we'll tell the fellas (p.176), if you're not into daily maintenance, a close trim with nail scissors or your boyfriend's beard trimmer may be just the kind of manicuring you're looking for. Turn it into sex play by handing him the tools.

A Close Shave—This is an acquired art. The genitals are made of delicate tissue and don't take kindly to being hacked at with a sharp blade (go figure). You need to build up tolerance gradually: don't go from full bush to completely bare in one session for your partner's birthday (if the surprise factor is important, you're better off with a professional waxjob, see below). Trim first, getting as close to the skin as possible, then refine your shaving technique on the bikini line, which is less sensitive than other areas. Then take a break for a few days, see how your body reacts. Next, start working on the mons mound, gradually (i.e., over the course of a few sessions) turning the triangle into a smaller triangle, a landing strip, or a clean slate, if that's your cup of tea. Apply the shaving cream or gel a few minutes before you start to soften the hairs—or better yet, take a warm bath or shower first, and rub oil (almond, olive, baby) or hair conditioner over the whole area before applying shaving gel. Just make sure oil doesn't get inside any orifices, as that can lead to infection. A thick shaving gel is more manageable than foam and lets you see what you're doing. Go for something with aloe or conditioner, and avoid fragrances—a hypo-allergenic gel that's made for sensitive skin is your best bet. Add a new layer of gel for each razor stroke. And use a brand new razor for each shave: don't ever borrow your partner's! The fewer strokes you make, the less likely you are to end up with razor burn. Rinse the razor in warm water before each pass. Don't shave the same spot more than twice. Go first in the direction of hair growth, then switch to a new razor and shave against the grain. If it's your first time shaving this region, skip the against-the-grain part, only make one stroke over each area, and don't press the razor into the skin. So you'll miss a few hairs—you'll get them next time around. Be sure to pull the skin taut while you shave, especially around the labia. And please: watch the clit. If, at any stage, the skin gets sore, itchy, or irritated, stop everything until your crotch starts to feel more like itself again. When you're done, rinse off and pat—don't rub—dry. Apply a fragrance-free, hypoallergenic lotion. Then, hang around naked for a while (an hour or more if you can), and don't wear tight pants or tights for at least a day. Also, don't run off the to gym for a workout—all that sweat and friction are pretty much guaranteed to give you a nasty case of razor burn. If all this seems like too much hassle, just shave at night and then sleep in the buff. Between shaves, tweeze out ingrown hairs—it's not nearly as painful as it sounds. And use a loofah or body scrub in the shower—gently—to keep dead skin from building up over the hair follicles. The only way not to itch—and not to give your partner the sandpaper treatment—is to shave every day or two. Once you get into the groove, it should take only a few minutes each time. If you're not prepared to commit, then go for a wax Instead. Or enjoy the verdant muff. Or learn the hard way. Finally, not everyone can get a clean shave; some are just too damned sensitive down there. If that's you, go for a close trim instead and think of all the starving children in Africa before bemoaning your fate.

Depilatory Creams—Hair-removal creams from the drugstore that dissolve your hair at the surface are fine for neatening your bikini line for a day or so, but they shouldn't be used for the full monty—those aren't chemicals you want anywhere near your private parts.

Wax Off—It hurts like hell but it hurts a little less like hell each time you go back for more pain and suffering. (It hurts a little more like hell in the week before your period, FYI.) You'll need at least a week's hair growth to get waxed, but then you'll be fur-free for a few weeks. You'll probably have to follow up with a little tweezer action, since waxing makes you prone to ingrown hairs, though using a gentle exfoliator each day will discourage those pesky ingrowns. You could wax at home if you're not planning on getting tricky

with any nooks and crannies, though in general, we recommend leaving the wax to the professionals. By the way, if you want to surprise your honey with a Telly Savalas, you should allow 24 hours for the redness and swelling to subside. And if you're going for anything more invasive than a bikini line touch-up—like say, the Sphynx (named for the hairless Egyptian cat, it includes outer labes, inner labes, mons, anus, the whole kitten caboodle), or the Brazilian (like the Sphynx except for a small landing strip right above the clit), prepare to swallow a little pride: getting one of these means either hanging out doggie-style or lying on your back with your legs nearly behind your ears. Your gyno's got nothing on this!

Hygiene & TLC
The vagina can be a sensitive little thing, but there are some easy ways to nurture it—while these tips aren't guaranteed to ward off the vagina problems discussed below, they'll certainly help:

• Always pee right after sex if you're prone to infection. If you're especially prone, consider showering after, too.
• Like the men, wash at least once a day using a mild soap (no scents down there!) and dry off thoroughly afterward (though steer clear of talc, which has been linked to ovarian cancer). Bubble bath is a no-no for sensitive vaginas.
• Actually, any fragrances down there, from sanitary pads to sprays, are a bad idea.
• Synthetic underpants don't let you breathe down there, which may lead to infection; all-cotton is much friendlier. Sleeping or walking around the house bottomless is even better (though be warned that your man may find this behavior "romantic").
• Your mom was right: drink lots of water, don't eat too much sugar or refined carbs, and always wipe front to back.
• The right kind of lube for sex (p.129) can cut down on friction, which is the enemy of the sensitive vagina.
• Make sure you get regular gynecological exams and pap smears.
• And finally: just say no to douching. It upsets your natural vaginal balance, which may lead to infection.

Vagina Problems
Unfortunately, sometimes all the TLC in the world isn't enough to protect your vagina. In fact, we'll go out on a limb and say that at some point you will get an infection. Vaginitis is a blanket term for a number of unpleasantries, including yeast infections, trichomoniasis, and bacterial vaginosis, among others. The symptoms are all pretty similar: itchiness, inflammation, and atypical (for you) discharge and smell. The latter is why it's good to know what an average day in the life of your vagina looks and smells like—though know that this will change throughout your cycle and may be affected by a number of other factors, too, including medication, hydration, diet, and your sexual partner. Once you've ascertained that something is out of sorts, you'll need to see your doctor for an exact diagnosis and prescription—especially because these symptoms may also

indicate something more serious, like chlamydia or gonorrhea (pp.180–181). Don't be embarrassed—even nuns get vaginitis! Sometimes it's sexually transmitted, other times it's due to rough sex, irritating soap, antibiotics, the Pill, having your period… you know, life. Life is also frequently responsible for urinary tract infections (UTIs)—other culprits include a bad wiping technique, rough sex, a pinkie that visits the back door and then the front, and using oil-based lubes (p.129). If you have a UTI, you'll feel like you need to wee all the time, and when you do wee, it'll burn like hell. See your doctor for antibiotics and a decent painkiller (though there are some great over-the-counter options that can tide you over until your appointment).

Her Kegels
Just like in men, your various pelvic muscles wrap around your genitals internally (see the illustration on page 174)—the clitoris, urethra, perineum, vagina, anus, along the pelvic floor, everything. These muscles involuntarily contract when you climax; you can clench them yourself if you need to wee and there's a long line. And working them out regularly can improve your sex life and your sexual health. What's not to love? Sure, the exercises are a pain in the groin, but what other work-out program can be accomplished on your couch, at your desk, or while stuck in traffic? Let us count the ways we love Kegels: toned pelvic muscles increase blood flow to the region, making everything more sensitive (including your G-spot), which could lead to stronger orgasms—or even your very first orgasm. They can also increase lubrication, ward off incontinence later in life, improve vaginal tone after childbirth, and protect you from prolapse. Plus, like him, you may find that knowing how to relax your pelvic muscles improves anal play. Working the muscles when he's inside you is a treat you'll both love—try squeezing and releasing his penis during intercourse as if you're trying to pull him toward you. Your Kegel regimen is the same as his (p.177), though you might find the exercises easier with something to grip onto. If a penis is not readily available, try a dildo or a pelvic exerciser like Betty's Barbell. And hey, you may be one of the lucky women who actually gets turned on by doing her Kegels! In which case, consider your workout DIY foreplay, too.

Man Parts—

Believe it or not, you are the boss of your penis, no matter how much it might act up sometimes. But with great power, as they say, comes great responsibility. Here's how to wield it.

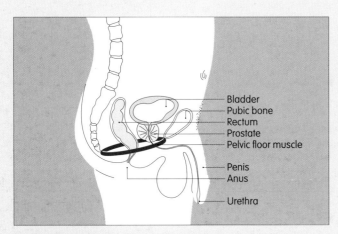

Pelvic Floor Muscles—The pink band shows your pelvic floor muscles wrapping around your internal genitalia. Exercising these muscles (see Kegels for Him, p.177) can enhance your erections and orgasms.

Labels on diagram:
- Bladder
- Pubic bone
- Rectum
- Prostate
- Pelvic floor muscle
- Penis
- Anus
- Urethra

The Great Size Debate Part II

Let's dispense with the size issue first, shall we? Because we're pretty sure that's the only reason you turned to this chapter. First, the good news: the importance of size—just like the size of many a man's member, ironically enough—has been wildly exaggerated. Studies have shown that the more a woman likes and knows you, the less important size becomes—in either direction. During a one-night stand, the sight of your extra-small or even (yes, really) extra-large willy may be a turn-off… but if you stick around, your number one guy will get a second chance at a first impression. But wait, there's more good news! The average erect penis is five to six inches long, and the average vagina is three and a half to six inches long. And most of the vagina's sensitivity is toward the opening, anyway. Which means that size is relative to the vagina in your life, and even a shorter-than-average penis is going to hold his own in an longer-than-average vagina. In fact, too much penis may bang against the cervix in an unpleasant manner, especially during doggy-style or woman-on-top positions. True, some women rave about the lovely filled-up sensation they get from a particularly wide penis—but we bet that the slimmer dongs see a lot more anal action! Can you handle still more good news? The standard male method for judging one's own penis size—looking down at your own member and then surreptitiously glancing at others in the locker room—is seriously flawed, because a) penises always look smaller when you look down on them, and b) smaller non-erect penises tend to benefit more from the growth spurt of an erection than do larger ones. Wait, there's more! Penile penetration isn't the be-all and end-all of great sex. But if you read the previous chapters, then you already knew that. And the only bad news? "Safe penis enlargement" is an oxymoronic crock of shit. Weights, surgery, pills, herbs, pumps, chants, the ancient art of "jelquing" (Google it)—these methods are at best ineffective and at worst, permanently disfiguring. If you really want to feel bigger, shave your pubes, lose some weight, wear a cock ring, or look at yourself in a mirror (not the one in the locker room). On a final size note: ladies, if your guy asks you if his penis is big enough, or if he's bigger than most guys you've slept with, it's perfectly acceptable to fib.

The Great Circumcision Debate

Supporters of snipping cite several studies that suggest circumcision reduces the number of penile infections, including STDs, while those in favor of foreskin argue that infections can be all but eliminated with basic hygiene and that circumcision doesn't guarantee you won't get an STD if you go condomless. Some are very attached to being trimmed, while others insist that normal, natural, nerve-rich tissue is unnecessarily removed during the procedure. But have you ever heard a guy, cut or uncut, say something like, "Sex is nice and all, but I sure wish it felt better on my penis"? Exactly. The procedure is on the decline in the States, but new research out of Africa (where AIDS and unprotected sex are both rampant), which has shown that

circumcision can reduce HIV infection in men by 50 percent, might just put it on the rise again. For most people, though, it's still just a matter of religious, social, or aesthetic preferences—preferences that, in our opinion, don't (and shouldn't) really affect your or your partner's enjoyment of sex. Once erect, a cut and an uncut penis are pretty much indistinguishable (which is not to say that every penis isn't special in its own way… it's just that penis personality is about more than foreskin). Sure, a woman might be slightly intimidated when first presented with the brand of penis she's personally unfamiliar with. But she's not "freaked out" or "disgusted" (and if she is, kick her to the curb)—she's simply a little confused as to whether or not she's meant to approach it differently. Show her how you like it—she'll appreciate the direction, and you can both move on. End of story.

Pubic Hair Care

Unless you wear blinders at the locker room, you've probably already figured out that ladies aren't the only ones who have a pubic hair care routine. And it's not just for gay men, either. Call it equal opportunity objectification. For one thing, a manicured lawn can make your tree stump look bigger. Or perhaps your girlfriend told you, "I will if you will." Two shaved sets of genitals rubbing up against each other can feel pretty cool. (Of course, two sets of genitals with five o'clock shadow rubbing up against each other can feel like Velcro.) Whatever your reasons, you have to groom even more carefully than the gals. The twin boys are housed in puckered, wrinkly skin that's damn near impossible not to nick with a razor. Same goes for the shaft. And just thinking about waxing your twig and berries makes us want to cry (most salons won't do it, in fact). Tweezers are no good, either—you guys just don't have enough breathing room down there to ward off infection. Which is why most guys just opt for a close trim. No blood spill, no razor burn, and—if you do it right—no itchy regrowth. Even if you are planning on shaving, it's a good idea to give yourself a trim first—it gets the area used to the attention, and makes it easier to shave later. Using either a sharp pair of manicure scissors or, for a really close crop, a beard trimmer, take off a little at a time until you find a look you like. Remember, pubic topiary is a very personal thing; there's no right or wrong way to trim. If you're using scissors, pull the hair away from your skin with fingers or a comb to avoid nicks. A very close cut will give you something approximating the look of a close shave, while a more wooly look will be less itchy as it grows out, especially if you don't cut the hairs a uniform length. Of course, what's old is always new again: going *au naturel* is perfectly acceptable (so long as you're tolerant of the same soft fluffy style on your partner).

Hygiene

Though a woman may be size-blind once she falls in love, cleanliness always matters. Wear clean underwear every day (turning your briefs inside-out doesn't count). Boxers provide more breathing room than briefs—and walking around the house naked is best of all (though be warned that she may not find this behavior "romantic"). Wash your willy at least once a day with soap and water, and definitely after working out or wearing tight trousers (you sexy beast). Focus especially just below the head, being sure to pull back the foreskin if you're uncircumcised. And dry off thoroughly before dressing—add powder if you're the sweaty type (not talc though, as that's bad for her bits). Do all this even if you're not expecting to get lucky—unless you like jock itch. If you *are* expecting to get lucky, why not hop in the tub together to get a head-start on the foreplay at the same time? We know: hygiene should go without saying. But given the number of otherwise upstanding citizens who don't wash their hands after a trip to the toilet, we have determined that it doesn't, in fact, go without saying.

Penis Problems

Penile predicaments vary from the benign (jock itch) to the unspeakable (broken penis). Fortunately for you, the former can be warded off with simple hygiene, as we discussed above, and the latter is incredibly rare. Here's your healthy penis cheat sheet:

Penis Curvature—Penises are unique, bless them, and not all of them stand to attention in quite the same way. Many curve to the left or the right—or in any other direction, for that matter. If you can still use yours for sex, then your curvature is considered completely normal. If you can't, see your doctor, please.

Blue Balls—This is when everything fills with blood but no happy ending is forthcoming. It might hurt, but there's a simple cure: self-administered manual release. Or just wait for the blood to drain out. She may offer to help out, but she's not obliged—your balls, your problem.

Erectile Dysfunction (E.D.)—Erection problems (e.g., maintaining one, getting one in the first place, etc) can be either psychological in nature (performance anxiety is a boner basher) or physical—as a result of, say, obesity, cardiovascular disease, or diabetes. We're not doctors, but we do know that if you exercise regularly, eat a healthy diet, avoid binge-drinking, quit smoking, and yes, masturbate regularly (it keeps life-giving oxygen flowing to the area), you're less likely to face E.D. later in life. If you're facing it now, see someone who *is* a doctor.

Premature Ejaculation—Officially, this means coming before or right at the moment of penetration. Most of the time, this is in your head. We don't mean you're imagining it, we just mean the solution is probably in your hands—literally. Occasional premature ejaculation is pretty much universal, and nothing to worry about, but if it's persistent and bothersome, then it might be time for a little penis re-education. We're pretty sure you know what it feels like right when you're about to come, but do you know what it feels like right before that? (Working on your Kegels, see below, will help.) Once you've identified this

moment, you can start to work around it. During masturbation, try letting go and pausing for air; once you've mastered this, you can try the same thing during mutual masturbation—first your hands, and then hers. And eventually, you'll be able to do the same thing during sex—use that moment to switch positions or take a cunnilingus break. The good news is that most women would kill for a guy who needs to take regular breaks to focus on her! If none of this helps, please don't self-medicate with one of those desensitizing creams. A numb penis is fun for no one, especially when the cream spreads to her parts. Talk to your doc instead.

Retarded Ejaculation—The opposite of the above, sometimes as a result of booze or medication (e.g., antidepressants), and sometimes as a result of stuff going on in your head. Again, as an occasional occurrence, this is a universal affliction, but if it's more serious, practice during masturbation (focusing on the pelvic muscles) may help. If not, your doctor or therapist needs to be brought into the loop.

Broken Penis—Despite containing no bones, penises can break. It's most likely to happen if an erect penis hits something rigid (like a headboard or pubic bone) with extreme force. Are you hiding under your bed yet? Don't worry, it's not something that happens easily or often. That said, if a position feels wrong (oh, you'll know) then stop immediately. And if something feels really wrong—meaning, you hear a cracking sound, you're in agony, your penis is suddenly bending in a funny direction, blood is shooting out—then head to the ER immediately. Surgery may well be able to fix the problem, but not always. So to be safe, don't treat your dick like a battering ram (she'll probably appreciate that for her own sake, too). And when under the influence, best to stick to slow and gentle love makin' in the missionary position.

Prostate Cancer—Let's end on a more cheery note, shall we? Studies have shown that regular "flushing of the prostate" via ejaculation can decrease a man's risk for prostate cancer. But just because you're a life-long masturbator, doesn't mean you can forgo regular check-ups, including the dreaded doctor poke. But hey, if you study your anatomy (p.43), learn how to relax your backdoor area (p.117), and strengthen your pelvic floor muscles (see immediately below), then it'll make those visits a lot more bearable.

Kegels for Him

Like Men Without Hats almost said, "you can Kegel if you want to!" Your pelvic muscles wrap around your genitals internally (see the illustration on the opposite page), just like hers do, and you can strengthen them with these exercises named after the doc who invented them, just like she can. Your mileage may vary (especially depending on how dedicated you are to the regimen), but some guys find that pumping up their pelvic muscles leads to stronger, more fully inflated erections, more stamina during intercourse, more intense orgasms and ejaculation, and even the ability to

come without, well, coming (you'll need to study Taoist sex separately for that). And because these muscles wrap around everything, knowing how to relax them may also help you enjoy anal play more. Like women, you can feel your pelvic muscles when you stop the flow of urine (try not to tense your abs or bum at the same time). You can work on these muscles while reading, driving to work, or watching porn: squeeze, hold, release, repeat, gradually building up—just like at the gym—until you can hold for 10 seconds. Eventually you should be able to repeat this 10 times, up to three times a day. Experiment with short-burst, quickie squeezes, too. Then, try relaxing and contracting these muscles during masturbation and intercourse, especially right before you come and during slow, close sex like the CAT position (p.106). It's all about getting in touch with your penis… like you needed the excuse.

STDs—

Got an STD? You're in good company: more than half us will eventually get some kind of STD. Some of the nicest, most upstanding, militant-about-protection people we know (including yours truly) have, or once had, an STD, so welcome to the club! Unless you're willing to "save yourself" for marriage (with someone who's also avoided all genital contact with others), then exposure to some kind of STD along the way is almost unavoidable. And there's no shame in that. The only shame is in not being educated or forthcoming enough about what you have, might have, or could get.

Your STD education begins on the next few pages, continues with asking your doctor questions (including "Can you test me for X, Y, and Z), and is supplemented by the resources on p.188.

Once armed with good information and an accurate, up-to-date bill of health, you need to have the Tough Talk with any potential new partners before the pants come off. We recommend doing it over a glass of wine when it's fairly clear where the relationship is heading. Don't wait until you're half-naked in bed. And don't wait until you're ready to stop using condoms, either—condoms don't provide 100 percent protection against some STDs, including herpes (p.179) and genital warts (p.179), and thus they shouldn't be considered a replacement for this conversation. You could start with the simple, straightforward truth: "So, this might be a little forward, but do you want to have sex with me?" If the answer is in the affirmative, say, "Oh good, me too. So let's just get the awkward stuff out of the way now!" Offer up your own sexual history first—past or current STDs, abnormal pap smears, when you were last tested—and explain that you're sharing these things because you think it's important to be honest, and you'd like to hear their side, too. Make it clear that you're not going to pass judgment or get mad, you just think it's good to be informed.

If you do have an STD, what you offer up depends on the kind you have. Those that can be cured completely, like bacterial and parasitic infections, need not be mentioned as long as you *resist all temptation* until treatment is successful and complete. However, we believe that the more the realities of STDs are discussed openly, the better off we'll all be as fuck buddies. If you have something more enduring, like a viral infection, then you've got to come clean. You could say, "Before we sleep together, I want to tell you that I have [*name of your STD*]." Give facts that will help your partner determine their risk—how it's transmitted, what percentage of people have it, what precautions you can take together, etc. Ask if they have any questions. Read on and do your homework so you're prepared with answers. Say, "If you want to take some time and think about it, here's a place where you can find out more." They may well be freaked out, but answering all their questions calmly and matter-of-factly should help. Steer clear of defensive comebacks like, "Oh yeah, well I bet your last partner had every STD in the book but was just too chicken-shit to tell you!" If they run before asking a single question, they weren't worth your time anyway—the good people of this world will appreciate your honesty. We know this sounds like something your mom would say, but your mom knows a thing or two about a thing or two.

And if your partner's the one who spills the beans about an STD? Whether or not you sleep with them is up to you—the information in this chapter will help you determine your risk—but at the very least, you owe your date an open mind and a friendly, nonjudgmental conversation. Remember, honesty in bed should be encouraged and even

rewarded, not punished! Besides, you're probably better off with someone who's upfront about their history, rather than someone who skirts the truth—or is ignorant of it. Most STDs have no symptoms, which means it's very easy to carry and spread an infection without knowing it. (This is why some clinics and organizations prefer the term "STI" (sexually transmitted infection), because they feel that "disease" implies symptoms, not to mention horribleness.) If both of you think you're in the clear, then we think it's incredibly romantic to get tested together before screwing each other silly—or, at the very least, before going condom-free. This cautious approach says, "I'm into you enough to care about your long-term health and I'm into you enough to wait until we're sure." Hey, it's certainly a lot more romantic than giving or getting genital herpes. And ladies, just in case you needed an added incentive to speak up, you should know that your risk of contracting an STD is way higher than his (with HIV, for example, your risk of getting it from him is twice as great as the reverse).

If you're single but, you know, "active", you should be getting tested and checked anyway at least once—ideally, twice—a year for HIV, syphilis, hepatitis B, chlamydia, gonorrhea, visible genital warts caused by HPV, and herpes sores. And all women, regardless of their relationship status, should also get an annual pap smear to check for evidence of abnormal cervical cell changes caused by other strains of HPV.

By the way, some clinics and websites offer anonymous partner notification if you discover, after the fact, that you have an STD, and just can't face calling up that one-night stand. Telling someone yourself is always preferable, however, because a) the more information they have, the easier it will be to treat their STD, b) they may well file that email as spam, and c) anonymous notification is just cold! But if it's this or nothing, they deserve to know one way or another.

We're not going to sugar-coat it: sharing your sexual health history will always be awkward as hell. But if you can pull it off, the rewards are sweet, because the more you share in the warm-fuzzy sense, the less you're likely to share in the contagious sense. And hey, just think how easy the "Are you into spanking?" conversation (see pp.166–167) will be after this one!

VIRAL STDs

Viral STDs include the four H's: HIV, herpes, HPV, and the hepatitis family. Most of them don't have vaccines and none of them have cures, so once you've got one, you're typically stuck with it for life. But before you sign up for missionary school, it's not all bad news: while not curable, these viruses are, for the most part, pretty manageable. In other words, with the right treatment and care, we see plenty of hot monkey loving in your future.

HIV—

The good news is, HIV is increasingly manageable—new and improved drugs mean that more and more people are living with the HIV virus without it progressing to the typically fatal acquired-immunodeficiency-syndrome stage (i.e. AIDS). The bad news is, the infection rate is not slowing down. An estimated one million people in the U.S. are currently living with HIV, and at least a quarter of them are ignorant of this fact. And each year, another 40,000 will get infected, but only half will know it. So don't skip this section.

Symptoms & Diagnosis—It takes an average of 10 years for symptoms to show up, but you're contagious from the moment you're infected. Most early symptoms could be mistaken for the flu or other generic illnesses, so the only way to be sure is to get tested. Later, more obvious symptoms include bruising and purple growths on the skin or mouth. HIV also weakens your body's ability to fight off diseases, leaving you vulnerable to "opportunistic" hazards such as pneumonia, cancer, and tuberculosis. The final stage of HIV is AIDS, which is officially defined as having at least one opportunistic infection and/or a T-cell count below 200 (that's how they measure your immune system). HIV can take anywhere from one to six months to show up on the standard blood test, though some newer, fancier tests can detect it sooner.

Treatment—There's no cure, but anti-viral drug cocktails can help reduce the amount of HIV in your bloodstream—in some cases, the drugs reduce the virus to practically undetectable levels. Doctors can also treat your opportunistic diseases.

Transmission—Infected vaginal fluids, semen (including pre-ejaculate), blood (including menstrual blood), or breast milk needs to get into your bloodstream. Unprotected anal or vaginal intercourse will do nicely. Less likely but still possible: oral sex, shared toys, intense French-kissing (i.e with broken skin). The virus can't survive outside the human body, so tongue-free kissing, hand-holding, hugging, sharing a glass—pretty much anything you might do with a platonic friend—are all fine. By the way, having another STD usually increases the chance of HIV transmission.

Prevention—Put on a condom or female condom as soon as you get naked. Get tested together. (See note on p.176 about circumcision and HIV.)

If You Have It—First off, you'll need counseling. Once diagnosed, you'll need to tell everyone you've had sex with in at least the last decade (unless you know exactly when you contracted it)—your doc should tell you how far back to go. And obviously you'll need to tell all potential partners so they can decide for themselves how much risk they're willing to take on. Condoms are much more effective against HIV than they are when it comes to herpes and HPV, though of course it's a very different level of risk you're talking about. (Even if you both have HIV, you should still use condoms, as you could be infected with different strains that are resistant to different drugs, making it harder to manage the infection.) In the meantime, please note how many pages of this book are dedicated to fun things you can do in bed besides intercourse.

Herpes—
Herpes is one of the popular kids. There are two types: herpes simplex virus 1 (HSV-1), which is usually found above the neck (mouth, nose, lips, eyes) and herpes simplex virus 2 (HSV-2), which is usually found below the waist (vagina, vulva, cervix, penis, buttocks, anus). That said, both types have been found in both places. When herpes shows up above the neck, it's referred to as oral herpes or cold sores; below the waist, it's called genital herpes.

Symptoms & Diagnosis—Most people who have herpes never get (or never notice) symptoms—though they can still spread the virus. For the symptomatic minority: about two to 20 days (though it occasionally takes years, especially in guys) after exposure to the virus, you'll experience a tingling feeling on either your mouth or your genitals, wherever the exposure occurred. After a day or so, this tingling will turn into painful blisters, which will become oozing sores, which will eventually scab over, and, two to three weeks later, heal. The first outbreak is typically the most severe and may be accompanied by a fever and swollen glands. Some people will never get another outbreak; others will get them regularly, maybe every few months—though the severity and frequency of attacks should lessen as time goes on. And after five or six years, most people will be done with outbreaks for good—though they'll be a carrier, and potentially contagious, for life. Your doctor will analyze your sores to confirm the herpes diagnosis. There is a blood test, though most tests don't distinguish between HSV-1 and HSV-2 and most clinics don't offer it.

Treatment—There's no cure, but you can manage it with medication prescribed by your doctor: you can either take it just when you feel the dreaded tingle, to help the attack be shorter and less severe, or you can take it daily, which will help reduce the frequency of attacks.

Transmission—As with HPV (see below), skin-on-skin contact is all it takes, so any kind of naked rubbing or grinding can spread genital herpes, and any kind of kissing can spread oral herpes. Also, oral sex is the fastest way to convert your oral herpes into your partner's genital herpes (and vice versa). Fingers and toys can also shuttle the virus between genitals or mouth and genitals, but toilet seats, etc., tend to be fairly safe because the virus doesn't survive long off the body. You should also be aware that you can spread herpes across your own body, e.g. genitals to butt or mouth to eye, etc.—though it's unlikely you'll spread your own oral herpes to the genitals and vice versa because of the way your antibodies work. But having oral herpes definitely does not protect you from other people's genital herpes! Herpes is most contagious during an outbreak, but most herpes sufferers will also occasionally be contagious between outbreaks, and unfortunately there's no way to know exactly when those times are.

Prevention—During an outbreak—i.e., from the first tingle to when the sores are healed—keep your pants on (or no kissing). Between outbreaks, that daily medication we mentioned will probably make you less contagious, too. Taking a lysine

supplement (it's in the vitamin aisle) may also help ward off attacks. And the following are all potential triggers for an outbreak: stress, lack of sleep, sun exposure, nuts, soda, coffee, tea, chocolate, your period, and irritating stubble, whether from your partner's face or genitals.

If You Have It—No matter how many years it's been since your last outbreak, tell every partner before you get naked—yes, even the one-night stands, and even if you're going to use protection. Here's their risk: If the two of you have sex for a year (except for during outbreaks, duh), their chance of contracting genital herpes is roughly one in 10, depending on whether you use protection and how long you go between outbreaks (the more time that passes, the less likely you are to be contagious between outbreaks). And taking medication may lower those odds still further. If you're a man with genital herpes, your girlfriend may be better protected with a female condom than an old-school one on you. Finally, HSV-1 (i.e. most oral herpes) tends to be much less contagious between outbreaks. That said, it's still best to tell a partner you have oral herpes before the first kiss.

HPV—
HPV is one of the most—if not *the* most —popular STDs out there, though its popularity should start to shrink over the coming years, thanks to a new vaccine. There are about 100 different strains of HPV, and about 30–40 of the strains are sexually transmitted. And these fall into two basic groups: strains that cause genital warts, and are considered "low risk" HPV because they don't have any serious long-term effects, and strains that cause abnormal cervical cell changes (invisible to the human eye), some of which are considered "high risk" because they can lead to cervical cancer. Basically, unless you married your virgin high school sweetheart, then chances are you've been exposed to the virus and probably even have the virus. It's incredibly pervasive, but in most people it's asymptomatic and is often cleared by your own immune system—which means that docs today tend to be much less stringent about the "fess up" policy when it comes to HPV.

HPV 1: Genital Warts—
Symptoms & Diagnosis—Painless warts, either alone or in clusters, can appear for the first time anywhere from a few weeks to a few months after exposure, on the penis, balls, vulva, vagina, cervix, anus, urethra, and general groin area (and, rarely, on lips, tongue, or mouth). That said, most people show no symptoms—but are still contagious. Your doctor will confirm the diagnosis by visually examining the warts (because what you think is genital warts could be another STD). Some people will get only one outbreak of warts, while others may have recurring outbreaks for a few years or more. While you are most contagious when you have visible warts, you can still spread the virus at other times (and besides, you may have internal warts and not know it).

Treatment—You can't cure the virus, you can only treat the warts—though most people's immune systems will rid their body of the virus after about

18 months. Your doctor will decide on the best way to treat your warts, whether it's surgery, topical chemicals, freezing, burning, or laser—and this will usually be done right there in the office. If you're suffering from repeat outbreaks, your doc may also prescribe you medicine to help reduce them. By the way, never treat your genital warts with over-the-counter wart medicine.

Transmission—Any kind of skin-to-skin contact down there will do it: dry-humping, fingers going between genitals, vaginal or anal intercourse with or without a condom (condoms provide *some* protection, however, so it's still worth wearing one). It's possible to spread the virus via oral sex, too, but the risk is very low. Warts on your hands or feet are usually a different strain of HPV, though, and are unlikely to give you genital warts.

Prevention—The great news is, there's a new vaccine that offers protection against the two strains of HPV that cause 90 percent of all genital warts (unfortunately it's only for women right now). Ask your doctor if it's right for (and available to) you. Other than that, always ask questions before getting naked, keep your body count low, and put on a condom before naked body parts get near each other (a female condom may provide even more coverage).

If You Have It—There's no way of knowing if you're one of the unlucky few who's stuck with the virus for life, so you should always tell your partner. However, if you haven't had an outbreak in more than 18 months, you can reassure them that their risk of contracting it is fairly low, and gets lower as each year passes without an outbreak.

HPV 2: Abnormal Cell Changes—

Symptoms & Diagnosis—Only your doctor will be able to detect the cervical cell changes that may result from HPV in some women—hence the importance of an annual pap smear. These changes may not show up until years after exposure to the virus, so there's generally no way of knowing when or from whom you contracted HPV. If the doctor spots changes to be concerned about, they will send off a sample for further tests. A swab test specific for HPV does exist for women only, however it's rarely done because a) it's expensive, and b) it doesn't make much difference to know you have it if it's is not causing you cervical problems (and that's what the pap smear is for). There is no reliable test for men.

Treatment—Some cell abnormalities go away on their own, some don't—your doctor will make the call about whether to just keep an eye on you via regular pap smears or remove the cells via surgery, freezing, burning, or laser. If the cell changes are more advanced, they will often do a biopsy to rule out cancer, because women with HPV are 10 times more likely to develop cervical cancer. The good news is that it takes years (if ever) for abnormal cells to lead to cancer, so as long as you're getting annual pap smears, you'll catch the virus in time. Other related cancers are much more rare, and include vulva, penis, anus, and oral cancers. After about seven years of normal pap smear tests, it's generally assumed your immune system has defeated the virus.

Transmission—Just like with genital warts, any kind of skin-to-skin contact can do it. And new research suggests that oral sex can spread HPV and lead to oral cancer, especially in guys.

Prevention—In addition to warding off most genital warts, the new HPV vaccine also protects women from the two strains of HPV that cause 70 percent of the cases of cervical cancer. And while a pap smear won't prevent HPV, it will help catch it before it turns cancerous. As with genital warts, skin-to-skin contact is all it takes to pass the virus on, therefore condoms offer only limited protection. So ask questions before so much as grinding naked and don't smoke (it increases your cancer risk, duh). Guys will likely never know whether or not they have HPV. Which means that all of us—both men and women—can ask questions until we're blue in the face, but we're still increasing our risk every time we sleep with someone new.

If You Have It—Ladies, always tell your partner—but if you've had a year of normal pap smears, you can tell them that the risk of contagion is very low. Guys, if you know that a woman you've slept with in the past had HPV, that's something good to mention, too. But everyone should feel free to remind their partners (in a friendly way) that most sexually active people will have slept with someone with HPV (if not had HPV themselves) at some point in their lives.

Hepatitis—

This virus comes in flavors A, B, C, D, and E—they all affect the liver, but only A and B are sexually transmitted. B is both the most common and the most worrisome.

Hep A—

Symptoms & Diagnosis—About 15–50 days after infection you may get any of the following: flu-like symptoms, abdominal and joint pain, dark urine, and jaundice. A blood test can confirm diagnosis.

Treatment—There's no treatment (except bed rest), but the symptoms will eventually go away on their own—typically within five weeks, though occasionally they may linger for up to a year. Once your symptoms are gone, you're immune and can also no longer pass on the virus. An injection of antibodies within a fortnight of exposure may prevent you from getting sick at all.

Transmission—When you ingest infected blood or poop, even in microscopic quantities, e.g., by going down on or rimming someone who's infected, or by eating in less than hygienic restaurants with infected employees.

Prevention—There's a vaccine! Also, use barrier protection for oral sex and rimming.

If You Have It—For as long as you still have symptoms, you need to tell all partners. Even once you're no longer contagious, it's still good to tell: it just sets the stage for an honest conversation.

Hep B—

Symptoms & Diagnosis—The initial symptoms, which show up six to 12 weeks after exposure, are the same as hep A, plus you may experience hives and arthritis, though about half will be symptom-free. Hep B can sometimes turn chronic, eventually causing cirrhosis, liver cancer, liver failure, and death. A blood test can confirm the initial diagnosis, sometimes as early as three weeks after exposure, though it usually takes at least a couple of months for the virus to show up in the blood. Further tests can tell you if it's chronic.

Treatment—As with hep A, there's no treatment besides an injection of antibodies and the vaccine within a fortnight of exposure, which may prevent illness. Most symptoms will go away within a few months, however, and 90–95 percent of adults who contract hep B will eventually recover and no longer be contagious. If hep B turns chronic (your doc will monitor you), there are medications you can take for your liver.

Transmission—When infected semen (including pre-come), vaginal fluids, blood (including menstrual blood), fecal matter, or saliva gets into someone's mucous membranes (vagina, labia, urethra, urethral opening, anus, mouth, eyes, and broken skin). In terms of behavior this means: unprotected or protected vaginal or anal intercourse, oral sex, rough kissing or biting. Hep B is 100 times more concentrated in blood than HIV, meaning it's way more contagious. Hugging, shaking hands, or sharing food won't spread it.

Prevention—There's a vaccine! Condoms will reduce the risk but won't remove it, so ask questions and get tested.

If You Have It—Tell all partners until your doctor tells you you're in the clear—and even then, it's nice to share.

BACTERIAL STDs

The very genial quality shared by all bacterial STDs—most famously, gonorrhea, chlamydia, pelvic inflammatory disease (PID), and syphilis, though there are numerous variations on these themes—is that they are pretty easily cured, usually with a round of antibiotics. The tricky thing is, many of them show no symptoms and can cause permanent damage if left untreated, so vigilance, regular testing, and safer sex are key. Once your doc pronounces you cured of any of the below, there's no obligation to tell future partners, though sometimes it's nice to, just to set an it's-good-to-share example.

Gonorrhea—

A.k.a. the clap, the drip, the dose, the strain.

Symptoms & Diagnosis—Most women show no symptoms; those who do may experience any of the following: green-yellow discharge, pain during sex, pain or burning when urinating, abdominal pain, tender vulva, abnormal bleeding. These symptoms can easily be confused for a UTI (p.175). Men are much more likely to show symptoms, including discharge from the urethra and pain or burning when urinating. Anal gonorrhea may cause itching, anal discharge, and pain during bowel movements, though most people are symptom-free. The same goes for oral gonorrhea—and any symptoms could be easily mistaken for a sore throat. Symptoms of all kinds usually show up within a few days of infection, though it can sometimes take up to a month. And for any form of gonorrhea, the symptoms could easily indicate any number of bacterial infections. In other words, the only way to know for sure is via an easy test at the doctor's office or health clinic. If untreated, gonorrhea can cause pelvic inflammatory disease (PID) in women (see below) or—much more rarely—infertility or urethral problems in men.

Treatment—A dose of antibiotics will clear you within a week; your partner should get treated simultaneously and you should lay off the sex until your doc gives you the all-clear. By the way, you may get treated for chlamydia at the same time, as the two frequently show up together.

Transmission—Most commonly, via unprotected oral, vaginal, or anal sex, as some exchange of body fluids is required. However, dry-humping or other non-penetrative rubbing can spread it too.

Prevention—Barrier protection helps (including during oral sex), though it isn't 100 percent guaranteed, so ask questions and get tested too. And ladies: get regular gyno checkups!

If You Have It—Once you're diagnosed, you should tell any partners from at least the past few months. And no sexual contact until your doc says you're cleared. At this point, there's no need to inform future partners.

Chlamydia—

The most common bacterial STD.

Symptoms & Diagnosis—Chlamydia is the STD least likely to show symptoms, and as with gonorrhea, women are far less likely to have symptoms than men. Any symptoms that do show up are almost identical to those of gonorrhea (except that in women, the vaginal discharge may not have such a yellow-green hue). Again, symptoms will usually show up within a few days. A doctor's test will confirm the diagnosis. Untreated, chlamydia can lead to PID in women and, rarely, infertility or urinary infection in men.

Treatment—Same deal as gonorrhea, just a slightly different antibiotic.

Transmission—Same as gonorrhea.

Prevention—Ditto.

If You Have It—Same deal.

Pelvic Inflammatory Disease (PID)—

PID, which affects only women, is usually the *result* of an STD, hence its inclusion in this section. Chlamydia and gonorrhea are the most common culprits, though any number of sexually transmitted bacterial infections, if left untreated, can cause it.

Symptoms & Diagnosis—PID is an infection that can spread to the uterus, fallopian tubes and ovaries, eventually causing ectopic pregnancy or infertility—and often there are no symptoms until it's too late. It's one of the leading causes of infertility in women, in fact. Symptoms—which can easily be confused for any number of other ailments—may include: abdominal pain, pain during sex, abnormal vaginal bleeding, pain or burning during urination, nausea or vomiting, a fever or the chills. The only way to know for sure is to get tested for STDs regularly and get a pap smear and vaginal exam at least once a year.

Treatment—If you catch it in time, antibiotics will do it. If the infection has progressed dramatically, you may need surgery to repair the damage. Your current partner should also be tested for STDs

and treated if necessary, as he may have an STD that led to your PID.

Transmission—PID is the result of an untreated STD. Less commonly, untreated vaginal infections (p.175) can also be to blame.

Prevention—Get screened routinely, especially for chlamydia and gonorrhea, and follow the prevention tips for those STDs. Pay attention to your body so you're aware of any vaginal infections (p.175). Get annual gyno checkups. Always use barrier protection. Never douche—it can spread the infection further. So can IUDs (p.185), so don't use one unless you're in a monogamous long-term relationship and have both been tested. By the way, once you've had PID, you're more likely to get it again, and the more times you get it, the more likely it is to lead to complications like infertility.

If You Have It—Lay off sex until your doc says the antibiotics have done the job. And if an STD was the culprit, check in with current or recent partners to let them know they should get tested, too.

Syphilis—

Syphilis is often thought of as an STD from the olden days, rumored to have killed historical figures from Baudelaire to Manet, Capone to Lenin. And it's true that it's one of the least common STDs and was on the wane for years. However, in the past few years in the U.S. the syphilis rate has started to rise again.

Symptoms & Diagnosis—Syphilis symptoms show up in four phases that sometimes overlap. The worst symptoms, when the disease starts to attack major organs, take years or even decades to appear. For most of the time, however, you'll have no symptoms at all. Phase one, within three months of infection: swollen glands and painless sores or ulcers on the genitals, anus or, rarely, the mouth (if the sores are internal you probably won't notice them). These sores usually go away without treatment, but you're still infected and contagious. Phase two is usually within six months and may feature flu-like symptoms and a non-itchy reddish-brown rash, especially on your palms or soles. Again, this will often clear, though the syphilis is still there. Later phases, within two to 30 years, may include blindness, paralysis, insanity, and death. A doctor confirms the diagnosis by examining the sores or doing a blood test three months or more after infection.

Treatment—Antibiotics for you and your partner will smite it in the early phases. The later phases are often untreatable, but unless you live in a cave, you shouldn't get to that point.

Transmission—It's most contagious when sores are present, via unprotected vaginal, anal, or oral sex. Kissing can also spread it, as can naked rubbing, if sores or rashes come into contact with mucous membranes or broken skin. And an infected woman can pass it to the fetus during pregnancy.

Prevention—Wrap up, ask questions, get tested regularly.

If You/Your Partner Has It—Get treated with your partner, tell any recent partners, and hold off on sex til the doc says you're cured. After that, it's your choice whether to tell or stay mum.

PARASITIC STDs

Parasitic STDs like crabs and scabies score high in the gross-out factor but they're usually nothing to worry about, as they're almost impossible not to notice and they're cured quickly, easily, and permanently. Yeast infections and trichomoniasis (p.175) are also classified as parasitic infections.

Crabs—

A.k.a. pubic lice.

Symptoms & Diagnosis—Excruciating itching in the genitals or anus about five days after infection. Plus you may notice lice and/or nits (the egg sacs) in your pubic hair. You can probably self-diagnose with a magnifying glass (they look just like beach crabs but tiny), though a doctor can confirm if you're unsure.

Treatment—Medicated shampoo is available over the counter. Any partners and roommates should be treated, too. Then remove all crabs and nits with a comb or fingernails; wash all clothes, bedding, and towels in hot water and dry on a hot cycle; and vacuum the floor and any couches, etc.

Transmission—Dry humping works as well as sex, as the crabs just need to jump from one pube to another. They can also jump to eyelashes and a beard during oral sex, and to armpit hair during, er, armpit sex? They don't really attach to head hair and are different from head lice. Crabs can live for up to 24 hours off the human body, so you can also get them by sharing bedding or a towel with someone who's infected.

Prevention—Ask questions and look before rubbing naked against someone.

If You Have It—Treat yourself and all partners and roomies and stay fully clothed til everyone's in the clear. Once it's gone, no need to tell, though you have to admit, it's kind of a funny story…

Scabies—

Symptoms & Diagnosis—Itching, especially at night, and red-brown bumps in small curling lines (this is the eggs being laid under your skin). It can take four to six weeks for these symptoms to show up, and the scabies can appear anywhere on your body, but especially in the pubic and groin area, between fingers and toes, and in the beds of elbows and knees. Scabies can be confused with any number of skin conditions such as poison ivy, so get a diagnosis from your doc.

Treatment—Prescription meds will clear you within 24 hours, though the itching may last for two weeks (but you'll no longer be contagious). Clothes and towels, etc., should be dealt with as with crabs.

Transmission—Any close human contact, though sexual contact is the most common way it's spread. No penetration or even grinding is necessary, however; just sharing a bed can do it.

Prevention—See crabs.

If you have it—Ditto.

Condoms & Dams—

The previous four pages present a water-tight case: unless you're in a long-term, monogamous relationship where you've been tested together and you trust each other not to stray, you should always be wrapping up. Male and female condoms and oral sex dams all cut down on skin-to-skin contact and the exchange of bodily fluids (ejaculate, pre-come, vaginal fluids, and saliva), which means that they provide an excellent defense against some STDs, like HIV, and a certainly-better-than-nothing defense against others, like herpes and HPV. And let's not forget about the birth control that condoms offer. We know that latex doesn't exactly smell like romance, but do you really want to sleep with someone who considers safety a mood-killer? We didn't think so.

Female Condoms

These days, female condoms should be available wherever male condoms are sold (unless you're in the habit of buying your rubbers at gas stations or from bar vending machines). Like male condoms, they protect against both STDs and pregnancy (in a year of perfect use, female condoms have a five percent failure rate for pregnancy).

Why to Put One On—Female condoms are pricier than their male cousins and move around more, meaning they make a slight crinkly noise during sex. But here are some good reasons to try one out anyway:

- It's made of polyurethane, which is great for sensitivity and works with any lube.
- It can be inserted up to eight hours before sex. Let's hear it for "spontaneity"!
- He doesn't have to be erect before going in and he doesn't have to pull out as soon as he's ejaculated.
- No constriction of his nerve endings.
- The outer ring covers her outer labia, which may provide better protection against STDs and may also pleasantly stimulate her labia and clitorial head.
- Great option during your period if either of you is a little squeamish about period sex.
- One size fits all!

How to Put One On—It'll take a bit of practice to get this right, so we recommend a solo run first. Detailed instructions come in every packet, but here are the basics:

01 It's shaped like a bag with a ring on either end. Lubricate the closed end and squeeze the sides of the inner ring to insert it like a tampon. Push it in as far as it will go, until it reaches the cervix.

02 The outer ring (i.e., the open end) should protrude about an inch from the vagina.

03 Add lube (any kind!) to his penis or inside the female condom.

04 Never use a female and male condom together: they'll stick to each other and slide right off.

05 To remove, twist the outer to ring to close it off and pull out gently.

Oral Sex Dams

If you're reading this section, congratulations! Most sexual creatures have an uncanny ability to convince themselves that oral sex is not a potential health hazard. And while it's admittedly less risky than intercourse when it comes to the transmission of most STDs, "less" isn't "zero": you've still got to watch out for herpes, HPV, HIV, gonorrhea, chlamydia, and syphilis (and who wants to eat pubic lice?). Most erotic shops sell oral sex dams, made out of either latex or polyurethane (the latter is much friendlier on the taste buds), but a piece of hefty plastic wrap should do the job just as well. Add lube to the side where your tongue won't be, then place over your partner's genitals, depending on whether cunnilingus (p.68) or analingus (p.120) is on the menu. Hold it in place while you kiss, lick, suck, etc—or commandeer a garter belt to help out. Or, if you're using plastic wrap, wrap it around like some kinky bondage (p.158). And no matter how "green" you want to be, dams are single-use-only, please.

Male Condoms

Affordable, readily available, effective—how can you not love condoms? Male and female condoms are the only form of birth control that also help protect you from STDs. (If you're looking to compare the male condom to the methods on p.185: in a year of perfect use, they have a failure rate of only two percent.) And with today's design advances, condom sex no longer has to feel like clapping with gloves on. That said: gentlemen, if your penis still tends to have a less than enthusiastic response to wearing a raincoat, then practice by masturbating with a condom (don't complain, this is masturbation we're talking about). And ladies, you should always have opinions on the matter and supplies on hand, too.

Find the right condom for you by test-driving a selection. Size does matter: the better the fit, the safer (i.e., less breakage and slippage) and more comfortable the condom will be for both of you. If you're allergic to latex or just want a new sensation, try polyurethane condoms, which,

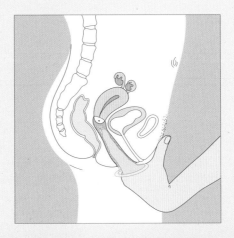

Inserting a Female Condom—This is the correct position for a female condom—the top ring should cover the cervix and the bottom ring should be outside the vaginal entrance. Read the detailed instructions above.

as compared to latex, are thinner, better at conducting heat, tasteless (no more rubber-flavored blowjobs!), more transparent, and compatible with any kind of lube, even oil. (And you should definitely use lube, because though polyurethane is stronger than latex, it's less elastic.) Avoid animal skin condoms (e.g., lambskin), as they don't protect against HIV. The more gimmicky a condom (glow-in-the-dark, "gold," novelty packaging), the more likely it is to let you down. So invest a little extra money in high-quality condoms—they're usually the ones that are ultra-thin yet strong, with extra bunching material or textures specifically designed to increase sensation for one or both of you.

Other important condom advice:
- Make sure the penis is fully erect before attempting to put on a condom.
- You can buy condoms with built-in lube, but avoid those with spermicide: this usually means Nonoxynol-9, which has been proven to cause irritation and potentially increase your risk of STD transmission.
- Should the condom roll up a bit during play, immediately put it back in place. Should it come off, remove entirely, and begin again with a brand new one (no skimping!).
- Immediately after ejaculation, before any softness sets in, hold the bottom of the condom in place at the base of the penis while the two of you disengage. Wrap up discreetly and throw in the wastebasket—do not flush!

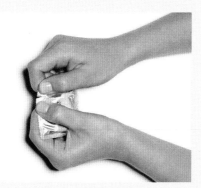

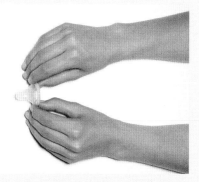

How to Put On a Condom Perfectly—

Step 1—Open the wrapper along one side of the foil with relish, but not with your teeth. Remove the condom gingerly from the package, taking care not to poke the material with fingernails or jewelry.

Step 2—Hold the condom the right way round. If you're not sure which side of the rolled-up condom should be placed against the penis, you can blow gently into the reservoir tip—this will help you determine if the roll is on the outside (it should be).

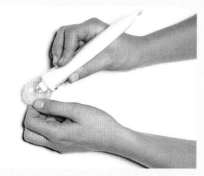

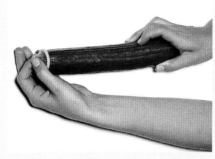

Step 3—Add two or three drops of water-based or silicone lubricant (never use oils with latex condoms!) into the reservoir tip. Lube will make it easier to roll down, and increase sensation for him. Do not skip this step!

Step 4—With one hand, pinch just below the reservoir tip, holding it against the top of the penis before any genital contact is made, because pre-ejaculate is a transmission fluid for STDs (as well as for pregnancy). Pinching the tip will make sure there's enough space for the semen to collect and prevent the condom from getting over-stretched.

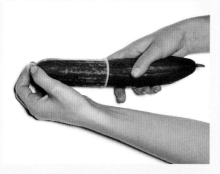

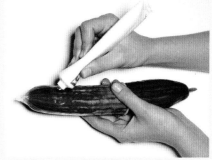

Step 5—With the other hand, roll the condom down smoothly and slowly all the way to the base, making sure there are no air bubbles along the shaft… and making sure this feels *good*.

Step 6—Lovingly add more lubricant to the outside for the woman's pleasure. Enjoy!

Birth Control Beyond Condoms—

Unfortunately, the following pages are "Ladies Only"—because besides male condoms and sterilization, the scientific community has yet to develop a decent range of birth control options for men. And so the brunt of the responsibility (and often the cost) rests squarely on the shoulders of women. Fortunately, it's given the gals a lot of freedom and independence over the past several decades. But don't mistake that freedom for a license to forgo condoms if you're playing the field. Unless you're in a long-term, monogamous relationship where you're positive your partner is holding up his end of the deal, you've been tested for all STDs together, and you've happily agreed to bump bare uglies, then the following options should be considered as back-up methods only.

Birth control falls into five categories: behavioral, over-the-counter, prescription, emergency, and permanent. We're assuming you're keeping your childbearing options open for the future, so we'll discuss only the first four here.

Behavioral—Abstinence, outercourse, and continuous breastfeeding don't really jibe with the overall theme of this book, so we'll skip them here. Two behavioral methods that actually involve intercourse are withdrawal and fertility awareness, but in our opinion, they're just too risky to rely on. However, being in tune with your menstrual cycle and when you ovulate can help reinforce your primary method of birth control, by ensuring you don't engage in risky behavior at high-risk times of the month. (If you need a refresher course on when those times are—sex ed class was a long time ago, we know—check out a site like Ovusoft. com for some tips.)

Over-the-Counter—In addition to male and female condoms (pp.182–183), barrier methods like the Sponge and spermicides (see chart) prevent sperm from hooking up with an egg. They can be purchased at your local pharmacy without a prescription and they're typically used once per session, i.e., when you need them, which makes them convenient—plus, you can stop at any time. And, unlike most prescription methods, they're non-hormonal.

Prescription—You'll need a doctor to prescribe these methods, which usually work continuously over a period of time. All except diaphragms, caps, and shields (see chart) are hormonal. Hormonal methods, which tend to be slightly more effective than other types of birth control, include the Pill, the Patch, the Ring, the Shot, the Implant, and IUDs (see chart).

Emergency—Emergency contraception is a hormonal method of preventing conception up to five days after the unprotected sex occurs. It's basically just an intense dose of the Pill, though it's not something you can go DIY on. Emergency contraception can be a safety net in case the condom breaks, or he doesn't quite manage to pull out, or you forgot to take your Pill, or—shame on you—you just neglected to use any protection. If you're 18 or older you can buy it without a prescription from your local pharmacy (men too!). Just ask your pharmacist for Plan B. Under 18, you'll need a prescription—see ec. princeton.edu to find a provider near you (and actually, even if you're older than 18, getting a prescription often means your state will cover the cost for you.) The sooner you take it, the more effective it's likely to be, so it's not a bad idea to have a supply on hand. Another, much less common, form of emergency contraception is an IUD, inserted by your doctor, which you can then keep in place as a form of ongoing birth control. And no matter what anyone may try to tell you, neither method is an abortion. *Emergency contraception doesn't end a pregnancy, it simply prevents a pregnancy from ever taking place, just like all the methods in the chart that follows.*

The birth control options on the following page barely scratch the surface—you'll need to talk to your doctor to figure out exactly which method is right for you. As you peruse the various methods, bear these questions in mind: do I want to avoid hormones or might they benefit me? Do I want fewer periods or none at all? How good am I at maintenance and up-keep? Which is more important to me, spontaneity in the moment or being able to switch methods at any time?

Birth Control Options—

What it is—	How it works—	How well it works—	Is it for you?
The Sponge (over-the-counter/ barrier)	You can insert it hours ahead of time and can wear it for for up to 30 hours after insertion, during which time you can have sex as many times as you like.	If you use it correctly every time and you've never given birth, failure rate over one year is nine percent.	Neither partner usually feels it and it need not interrupt the flow of sex. Plus it's hormone-free, which is great if you found that the Pill sapped your libido. You need to be comfortable getting *in there* to insert it, though. Plus, it may cause vaginal irritation and odor. And it's incredibly ineffective if you've already had kids. Finally, because it contains Nonoxynol-9 (which may increase STD transmission), this may not be a great back-up method to condoms if you're playing the field.
Spermicide (over-the-counter/ barrier)	Creams, jellies, film, foam, and suppositories inserted deeply into the vagina before you do it, either on their own or with the Sponge or a diaphragm, cap, or shield.	If you use it correctly every time, failure rate over one year is 15 percent.	That failure rate is too high to make it work as a stand-alone method—but it's a decent back-up method to use, but only in a long-term monogamous relationship, as Nonoxynol-9 (the main ingredient in most spermicides) increases the risk of STD transmission. You have to wait 10 minutes after inserting some products before intercourse (foreplay time!) and they're only effective for one hour after insertion (not too much foreplay!).
The Pill (prescription/ hormonal)	You take a Pill once a day. With the classic version, you stop taking the Pill for one week a month to get your period, but some newer versions allow you to choose how many times a year you'd like Aunt Flow to visit—12, three, once, or not at all.	If you take it correctly, failure rate over one year is less than one percent.	Not if you smoke. It can also dull the libido and lead to depression in some women. On the other hand, if you experience heavy or painful periods, the Pill may provide some relief. It also reduces your risk of ovarian and endometrial cancers and, on a lighter note, may clear up your acne.
The Patch (prescription/ hormonal)	You stick a thin, beige, plastic patch to your skin (e.g. your stomach or bum) once a week; it releases hormones to protect against pregnancy.	If you use it correctly every time, failure rate over one year is less than one percent.	Yes, if you can't remember to take a Pill every day. Other than that, the pros and cons are pretty similar to the Pill.
The Ring (prescription/ hormonal)	You insert a small, flexible ring into the vagina once a month; it releases hormones to prevent pregnancy.	If you use it correctly every time, failure rate over one year is less than one percent.	Yes, if you can't remember to take a Pill every day. No, if you're prone to vaginal infections, as the Ring can increase your risk. Other than that, the pros and cons are similar to the Pill.
The Shot, usually Depo-Provera (prescription/ hormonal)	You visit your doctor once every three months for an injection of hormones that prevents pregnancy.	If you get the shot consistently for a year, failure rate is 0.3 percent.	Yes, if you won't remember a daily Pill. No, if you might want to get pregnant soon, as it can take a year or so for your cycle to return to normal. Plus, its widely reported side effects—in particular breakthrough bleeding or extended, very heavy periods—mean that it's never become the popular kid that the Pill is. Especially because, if you change your mind, the side effects will last for months, until the injection wears off.
The Implant (prescription/ hormonal)	Your doctor inserts a thin, flexible plastic implant about the size of a matchstick under the skin of the upper arm. You can wear it for up to 5 years.	Studies have not been released yet for the new-and-improved Implant, but it's estimated that it's 99.9 percent effective for up to three years.	Perhaps, if you're looking for a long-term option and your health care center offers it (not all do). And unlike the Shot, you can get pregnant shortly after the Implant is removed. Unfortunately it has similar reported side effects to the Shot.
Intrauterine Device (IUD) (prescription, either hormonal or non-hormonal)	Your doctor inserts a small T-shaped device into your uterus; a thin string hangs down through the cervix into the vagina. You can wear it either up to 12 years (the non-hormonal copper version) or five years (the hormonal version).	During the first year of continued use, failure rate is less than one percent.	It's the most popular reversible method worldwide and you can get pregnant very soon after it's removed. But not a great option if there's a chance you might be "getting back out there" in the near future, as wearing an IUD can increase your risk of PID (p.181).
Diaphragm, cap, or shield (prescription, non-hormonal)	Your doc will fit yours to your cervix so that it correctly blocks the opening to the uterus. You insert it, along with spermicidal cream or jelly, before intercourse and remove it afterward.	If you use a diaphragm correctly for a year, failure rate is six percent. Perfect use figures aren't available for caps and shields, but their typical use rates aren't good enough for us to recommend them as stand-alone options.	Not if you're prone to vaginal infections or UTIs, as this method can increase your susceptibility. And not if you're squeamish about the insertion and removal. You also can't use any of these during your period. But like the Sponge, you can't usually feel it, and you can insert it hours ahead of time.

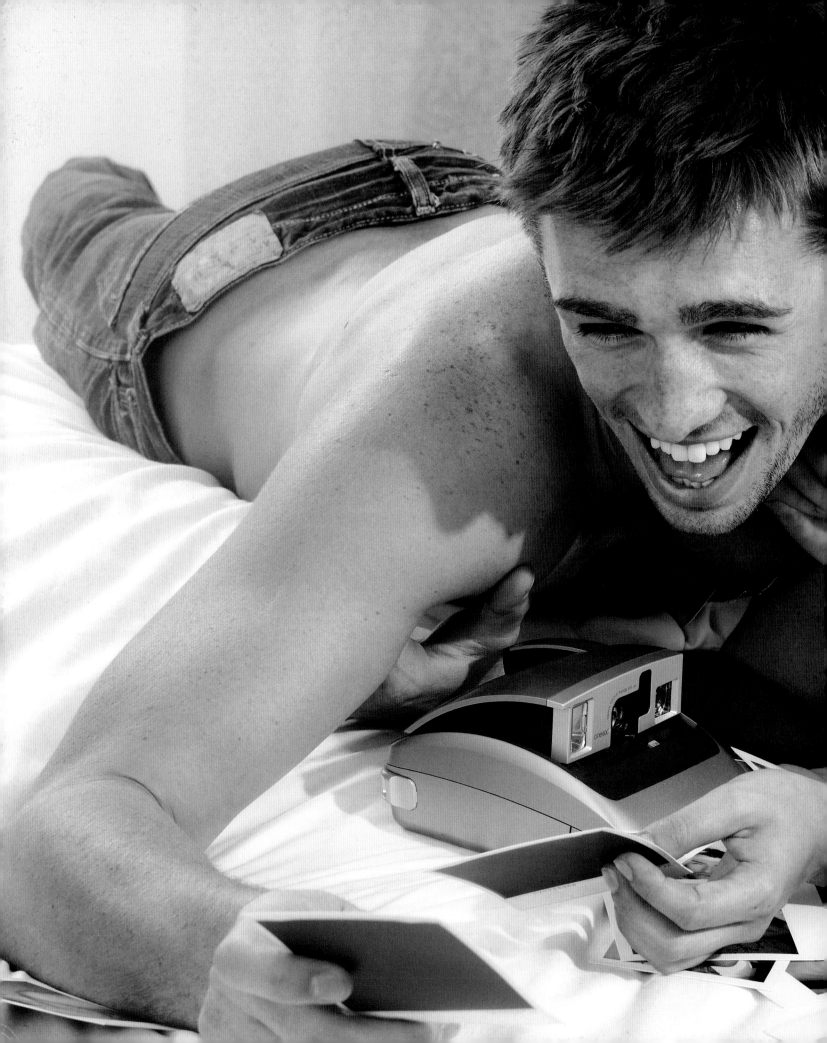

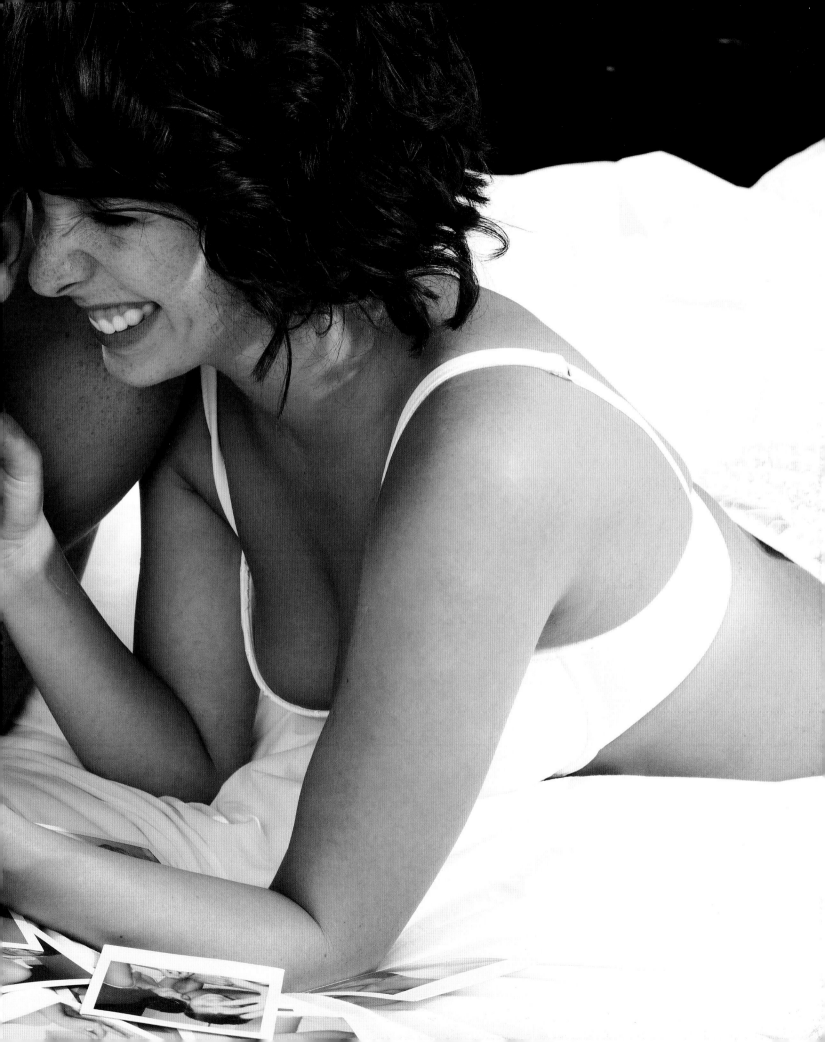

Resources—

These are a few of our favorite sex-related websites and books (in addition to the recommendations sprinkled throughout the chapters).

Surfing—

DailyBedpost.com (Sex & sexual health news, advice, and gossip)
PuckerUp.com (Online home of Tristan Taormino, "Anal Advisor")
JanesGuide.com (Comprehensive index of sex-related websites)
Sexuality.About.com (Guide to sex on the Web)
The-Clitoris.com (All about the clitoris and female sexuality)
Sexuality.org (Info on everything from safer sex to multiple male orgasms)
GoAskAlice.columbia.edu (Sex advice on every topic under the sun)
EC.Princeton.edu (All about emergency contraception)
CDC.gov (Centers for Disease Control & Prevention)
ASHASTD.org (Comprehensive guide to STIs/STDs)
FWHC.org (Feminist Women's Health Center)
PlannedParenthood.org (Sexual health and birth control resource)
Avert.org (AIDS & HIV information)
RopeFashions.com (All about rope bondage)
KinkyRopes.com (More about rope bondage)

Shopping—

Babeland.com
GoodVibes.com
A-Womans-Touch.com
TantusDirect.com
VixenCreations.com
ToysJustForBoys.com
ErosBoutique.com
ExtremeRestraints.com
Condomania.com
KikiDM.com
ShiriZinn.com
KamaSutra.com
Lelo.com
Natural-Contours.com
VeganErotica.com
StormyLeather.com
JapanRope.com
Stockroom.com
Sub-Shop.com

Reading—

A New View of a Woman's Body
(Feminist Press, 1991) By Federation of Feminist Women's Health Center

The Clitoral Truth
(Seven Stories Press, 2002) By Rebecca Chalker

Women: An Intimate Geography
(Anchor Press, 2000) By Natalie Angier

Our Bodies, Ourselves
(Touchstone, 2005) By Boston Women's Health Collective

Sexual Health for Men: The Complete Guide
(Perseus Publishing, 2000) By Richard F. Spark

Are We Having Fun Yet?: The Intelligent Woman's Guide to Sex
(Hyperion, 1997) By Marcia Douglass, Ph.D., & Lisa Douglass, Ph.D.

The New Good Vibrations Guide to Sex
(Cleis Press, 1997) By Anne Semans & Cathy Winks

Guide to Getting It On!
(Goofy Foot Press, 2006) By Paul Joannides

Sensuous Magic: A Guide to S/M for Adventurous Couples
(Cleis Press, 2001) By Patrick Califia

The Good Vibrations Guide: The G-Spot
(Down There Press, 1998) By Cathy Winks

Getting Off: A Woman's Guide to Masturbation
(Seal Press, 2007) By Jamye Waxman

Erotic Massage
(Dorling Kindersley, 2004) By Anne Hooper

Kama Sutra for Her/for Him
(Dorling Kindersley, 2004) By Anne Hooper

The Bedside Kama Sutra
(Fair Winds Press, 2001) By Linda Sonntag

Taoist Secrets of Love: Cultivating Male Sexual Energy
(Aurora Press, 1984) By Mantak Chia

She Comes First: The Thinking Man's Guide to Pleasuring a Woman
(Collins, 2008) By Ian Kerner

Sex Tips for Straight Women from a Gay Man
(Thorsons, 2005) By Dan Anderson and Maggie Berman

Anal Pleasure and Health
(Down There Press, 1998) By Jack Morin, Ph.D.

The Ultimate Guide to Anal Sex for Women
(Cleis Press, 2006) By Tristan Taormino

The Ultimate Guide to Sexual Fantasy
(Cleis Press, 2004) By Violet Blue

The Claiming of Sleeping Beauty series
(Plume, 1999) By Anne Rice writing as A. N. Roquelaure

Sweet Life: Erotic Fantasies for Couples
(Cleis Press, 2001-2003) Edited by Violet Blue

Naughty Spanking Stories from A to Z
(Pretty Things Press, 2004) Edited by Rachel Kramer Bussel

My Secret Garden
(Quartet Books, 2001) By Nancy Friday

Best Bondage Erotica
(Cleis Press, 2005) Edited by Alison Tyler

Best Fetish Erotica
(Cleis Press, 2005) Edited by Cara Bruce

Come Hither: A Commonsense Guide to Kinky Sex
(Fireside, 2000) By Gloria G. Brame

Erotic Bondage Handbook
(Greenery Press, 2000) By Jay Wiseman

SM 101: A Realistic Introduction
(Greenery Press, 1998) By Jay Wiseman

Watching—

Whipsmart: A Good Vibrations Guide to Beginning S/M for Couples
(Good Vibrations/SexPositive Productions)

Index—

Index—

Index/Acknowledgements—

From Em & Lo—

Thanks to the gang at DK for plying us with pink champagne until we agreed we could pull this off, especially: Gary June, Stephanie Jackson, Sharon Lucas, Peter Jones, Peter Luff, Kesta Desmond, Sara Robin, Abe Chang, and Rachel Kempster. Thanks to Paul West, Paula Benson, and Becky Johnson at Form® for making it all look so good (right down to the angle of every leg and the placement of each bondage knot). Thanks to Rankin for making us seem hipper than we deserve to be by association. Thanks to our fearless research interns Daphne Larose, Haley Yarosh, and Lisa Marie Basile—we owe you all a second round. Ira Silverberg, thanks for having our back. And thanks, as always, to Joey and Rob for bearing with two sex writers who don't practice what they preach quite as often as they should.

DK would like to thank—

Adam Brackenbury for retouching work
Julie Telfer for styling

www.AnnSummers.com for supplying "The Minx" by Shiri Zinn on page 131. (Enquiries: 0845 456 2399 and www.shirizinn.com.)

www.sh-womenstore.com for supplying harnesses, "The Laya" and rocking G-spot toys ("the Rock Chick". Enquiries: 020 7613 5458 or shop@sh-womenstore.com.)

www.LoveHoney.co.uk for supplying all other toys (Enquiries: 0800 915 6635.)

Master U, London-Vauxhall, for supplying bondage advice (masteru.com)

LONDON, NEW YORK, MUNICH, MELBOURNE, DELHI

Senior Art Editor—Sara Robin
Senior Editor—Peter Jones
Managing Art Editor—Kat Mead
Executive Managing Editor—Adèle Hayward
Production Editor—Ben Marcus
Senior Production Editor—Luca Frassinetti
Creative Technical Support—Sonia Charbonnier
Production Controller—Mandy Inness
Art Director—Peter Luff
Category Publisher—Stephanie Jackson
US Editors—Shannon Beatty, Charles Wills

Photography—Rankin (www.rankin.co.uk)

Art Direction—Paul West & Paula Benson, Form® London
Design—Paul West, Paula Benson & Becky Johnson,
Form® London (www.form.uk.com)
Project Editor—Kesta Desmond
Illustrator—André Metzger

First American edition, 2008

Published in the United States by
DK Publishing
375 Hudson Street
New York, NY 10014

08 09 10 11   10 9 8 7 6 5 4 3

SD353—014—May 2008

Published in Great Britain by Dorling Kindersley Limited.

A catalog record for this book is available from the Library
of Congress.

ISBN 978-0-7566-5790-1

DK books are available at special discounts when purchased
in bulk for sales promotions, premiums, fund-raising, or
educational use. For details, contact: DK Publishing Special
Markets, 375 Hudson Street, New York, New York 10014 or
SpecialSales@dk.com.

Color reproduction by MDP, England
Printed and bound in Hong Kong by Toppan

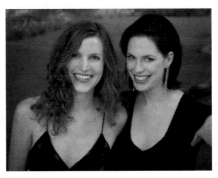

Sophisticated, sassy, and experts in everything sexual, **Em & Lo**
describe their writing as informative but fun, opinionated but
non-judgmental, sexy but never sleazy. They are the authors
of Nerve's bestselling positions book, *Position of the Day:
Sex Every Day & Every Way* and the sex manual *The Big Bang*,
which *Time* described as "this generation's smarter, funnier,
and raunchier version of *The Joy of Sex*." Their most recent
books are *Rec Sex: An A-Z Guide to Hooking Up*. *Sex Toy: An
A-Z Guide to Bedside Accessories*, and *Buh Bye: The Ultimate
Guide to Dumping and Getting Dumped*.

Form® is an award-winning London-based graphic design
and branding agency co-founded by Paul West and Paula
Benson in 1991. Form's work in design for print, web, and
moving image embraces many areas of contemporary culture
including music, entertainment, media and design-led brands
as well as books, brochures, and events.